Pediatric Fractures

Pediatric Fractures

Editor
Christiaan J. A. van Bergen

MDPI • Basel • Beijing • Wuhan • Barcelona • Belgrade • Manchester • Tokyo • Cluj • Tianjin

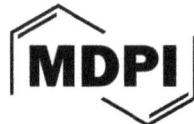

Editor
Christiaan J. A. van Bergen
Orthopedic Surgery
Amphia Hospital & Erasmus MC
Breda & Rotterdam
The Netherlands

Editorial Office
MDPI
St. Alban-Anlage 66
4052 Basel, Switzerland

This is a reprint of articles from the Special Issue published online in the open access journal *Children* (ISSN 2227-9067) (available at: www.mdpi.com/journal/children/special_issues/pediatric_fractures).

For citation purposes, cite each article independently as indicated on the article page online and as indicated below:

LastName, A.A.; LastName, B.B.; LastName, C.C. Article Title. *Journal Name* **Year**, *Volume Number*, Page Range.

ISBN 978-3-0365-6142-4 (Hbk)
ISBN 978-3-0365-6141-7 (PDF)

© 2023 by the authors. Articles in this book are Open Access and distributed under the Creative Commons Attribution (CC BY) license, which allows users to download, copy and build upon published articles, as long as the author and publisher are properly credited, which ensures maximum dissemination and a wider impact of our publications.

The book as a whole is distributed by MDPI under the terms and conditions of the Creative Commons license CC BY-NC-ND.

Contents

Christiaan J. A. van Bergen
Pediatric Fractures Are Challenging from Head to Toe
Reprinted from: *Children* **2022**, *9*, 678, doi:10.3390/children9050678 1

Christiaan J. A. van Bergen
Advances in Pediatric Fracture Diagnosis and Treatment Are Numerous but Great Challenges Remain
Reprinted from: *Children* **2022**, *9*, 1489, doi:10.3390/children9101489 5

Fabio Verdoni, Martina Ricci, Cristina Di Grigoli, Nicolò Rossi, Michele Davide Maria Lombardo and Domenico Curci et al.
Effect of the COVID-19 Outbreak on Pediatric Patients' Admissions to the Emergency Department in an Italian Orthopedic Trauma Hub
Reprinted from: *Children* **2021**, *8*, 645, doi:10.3390/children8080645 9

Ya-Chih Yang, Tsung-Han Hsieh, Chi-Yuan Liu, Chun-Yu Chang, Yueh-Tseng Hou and Po-Chen Lin et al.
Analysis of Clinical Outcome and Predictors of Mortality in Pediatric Trauma Population: Evidence from a 10 Year Analysis in a Single Center
Reprinted from: *Children* **2021**, *8*, 688, doi:10.3390/children8080688 17

Paul Andrei Țenț, Raluca Iulia Juncar, Abel Emanuel Moca, Rahela Tabita Moca and Mihai Juncar
The Etiology and Epidemiology of Pediatric Facial Fractures in North-Western Romania: A 10-Year Retrospective Study
Reprinted from: *Children* **2022**, *9*, 932, doi:10.3390/children9070932 29

Pei-Ju Hsieh and Han-Tsung Liao
Outcome Analysis of Surgical Timing in Pediatric Orbital Trapdoor Fracture with Different Entrapment Contents: A Retrospective Study
Reprinted from: *Children* **2022**, *9*, 398, doi:10.3390/children9030398 39

Lisa van der Water, Arno A. Macken, Denise Eygendaal and Christiaan J. A. van Bergen
Pediatric Clavicle Fractures and Congenital Pseudarthrosis Unraveled
Reprinted from: *Children* **2022**, *9*, 49, doi:10.3390/children9010049 47

Florian Freislederer, Susanne Bensler, Thomas Specht, Olaf Magerkurth and Karim Eid
Plate Fixation for Irreducible Proximal Humeral Fractures in Children and Adolescents—A Single-Center Case Series of Six Patients
Reprinted from: *Children* **2021**, *8*, 635, doi:10.3390/children8080635 59

Tu Ngoc Vu, Son Hong Duy Phung, Long Hoang Vo and Uoc Huu Nguyen
Diagnosis and Treatment for Pediatric Supracondylar Humerus Fractures with Brachial Artery Injuries
Reprinted from: *Children* **2021**, *8*, 933, doi:10.3390/children8100933 69

Sietse E. S. Terpstra, Paul T. P. W. Burgers, Huub J. L. van der Heide and Pieter Bas de Witte
Pediatric Supracondylar Humerus Fractures: Should We Avoid Surgery during After-Hours?
Reprinted from: *Children* **2022**, *9*, 189, doi:10.3390/children9020189 81

Maximiliaan A. Poppelaars, Denise Eygendaal, Bertram The, Iris van Oost and Christiaan J. A. van Bergen
Diagnosis and Treatment of Children with a Radiological Fat Pad Sign without Visible Elbow Fracture Vary Widely: An International Online Survey and Development of an Objective Definition
Reprinted from: *Children* **2022**, *9*, 950, doi:10.3390/children9070950 . . . . **93**

Lisette C. Langenberg, Kimberly I. M. van den Ende, Max Reijman, G. J. (Juliën) Boersen and Joost W. Colaris
Pediatric Radial Neck Fractures: A Systematic Review Regarding the Influence of Fracture Treatment on Elbow Function
Reprinted from: *Children* **2022**, *9*, 1049, doi:10.3390/children9071049 . . . . **101**

Kyra Hermans, Duncan Fransz, Lisette Walbeehm-Hol, Paul Hustinx and Heleen Staal
Is a Parry Fracture—An Isolated Fracture of the Ulnar Shaft—Associated with the Probability of Abuse in Children between 2 and 16 Years Old?
Reprinted from: *Children* **2021**, *8*, 650, doi:10.3390/children8080650 . . . . **115**

Femke F. Schröder, Feike de Graaff and Anne J. H. Vochteloo
Patient-Specific Guided Osteotomy to Correct a Symptomatic Malunion of the Left Forearm
Reprinted from: *Children* **2021**, *8*, 707, doi:10.3390/children8080707 . . . . **123**

Jack Zhang, Naveenjyote Boora, Sarah Melendez, Abhilash Rakkunedeth Hareendranathan and Jacob Jaremko
Diagnostic Accuracy of 3D Ultrasound and Artificial Intelligence for Detection of Pediatric Wrist Injuries
Reprinted from: *Children* **2021**, *8*, 431, doi:10.3390/children8060431 . . . . **131**

Hanneke Weel, A. J. Peter Joosten and Christiaan J. A. van Bergen
Apophyseal Avulsion of the Rectus Femoris Tendon Origin in Adolescent Soccer Players
Reprinted from: *Children* **2022**, *9*, 1016, doi:10.3390/children9071016 . . . . **141**

Alexandru Herdea, Vlad Pencea, Claudiu N. Lungu, Adham Charkaoui and Alexandru Ulici
A Prospective Cohort Study on Quality of Life among the Pediatric Population after Surgery for Recurrent
Patellar Dislocation
Reprinted from: *Children* **2021**, *8*, 830, doi:10.3390/children8100830 . . . . **149**

Zenon Pogorelić, Viktor Vegan, Miro Jukić, Carlos Martin Llorente Muñoz and Dubravko Furlan
Elastic Stable Intramedullary Nailing for Treatment of Pediatric Tibial Fractures: A 20-Year Single Center Experience of 132 Cases
Reprinted from: *Children* **2022**, *9*, 845, doi:10.3390/children9060845 . . . . **157**

Stephanie Choo and Julia A. V. Nuelle
NSAID Use and Effects on Pediatric Bone Healing: A Review of Current Literature
Reprinted from: *Children* **2021**, *8*, 821, doi:10.3390/children8090821 . . . . **169**

Maxwell Luke Armstrong, Nicholas Smith, Rhiannon Tracey and Heather Jackman
The Orthopedic Effects of Electronic Cigarettes: A Systematic Review and Pediatric Case Series
Reprinted from: *Children* **2022**, *9*, 62, doi:10.3390/children9010062 . . . . **179**

Wouter Nijhuis, Marjolein Verhoef, Christiaan van Bergen, Harrie Weinans and Ralph Sakkers
Fractures in Osteogenesis Imperfecta: Pathogenesis, Treatment, Rehabilitation and Prevention
Reprinted from: *Children* **2022**, *9*, 268, doi:10.3390/children9020268 . . . . **189**

Viridiana Ramírez-Vela, Luis Antonio Aguilar-Pérez, Juan Carlos Paredes-Rojas, Juan Alejandro Flores-Campos, Fernando ELi Ortiz-Hernández and Christopher René Torres-SanMiguel
Bone Fractures Numerical Analysis in a Femur Affected by Osteogenesis Imperfecta
Reprinted from: *Children* **2021**, *8*, 1177, doi:10.3390/children8121177 . . . . **199**

Joseph R. Fuchs, Romie F. Gibly, Christopher B. Erickson, Stacey M. Thomas, Nancy Hadley Miller and Karin A. Payne
Analysis of Physeal Fractures from the United States National Trauma Data Bank
Reprinted from: *Children* **2022**, *9*, 914, doi:10.3390/children9060914 . . . . **215**

Amber Carlijn Traa, Ozcan Sir, Sanne W. T. Frazer, Brigitte van de Kerkhof-van Bon, Birgitte Blatter and Edward C. T. H. Tan
Levels of Physical Activity in Children with Extremity Fractures a Dutch Observational Cross-Sectional Study
Reprinted from: *Children* **2022**, *9*, 325, doi:10.3390/children9030325 . . . . **225**

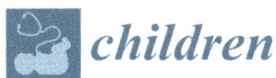

Editorial

Pediatric Fractures Are Challenging from Head to Toe

Christiaan J. A. van Bergen

Department of Orthopedic Surgery, Amphia Hospital, P.O. Box 90150, 4800 RK Breda, The Netherlands; cvanbergen@amphia.nl; Tel.: +31-76-5955000

Fractures are extremely common in children. The fracture risk is 40% in boys and 28% in girls. Although many pediatric fractures are frequently regarded as "innocent" or "forgiving", typical complications do occur in this precious population, e.g., premature physeal closure and post-traumatic deformity, which could potentially cause life-long disability.

Despite the high incidence of pediatric injuries, there is still much debate on optimal treatment regimes. Although nonoperative and surgical treatment techniques have developed enormously during the past decades, current management is still more eminence-based rather than evidence-based because of the limited scientific evidence. For example, the recently developed comprehensive Dutch clinical practice guideline on diagnosis and treatment of the most common pediatric fractures included almost solely "low" or "very low" level recommendations, based on the Grading of Recommendations Assessment, Development, and Evaluation (GRADE) criteria. The only exceptions were some forearm fracture recommendations, which received "moderate" GRADEs. There is a clear lack of data and a need for higher-level science in pediatric trauma.

The main goal of this Special Issue in *Children* was to help fill the gap of undiscovered knowledge and improve the scientific understanding of pediatric fractures and related subjects. A great variety of topics were covered in the 14 high-quality original and review papers that have been published so far.

Two studies dealt with general aspects related to acute pediatric trauma. To start with a contemporary hot topic, Verdoni et al. [1] studied the effect of COVID-19 on pediatric emergency department admissions in Italy. Compared to 2019, they found a striking 87% reduction of admissions during the initial COVID period in their observational cohort study. The proportion of children diagnosed with a fracture was significantly higher during the pandemic. In addition, a trend was observed towards more severe injuries and more home-related injuries.

To analyze predictors of mortality in pediatric trauma, Yang et al. [2] retrospectively studied a large population of 1265 children in a trauma center in Taiwan over a 10-year period. The (pediatric age-adjusted) shock index was used in an attempt to predict intensive care admission, surgery and mortality. Interestingly, they found that the index was able to predict the mortality and injury severity in their pediatric trauma population.

In addition, numerous articles investigated specific pediatric fractures, including their diagnosis, treatment, complications and outcomes. In line with the epidemiology of fracture localizations in children, most papers reported on the upper extremity. Many interesting papers were published, from head to toe:

Van der Water et al. [3] provided a comprehensive review on pediatric clavicle fractures and congenital pseudarthrosis. Their article provides useful tools to diagnose, differentiate, and treat both entities.

Plate fixation for proximal humerus fractures was investigated in a small case series by Freislederer et al. [4] from Switzerland. Although closed reduction and K-wire fixation remains the preferred technique for this condition, their series shows that open reduction and plate fixation is a good alternative in cases where closed reduction is unsuccessful.

Supracondylar humerus fractures are very common in children and are sometimes accompanied by brachial artery injuries. Vu et al. [5] described an impressive series of

Citation: van Bergen, C.J.A. Pediatric Fractures Are Challenging from Head to Toe. *Children* **2022**, *9*, 678. https://doi.org/10.3390/children9050678

Received: 25 February 2022
Accepted: 2 April 2022
Published: 6 May 2022

Publisher's Note: MDPI stays neutral with regard to jurisdictional claims in published maps and institutional affiliations.

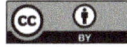

Copyright: © 2022 by the author. Licensee MDPI, Basel, Switzerland. This article is an open access article distributed under the terms and conditions of the Creative Commons Attribution (CC BY) license (https://creativecommons.org/licenses/by/4.0/).

50 pediatric patients with this unfortunate combination of injuries. They showed that doppler sonography could not reliably identify the vascular lesions, most cases only had vasospasms, and the treatment remained difficult.

In order to investigate when to operate these injuries, Terpstra et al. [6] reviewed the literature on the question of whether there is a benefit of after-hour surgery for supracondylar humeral fractures. Although the included studies showed no differences in functional outcomes, the authors could carefully conclude that surgery during office hours has some advantages with regards to the quality of reduction and fixation.

Next, Hermans et al. [7] investigated the possible association between child abuse and isolated ulnar shaft fractures, as these fractures can result from a direct impact to the forearm when protecting the head. In this retrospective case series of 36 patients from the Netherlands, none of the children were referred to a child protective team. Therefore, a possible association could not be shown.

Forearm fractures may malunite, leading to rotational deficits. Schröder et al. [8] described an interesting case of a patient-specific 3D-guided osteotomy for a malunited forearm, which effectively restored the full range of motion.

With the aim of reducing exposure to radiographic radiation, Zhang et al. [9] in their innovative Canadian study investigated the use of 3D ultrasound and artificial intelligence to diagnose pediatric wrist fractures. The results were remarkable, with very high sensitivity and specificity of the ultrasound scans and a perfect agreement between human judgement and artificial intelligence, suggesting that this technique can reliably rule out these fractures in the emergency room.

One lower limb study was included in this Special Issue. Quality of life after surgery for recurrent patellar dislocation was prospectively studied by Herdea et al. [10] from Romania. A total of 108 pediatric patients were treated by two different soft-tissue surgeries and assessed with the Pediatric International Knee Documentation Committee form. Medial patellofemoral ligament reconstruction led to better quality of life compared to medial imbrication.

After a fracture, the healing of bone in the skeletally immature may be influenced by several factors. Bone healing and the use of non-steroidal anti-inflammatory drugs were systematically reviewed by Choo and Nuelle from the USA [11]. Their analysis of the available literature suggests that the use of these drugs does not increase the risk of nonunion of long bones, although further work is needed with respect to the drug types, dosage and duration.

In another systematic review, Armstrong et al. [12] investigated the orthopedic effects of electronic cigarettes, as they observed delayed unions in their adolescent population using electronic cigarettes. They found no human studies and some experimental studies investigating this topic. Currently, the relationship between electronic cigarettes and bone fractures and healing remains poorly understood, which could be inspiration for further study.

Finally, two papers focused on children with brittle bones. Nijhuis et al. [13] provided a broad perspective on pediatric patients with osteogenesis imperfecta. Among other things, they presented some clear guidelines on the treatment of fractures in this vulnerable population, and underlined the importance of a multidisciplinary approach in dedicated expertise centers.

Ramírez-Vela et al. [14] from Mexico presented an innovative finite element model to study a femur affected by osteogenesis imperfecta. They showed that the highest levels of stress occur in comminuted fractures and the lowest levels in transverse fractures.

In conclusion, this Special Issue contains a great diversity of studies on a broad pediatric population in relation to fractures. Each paper contributes to our knowledge in its own way and helps improve care for our most valuable population. During the writing of this Editorial, more papers are on their way to further fill the current knowledge gaps and identify room for further study.

Funding: This research received no external funding.

Conflicts of Interest: The author declares no conflict of interest.

References

1. Verdoni, F.; Ricci, M.; Di Grigoli, C.; Rossi, N.; Lombardo, M.D.M.; Curci, D.; Accetta, R.; Viganò, M.; Peretti, G.M.; Mangiavini, L. Effect of the COVID-19 Outbreak on Pediatric Patients' Admissions to the Emergency Department in an Italian Orthopedic Trauma Hub. *Children* **2021**, *8*, 645. [CrossRef] [PubMed]
2. Yang, Y.; Hsieh, T.; Liu, C.; Chang, C.; Hou, Y.; Lin, P.; Chen, Y.; Chien, D.; Yiang, G.; Wu, M. Analysis of Clinical Outcome and Predictors of Mortality in Pediatric Trauma Population: Evidence from a 10 Year Analysis in a Single Center. *Children* **2021**, *8*, 688. [CrossRef] [PubMed]
3. Van der Water, L.; Macken, A.A.; Eygendaal, D.; van Bergen, C.J.A. Pediatric Clavicle Fractures and Congenital Pseudarthrosis Unraveled. *Children* **2022**, *9*, 49. [CrossRef] [PubMed]
4. Freislederer, F.; Bensler, S.; Specht, T.; Magerkurth, O.; Eid, K. Plate Fixation for Irreducible Proximal Humeral Fractures in Children and Adolescents—A Single-Center Case Series of Six Patients. *Children* **2021**, *8*, 635. [CrossRef] [PubMed]
5. Vu, T.N.; Phung, S.H.D.; Vo, L.H.; Nguyen, U.H. Diagnosis and Treatment for Pediatric Supracondylar Humerus Fractures with Brachial Artery Injuries. *Children* **2021**, *8*, 933. [CrossRef] [PubMed]
6. Terpstra, S.E.S.; Burgers, P.T.P.W.; van der Heide, H.J.L.; de Witte, P.B. Pediatric Supracondylar Humerus Fractures: Should We Avoid Surgery during After-Hours? *Children* **2022**, *9*, 189. [CrossRef] [PubMed]
7. Hermans, K.; Fransz, D.; Walbeehm-Hol, L.; Hustinx, P.; Staal, H. Is a Parry Fracture—An Isolated Fracture of the Ulnar Shaft—Associated with the Probability of Abuse in Children between 2 and 16 Years Old? *Children* **2021**, *8*, 650. [CrossRef] [PubMed]
8. Schröder, F.F.; de Graaff, F.; Vochteloo, A.J.H. Patient-Specific Guided Osteotomy to Correct a Symptomatic Malunion of the Left Forearm. *Children* **2021**, *8*, 707. [CrossRef] [PubMed]
9. Zhang, J.; Boora, N.; Melendez, S.; Hareendranathan, A.R.; Jaremko, J. Diagnostic Accuracy of 3D Ultrasound and Artificial Intelligence for Detection of Pediatric Wrist Injuries. *Children* **2021**, *8*, 431. [CrossRef] [PubMed]
10. Herdea, A.; Pencea, V.; Lungu, C.N.; Charkaoui, A.; Ulici, A. A Prospective Cohort Study on Quality of Life among the Pediatric Population after Surgery for Recurrent Patellar Dislocation. *Children* **2021**, *8*, 830. [CrossRef] [PubMed]
11. Choo, S.; Nuelle, J.A.V. NSAID Use and Effects on Pediatric Bone Healing: A Review of Current Literature. *Children* **2021**, *8*, 821. [CrossRef] [PubMed]
12. Armstrong, M.L.; Smith, N.; Tracey, R.; Jackman, H. The Orthopedic Effects of Electronic Cigarettes: A Systematic Review and Pediatric Case Series. *Children* **2022**, *9*, 62. [CrossRef] [PubMed]
13. Nijhuis, W.H.; Verhoef, M.; van Bergen, C.J.A.; Weinans, H.; Sakkers, R.J.B. Fractures in Osteogenesis Imperfecta: Pathogenesis, Treatment, Rehabilitation and Prevention. *Children* **2022**, *9*, 268. [CrossRef] [PubMed]
14. Ramírez-Vela, V.; Aguilar-Pérez, L.A.; Paredes-Rojas, J.C.; Flores-Campos, J.A.; Ortiz-Hernández, F.E.; Torres-San Miguel, C.R. Bone Fractures Numerical Analysis in a Femur Affected by Osteogenesis Imperfecta. *Children* **2021**, *8*, 1177. [CrossRef] [PubMed]

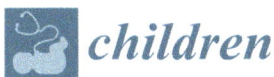

Editorial

Advances in Pediatric Fracture Diagnosis and Treatment Are Numerous but Great Challenges Remain

Christiaan J. A. van Bergen [1,2]

1 Department of Orthopaedic Surgery, Amphia Hospital, 4800 RK Breda, The Netherlands; cvanbergen@amphia.nl; Tel.: +31-76-5955000
2 Department of Orthopaedic Surgery and Sports Medicine, Sophia Children's Hospital, Erasmus University Medical Center, 3000 CA Rotterdam, The Netherlands

Broken bones are very common during childhood. Nevertheless, there are many uncertainties in the scientific understanding of these injuries, and the foundations of their diagnosis and treatment. The current Special Issue on pediatric fractures, therefore, aims to improve our knowledge on various specific fractures in otherwise healthy children, and offer research on general principles in certain populations such as osteogenesis imperfecta patients. The previous Editorial [1] discussed the first 14 articles published [2–15]. Subsequently, seven more high-quality original studies and one systematic review have been published in this popular Special Issue.

Two publications address pediatric facial fractures. Children's heads are relatively heavy compared to adults and, therefore, vulnerable to injury. Tent et al. [16] studied the etiology and epidemiology of pediatric facial fractures in Romania in a 10-year retrospective study. Of 142 children and adolescents with facial fractures, the majority were diagnosed in the 13–18 age group (79%) and in boys (88%). Most were caused by interpersonal violence, followed by falls and motor vehicle accidents. The mandible was the most affected bone. This study improves our understanding on facial fracture occurrence and provides targets for prevention.

A rare facial fracture that can be seen in children is an orbital fracture. Hsieh and Liao [17] from Taiwan and China retrospectively studied the optimal timing of surgery in 23 pediatric orbital trapdoor fractures. In a comparison between early (≤3 days) and delayed (>3 days) surgery, they concluded that operation within 3 days results in a shorter recovery interval for patients with extraocular rectus muscle entrapment.

Two more upper extremity studies have been published since the first Editorial [1]. Poppelaars et al. [18], from the Netherlands, investigated the radiological elbow fat pad sign without visible fracture in children. This sign is sometimes the only abnormal finding on radiography, and may be a clue to an occult fracture. In a large international survey amongst 133 colleagues, they found that further diagnosis and treatment of this population varied widely. Hence, more uniform protocols are required. A first step is to objectify the definition of a fat pad sign. They also performed radiographic measurements and compared those with the respondents' judgements on the presence or absence of a positive fat pad sign. A cut-off angle of 16 degrees with respect to the anterior humeral line indicated a positive anterior fat pad sign, while any visible posterior fat pad was found to be a positive sign.

One frequent cause of a fat pad sign is a radial neck fracture. Langenberg and colleagues [19] systematically reviewed the literature on pediatric radial neck fractures, particularly on the influence of fracture treatment on range of motion after at least 1 year. In total, 26 studies with a total of 551 children were included. Closed reduction without a fixation of fractures with less than 30 degrees of angulation led to an excellent range of motion. Interestingly, in fractures angulated at more than 60 degrees, Kirshner wire fixation

Citation: van Bergen, C.J.A. Advances in Pediatric Fracture Diagnosis and Treatment Are Numerous but Great Challenges Remain. *Children* **2022**, *9*, 1489. https://doi.org/10.3390/children9101489

Received: 29 August 2022
Accepted: 30 August 2022
Published: 28 September 2022

Publisher's Note: MDPI stays neutral with regard to jurisdictional claims in published maps and institutional affiliations.

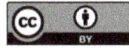

Copyright: © 2022 by the author. Licensee MDPI, Basel, Switzerland. This article is an open access article distributed under the terms and conditions of the Creative Commons Attribution (CC BY) license (https://creativecommons.org/licenses/by/4.0/).

resulted in a better range of motion than intramedullary retrograde fixation. Moreover, open reduction resulted in a loss of motion in the majority of cases.

Descending further in the human body, two studies investigated lower extremity injuries. Weel et al. [20], in a long-term retrospective study, obtained patient-reported outcomes of adolescent soccer players with avulsion fractures of the anterior inferior iliac spine at the origin of the rectus femoris. Of seven initially nonoperatively treated patients, one required surgical excision of a heterotopic ossification. Sports were resumed at 2 to 3 months after injury in all patients, and patient-reported outcomes in the long term were highly satisfactory.

Furthermore, a large Croatian study describes the results of an impressive number of 132 pediatric tibial fractures treated with elastic stable intramedullary fixation during a period of 20 years [21]. Fifteen complications occurred, of which six required reoperation due to the secondary angulation of the fracture. They concluded that elastic nailing is an effective technique with a low complication rate.

In addition, two general studies provide insight into a broad pediatric fracture population. Fuchs et al. [22] analyzed all physeal long-bone fractures registered in the United States in 2016. Almost 6% of pediatric long-bone fractures involved the physis. Out of these 3291 fractures, 59% were localized in the lower extremity, mostly the distal tibia. The majority were classified as Salter–Harris type 2. The peak age was 11 years for girls and 14 years for boys.

Finally, Traa et al. [23] addressed the physical activity of children with extremity fractures presenting at the emergency department in an observational cross-sectional study. In the children's population ($\leq$12 years), 56% were adequately physically active, while in the adolescent population (>12 years), only 43% were adequately physically active, with respect to the Global Recommendations on Physical Activity for Health. These data provide opportunities for injury prevention.

In conclusion, the Special Issue consists of 22 original and review articles, which together contribute to our understanding of pediatric fracture epidemiology, diagnosis, treatment and outcomes. However, many scientific questions are still unanswered and great challenges in this interesting population remain. Therefore, a second volume of this Special Issue has been launched and is open for contributions from researchers worldwide.

Funding: This research received no external funding.

Conflicts of Interest: The author declares no conflict of interest.

References

1. Van Bergen, C.J.A. Pediatric Fractures Are Challenging from Head to Toe. *Children* **2022**, *9*, 678. [CrossRef] [PubMed]
2. Verdoni, F.; Ricci, M.; Di Grigoli, C.; Rossi, N.; Lombardo, M.D.M.; Curci, D.; Accetta, R.; Viganò, M.; Peretti, G.M.; Mangiavini, L. Effect of the COVID-19 Outbreak on Pediatric Patients' Admissions to the Emergency Department in an Italian Orthopedic Trauma Hub. *Children* **2021**, *8*, 645. [CrossRef] [PubMed]
3. Yang, Y.; Hsieh, T.; Liu, C.; Chang, C.; Hou, Y.; Lin, P.; Chen, Y.; Chien, D.; Yiang, G.; Wu, M. Analysis of Clinical Outcome and Predictors of Mortality in Pediatric Trauma Population: Evidence from a 10 Year Analysis in a Single Center. *Children* **2021**, *8*, 688. [CrossRef] [PubMed]
4. Van der Water, L.; Macken, A.A.; Eygendaal, D.; van Bergen, C.J.A. Pediatric Clavicle Fractures and Congenital Pseudarthrosis Unraveled. *Children* **2022**, *9*, 49. [CrossRef]
5. Freislederer, F.; Bensler, S.; Specht, T.; Magerkurth, O.; Eid, K. Plate Fixation for Irreducible Proximal Humeral Fractures in Children and Adolescents—A Single-Center Case Series of Six Patients. *Children* **2021**, *8*, 635. [CrossRef]
6. Vu, T.N.; Phung, S.H.D.; Vo, L.H.; Nguyen, U.H. Diagnosis and Treatment for Pediatric Supracondylar Humerus Fractures with Brachial Artery Injuries. *Children* **2021**, *8*, 933. [CrossRef]
7. Terpstra, S.E.S.; Burgers, P.T.P.W.; van der Heide, H.J.L.; de Witte, P.B. Pediatric Supracondylar Humerus Fractures: Should We Avoid Surgery during After-Hours? *Children* **2022**, *9*, 189. [CrossRef]
8. Hermans, K.; Fransz, D.; Walbeehm-Hol, L.; Hustinx, P.; Staal, H. Is a Parry Fracture—An Isolated Fracture of the Ulnar Shaft—Associated with the Probability of Abuse in Children between 2 and 16 Years Old? *Children* **2021**, *8*, 650. [CrossRef]
9. Schröder, F.F.; de Graaff, F.; Vochteloo, A.J.H. Patient-Specific Guided Osteotomy to Correct a Symptomatic Malunion of the Left Forearm. *Children* **2021**, *8*, 707. [CrossRef]

10. Zhang, J.; Boora, N.; Melendez, S.; Hareendranathan, A.R.; Jaremko, J. Diagnostic Accuracy of 3D Ultrasound and Artificial Intelligence for Detection of Pediatric Wrist Injuries. *Children* **2021**, *8*, 431. [CrossRef]
11. Herdea, A.; Pencea, V.; Lungu, C.N.; Charkaoui, A.; Ulici, A. A Prospective Cohort Study on Quality of Life among the Pediatric Population after Surgery for Recurrent Patellar Dislocation. *Children* **2021**, *8*, 830. [CrossRef] [PubMed]
12. Choo, S.; Nuelle, J.A.V. NSAID Use and Effects on Pediatric Bone Healing: A Review of Current Literature. *Children* **2021**, *8*, 821. [CrossRef] [PubMed]
13. Armstrong, M.L.; Smith, N.; Tracey, R.; Jackman, H. The Orthopedic Effects of Electronic Cigarettes: A Systematic Review and Pediatric Case Series. *Children* **2022**, *9*, 62. [CrossRef] [PubMed]
14. Nijhuis, W.H.; Verhoef, M.; van Bergen, C.J.A.; Weinans, H.; Sakkers, R.J.B. Fractures in Osteogenesis Imperfecta: Pathogenesis, Treatment, Rehabilitation and Prevention. *Children* **2022**, *9*, 268. [CrossRef]
15. Ramírez-Vela, V.; Aguilar-Pérez, L.A.; Paredes-Rojas, J.C.; Flores-Campos, J.A.; Ortiz-Hernández, F.E.; Torres-San Miguel, C.R. Bone Fractures Numerical Analysis in a Femur Affected by Osteogenesis Imperfecta. *Children* **2021**, *8*, 1177. [CrossRef]
16. Tent, P.A.; Juncar, R.I.; Moca, A.E.; Moca, R.T.; Juncar, M. The Etiology and Epidemiology of Pediatric Facial Fractures in North-Western Romania: A 10-Year Retrospective Study. *Children* **2022**, *9*, 932. [CrossRef]
17. Hsieh, P.; Liao, H. Outcome Analysis of Surgical Timing in Pediatric Orbital Trapdoor Fracture with Different Entrapment Contents: A Retrospective Study. *Children* **2022**, *9*, 398. [CrossRef]
18. Poppelaars, M.A.; Eygendaal, D.; The, B.; van Oost, I.; van Bergen, C.J.A. Diagnosis and Treatment of Children with a Radiological Fat Pad Sign without Visible Elbow Fracture Vary Widely: An International Online Survey and Development of an Objective Definition. *Children* **2022**, *9*, 950. [CrossRef]
19. Langenberg, L.C.; van den Ende, K.I.M.; Reijman, M.; Boersen, G.J.; Colaris, J.W. Pediatric Radial Neck Fractures: A Systematic Review Regarding the Influence of Fracture Treatment on Elbow Function. *Children* **2022**, *9*, 1049. [CrossRef]
20. Weel, H.; Joosten, A.P.J.; van Bergen, C.J.A. Apophyseal Avulsion of the Rectus Femoris Tendon Origin in Adolescent Soccer Players. *Children* **2022**, *9*, 1016. [CrossRef]
21. Pogorelic, Z.; Vegan, V.; Jukic, M.; Munoz, C.M.L.; Furlan, D. Elastic Stable Intramedullary Nailing for Treatment of Pediatric Tibial Fractures: A 20-Year Single Center Experience of 132 Cases. *Children* **2022**, *9*, 845. [CrossRef] [PubMed]
22. Fuchs, J.R.; Gibly, R.F.; Erickson, C.B.; Thomas, S.M.; Miller, N.H.; Payne, K.A. Analysis of Physeal Fractures from the United States National Trauma Data Bank. *Children* **2022**, *9*, 914. [CrossRef] [PubMed]
23. Traa, A.C.; Sir, O.; Frazer, S.W.T.; van de Kerkhof-van Bon, B.; Blatter, B.; Tan, E.C.T.H. Levels of Physical Activity in Children with Extremity Fractures a Dutch Observational Cross-Sectional Study. *Children* **2022**, *9*, 325. [CrossRef] [PubMed]

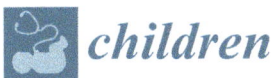

Article

Effect of the COVID-19 Outbreak on Pediatric Patients' Admissions to the Emergency Department in an Italian Orthopedic Trauma Hub

Fabio Verdoni [1], Martina Ricci [2], Cristina Di Grigoli [2], Nicolò Rossi [2], Michele Davide Maria Lombardo [2], Domenico Curci [1], Riccardo Accetta [1], Marco Viganò [1], Giuseppe Maria Peretti [1,3] and Laura Mangiavini [1,3,*]

1. IRCCS Istituto Ortopedico Galeazzi, 20161 Milan, Italy; verdonifabio@alice.it (F.V.); nicocurci73@gmail.com (D.C.); riccardo.accetta@grupposandonato.it (R.A.); marco.vigano@grupposandonato.it (M.V.); giuseppe.peretti@unimi.it (G.M.P.)
2. Residency Program in Orthopedics and Traumatology, University of Milan, 20122 Milan, Italy; martina.ricci@unimi.it (M.R.); cristina.digrigoli@unimi.it (C.D.G.); nicolo.rossi@unimi.it (N.R.); micheledavide.lombardo@unimi.it (M.D.M.L.)
3. Department of Biomedical Sciences for Health, University of Milan, 20133 Milan, Italy
* Correspondence: laura.mangiavini@unimi.it; Tel.: +39-026-621-4494

Citation: Verdoni, F.; Ricci, M.; Di Grigoli, C.; Rossi, N.; Lombardo, M.D.M.; Curci, D.; Accetta, R.; Viganò, M.; Peretti, G.M.; Mangiavini, L. Effect of the COVID-19 Outbreak on Pediatric Patients' Admissions to the Emergency Department in an Italian Orthopedic Trauma Hub. *Children* **2021**, *8*, 645. https://doi.org/10.3390/children8080645

Academic Editor: Johannes Mayr

Received: 9 July 2021
Accepted: 26 July 2021
Published: 27 July 2021

Publisher's Note: MDPI stays neutral with regard to jurisdictional claims in published maps and institutional affiliations.

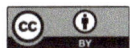

Copyright: © 2021 by the authors. Licensee MDPI, Basel, Switzerland. This article is an open access article distributed under the terms and conditions of the Creative Commons Attribution (CC BY) license (https://creativecommons.org/licenses/by/4.0/).

Abstract: Background: The rapid diffusion of Coronavirus disease (COVID-19) in Northern Italy led the Italian government to dictate a national lockdown from 12 March 2020 to 5 May 2020. The aim of this observational cohort study is to analyze the differences in the number of pediatric patients' admission to the Emergency Room (ER) and in the type and causes of injury. Methods: The pediatric population during the pandemic was compared to a similar group of patients admitted to the ER in 2019. Sex, age, triage color-code at admission, cause of trauma and presence of symptoms related to COVID-19 infection, discharge diagnosis and discharge modes were investigated. Results: The lockdown period led to a reduction of 87.0% in ER admissions with a particular decrease in patients older than 12 years old. Moreover, a trend towards more severe codes and an increase in home-related injuries were observed during the pandemic, whereas the diagnosis of fracture was less frequent in the pre-pandemic group ($p < 0.0001$). Conclusions: A significant decrease in the ER attendances was reported during the lockdown. A shift in the cause and type of injury was observed; only the most serious traumas sought medical care with a higher percentage of severe triage codes and fractures.

Keywords: COVID-19; pediatric trauma HUB; outbreak; ER admissions; pediatric fractures; pediatric injuries

1. Introduction

Coronavirus disease (COVID-19) is a worldwide public health challenge, declared a pandemic by the World Health Organization on 12 March 2020 [1]. Northern Italy was the most affected area within the whole country and has been struggling with COVID-19 since the end of February 2020 [2]. The government dictated measures of national lockdown; in Italy, from 12 March 2020 to 5 May 2020, people could leave their homes only for proved necessity, no recreational activities or sport were allowed and schools were closed. Hospitals were overwhelmed with COVID-19 patients and most of the wards were converted into ICU or infectious diseases care units, while deferrable surgeries and outpatient visits were suspended. Two regional referral centers specialized in traumas and orthopedics emergencies were identified in Milan, Italy, as the hubs for minor traumas or non-deferrable elective orthopedic surgeries [3].

Indeed, during the COVID-19 crisis, the necessity to reduce the risk of virus exposure and transmission and the need to maintain the quality of care provided to critical patients forced the healthcare system to discourage unnecessary admissions to the Emergency Room (ER) related to minor traumas and other ailments. Therefore, a reduction in patient flow to the ER during the pandemic period was noticed, especially in the pediatric population. We performed an observational cohort study on the ER admission of pediatric population (<16) before and after lockdown. The aim of this study was to analyze the number of pediatric patients' admission to the ER, the type and the possible causes of injury.

2. Materials and Methods

We conducted a retrospective study of prospectively collected data. Data collection has been performed on two groups, according to the STROBE guidelines [4]. The Pandemic Group (Pandemic Group—PG) was composed of consecutive patients, aged 0–16 years, admitted to the ER of our Orthopaedic Trauma Hub Centre between 12 March and 5 May 2020, the lockdown period. The Non-Pandemic Group (NG) was composed of all the ER pediatric admissions between 12 March and 5 May 2019. The investigated variables were sex, age, triage color-code at admission, declared cause of trauma and presence of symptoms related to COVID-19 infection, discharge diagnosis and discharge modes.

During ER admission, after checking for symptoms related to COVID-19 disease, the PG patients were assigned to a triage category by a nurse:

- White code: non-urgent patients;
- Green code: urgent but non-critical patients;
- Yellow code: fairly critical patients;
- Red code: very critical patients at danger of death.

Pediatric patients were defined as age $\leq$16 years old.

After triage, patients were evaluated by the attending orthopedic surgeon that provided the appropriate treatment and the most adequate ER discharge mode.

The place where the trauma has occurred was also analyzed based on the clinical history:

- Injuries at home;
- Injuries at school;
- Injuries at play areas;
- Road injuries;
- Unknown: cause of injury was not reported.

Our Institutional Board did not require any ethical approval for this kind of study. All procedures performed in studies involving human participants were in accordance with the ethical standards of the institutional and/or national research committee and with the 1964 Helsinki declaration and its later amendments or comparable ethical standards.

Statistical Analysis

The analyses were performed using Graphpad Prism v5.0 (GraphPad Software, San Diego, CA, USA). Numerical data are presented as median and interquartile range; categorical variables are reported as absolute frequency and percentage. Distribution of continuous variables was assessed by Shapiro–Wilk test. In accordance with the results of this test, the difference between the groups were assessed by Student *t* test or Mann–Whitney test for normally and non-normally distributed variables, respectively; Fisher's exact test was applied to categorical variables. Chi-square test for trends have been applied for ordinal categorical variables with more than 2 categories. A *p*-value < 0.05 was considered statistically significant.

3. Results

Our main finding was the decrease in the number of pediatric patients admitted to ER during the pandemic period: the NG counts for 790 cases, whereas the PG includes 103 patients, showing a reduction of 87.0% in the admissions. Data are reported in Table 1; a statistically significant difference between the two groups was found in the mean age of patients, that decreased from 11.4 ± 3.4 (NG) to 8.6 ± 4.6 years (PG) ($p < 0.0001$); in particular, the decrease relates to the percentage of patients older than 12 years in 2020, from 41.8% in NG to 22.3% in PG ($p < 0.0001$; OR 0.40, CI 95%: 0.25–0.65) (Table 2).

Table 1. Demographic differences between NG and PG.

	NG (2019)	PG (2020)
Number of patients *	790	103
Sex (Males/Females)	454/336 (ratio 1.35)	55/48 (ratio 1.15)
Mean age (years) *	11.4 ± 3.4	8.6 ± 4.6

* = statistically significant difference, $p < 0.0001$.

Table 2. Patients divided by age groups admitted to ER: differences between NG and PG.

Age (Years)	0–2	2–6	6–12	>12	Mean Age	SD	Median Age
NG (2019)	2.3%	6.5%	49.5%	41.8%	11.4	3.4	12
PG (2020)	14.6%	15.5%	47.6%	22.3%	8.6	4.6	9

Regarding the triage code assigned at admittance, a trend toward more severe codes (green and yellow) in the PG compared to NG was recorded ($p = 0.039$) (Figure 1); the diagnosis of fracture was less frequent in NG ($p < 0.0001$) with an Odds Ratio of 2.78 (CI 95%: 1.75–4.09), while the percentage of contusions changed from 19.1% in NG to 13.6% in PG, though no significant difference was detected ($p = 0.22$; OR= 0.67 CI95%: 0.37–1.20). Additionally, a change in the most common diagnoses was noticed: in the NG prevailed ankle sprains (14.2%), forearm fractures (9.4%) and sprains of the interphalangeal joints (8.0%), whereas in PG, forearm fracture was the most frequent trauma (26.2%), followed by elbow contusions (7.2%) and fingers fractures (6.8%). Complete data are reported in Figure 2.

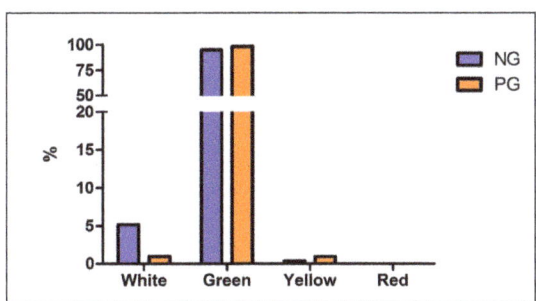

Figure 1. Triage code at ER admission: differences between NG and PG. Legend: NG: Non-pandemic Group PG: Pandemic Group.

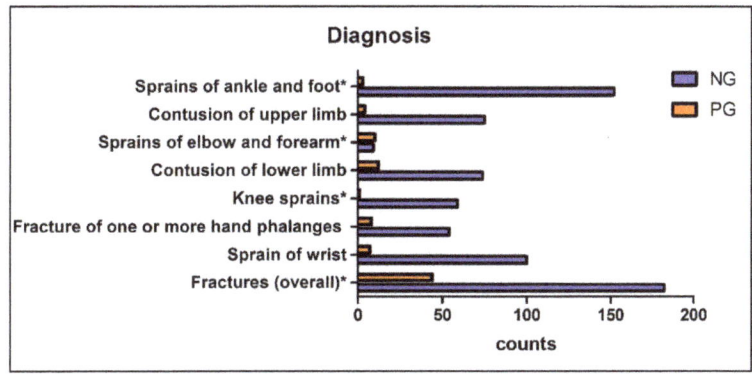

Figure 2. Most frequent diagnosis: differences between NG and PG. * = statistically significant difference. Legend: NG: Non-pandemic Group PG: Pandemic Group.

As far as the location of injuries, data were available for 474 patients out of 790 (60%) for the NG and for 69 patients out of 103 (67%) for the PG. As expected, during the pandemic period injuries at home were far more frequent (34.8% compared to 6.8% in NG), whereas in 2019, traumas mostly occurred during sport activities or at playgrounds (68.4%), followed by injuries at school (18.8%); all these differences are highly statistically significant ($p < 0.0001$). Detailed results are shown in Figure 3.

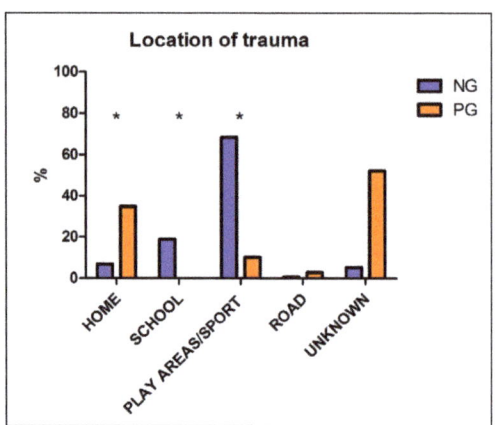

Figure 3. Place of traumas, differences between NG and PG. * = statistically significant difference, $p < 0.0001$. Legend: NG: Non-pandemic Group PG: Pandemic Group.

Surprisingly, no cases of suspected or confirmed COVID-19 infection were recorded in the PG at the investigated Emergency Room.

4. Discussion

Over the last few decades, ERs have known an important growth in patient flow. Thus, "Observatoire Regionale des Urgences Champagne—Ardennes" organization reported an increase in the number of admissions to the ERs in the Champagne-Ardennes state of France of 6.43% per year from 2008 to 2013 [5].

During the outbreak of COVID-19, patients were forced to postpone regular check-ups and non-urgent clinical or surgical procedures to avoid risks of COVID-19 transmission due to the overcrowding of the ERs and of the departments. At the same time, the government imposed a total lockdown in Italy and obligated people to stay at home except for proved necessities. Schools of any grade were closed and sport activities were prohibited. Our findings demonstrate that the lockdown led to 87% reduction in the overall ER pediatric patient flow of our Regional Trauma Hub. In normal conditions, unnecessary admissions contribute to the ER congestion with a long length of stay. Nevertheless, these issues resolved spontaneously during the pandemic. A similar decrease in ER patient's flow was reported in Canada, Taiwan and Hong Kong during the SARS epidemic (2003–2004), and this may be attributed to people's perception of the ER as a possible source of infection. As reported by Huang et al. [6], at the peak of the SARS epidemic, the reduction in daily ER visits reached 51.6% of pre-epidemic numbers ($p < 0.01$). In pediatric patients, the maximum mean decreases in number of visits were 80.0% ($p < 0.01$), 57.6% ($p < 0.01$) and 40.8% ($p < 0.01$), respectively. Moreover, this reduction persisted 3 months after the end of the epidemic. Man et al. [7] displayed a significant drop in the overall ER attendance following the outbreak of SARS; in particular, the trauma rate was significantly lower in 2003 than in 2002 ($p = 0.03$) due to the fear of virus exposure. In addition, during the SARS spread, as well as during the COVID-19 outbreak, most people preferred to avoid crowded areas; thus, recreational or sporting activities may have been less popular then before.

Consequently, a change in community behavior may also explain the drop in ER admission reported in the present study.

Moreover, Bhuvaneswari et al. [8] reported that the most common age group injured at home included patients younger than 12 years and toddlers. Similarly, our study demonstrates an important reduction of patients' age during the lockdown. As a matter of fact, we found an important reduction of patients older than 12 years old who visited the Emergency Department during the COVID-19 outbreak (41.8% in 2019 vs. 22.3% in 2020) (Table 2). This finding may be related to several elements. First, younger children are less aware of the risks of injury and they probably have a similar behavior during outdoor or indoor activities. Thus, they are exposed to traumas even in a domestic context. Furthermore, the closure of schools and play areas constricted at home many older children. Therefore, older children radically changed their behaviors, becoming more focused on board games, computer games and videogames, as they were not allowed to meet with their friends and play outdoors. This clearly represents a difference in the risk of injuries since all these indoor recreational activities did not expose them to traumas. Lastly, older children are more keen on competitive sports activities and contact sports that were prohibited during the national lockdown, and this clearly can explain the reduction of ER admissions of these subset of pediatric patients.

Farrell et al. [9] reported that during the SARS outbreak in 2003, ER visits declined by 21% (95% CI, 18–24%) over the 4-week study period. Conversely to what the present study shows, those authors found the greatest reduction involves both infant and toddler visits (69%; 95% CI, 58–79%) and these data did not recover the following year. This difference might be explained by the fact that our data are relative only to pediatric admissions in a Trauma Hub center specialized only in Orthopaedic surgery. Indeed, COVID-19 disease in neonates, infants and children has been reported to be significantly milder than their adult counterparts. Similarly, all the reported neonatal cases have been mild [10]. Concerning admissions to ER in our Center, no cases of COVID-19 were registered in children, whereas many adult patients diagnosed with COVID-19 were hospitalized at our institute.

During the COVID-19 pandemic, a spike in the purchase of home play equipment and trampolines has been registered. Consequently, the lockdown per se did not prevent all injuries [9]. Regarding the place and causes of trauma, Prakash et al. [11] reported that up to 63.9% children attending ER in ordinary times sustained injuries at home, followed by road accidents (26.2%), whereas school and play areas accounted only for 8.8% of traumas. Conversely, Sephton et al. reported a change in mechanism of injuries during the pandemic period. Indeed, authors showed that the proportion of sports-related injuries during the lockdown period fell from 6.2% to 3.6% [12]. Similarly, the present study demonstrated a big shift from non-domestic traumas (including both scholastic, sport and play areas injuries) to injuries occurred at home in the NG in comparison with the PG (respectively 6.8% and 34.8%). More specifically, our study showed 0% of scholastic traumas during the period of lockdown and only 10% of play area injuries, whereas in 2019 they counted for 18.8% and 68.4% of traumas, respectively. This shift is obviously due to the banning of both outdoor activities and sports performed in gyms and swimming pools. These measures led to a drop of patients presenting for non-urgent chronic reasons, sports-related injuries (sprains, contusions, dislocations) and minor road accidents. Therefore, fewer minor traumas such as sprains of knee reached our ER, as expected, and this finding explains the decreased percentages of non-urgent codes and a statistically significant tendency towards more serious triage codes in the PG. Moreover, we found that the fracture diagnosis was more frequent in the PG in comparison with the NG, confirming that only the most severe injured patients sought medical attention during the pandemic period. In addition, forearm fractures and elbow contusions were the most frequent traumas in the PG, consistently with the younger age of ER admissions as these type of injuries are more frequent in this subset of pediatric patients [13].

A recent study also reported an increase in domestic violence and child abuse, particularly in dysfunctional families during the pandemic period. This event might be related to restrictions, isolation, higher level of anxiety and stress with a relevant impact on risks of developmental delay and behavioral problems [14]. Nevertheless, our study did not show any increase in domestic violence and child abuse rate, probably because our institution is mainly an Orthopedic Trauma Hub and it lacks a psychological or psychiatric support for children and adolescents; thus, suspected child abuses were not recorded. A more extensive analysis involving other hospitals with a pediatric psychiatric service may confirm the results shown by Boo et al. [14].

The conclusions drawn from this study rely on data about an Orthopedic Trauma Hub that includes also a Pediatric Orthopedics service and may be different from the flow in other hospitals. Thus, we cannot comment on the pediatric patients' flow in the ER due to ailments other than traumas. Nevertheless, this is the first study revealing the epidemiologic effects that COVID-19 pandemic and lockdown measures had on pediatric patients' flow in an emergency department.

Moreover, our study indirectly demonstrated that the vast majority of ER admissions in normal conditions is due to non-urgent or deferrable conditions. Thus, this evidence-based analysis is fundamental to improving the strategies of care of the National Health System, to better employ the available resources and to reduce overcrowding in the ER that usually leads to long waiting time for patients and the risk of a lower standard of care.

5. Conclusions

A significant drop in the overall ER attendances in a Trauma Hub center was reported after the outbreak of COVID-19 pandemic. The fear of virus exposure in hospital undoubtedly acted as a significant deterrent. However, it is likely that the community precautions adopted during the lockdown, namely school closures and decreased sport activities, resulted in fewer injuries; thus, only the most serious traumas sought medical care, resulting in a higher percentage of severe triage codes and fractures.

Author Contributions: Conceptualization, F.V., G.M.P. and L.M.; methodology, M.R., C.D.G., N.R., D.C. and M.D.M.L.; software, M.V.; validation, F.V., G.M.P. and L.M.; formal analysis, M.V.; investigation, F.V., M.R., C.D.G., N.R., D.C., R.A. and M.D.M.L.; resources, F.V. and R.A.; data curation, M.R., C.D.G., N.R., M.V. and M.D.M.L.; writing—original draft preparation, F.V., M.R., C.D.G. and N.R.; writing—review and editing, G.M.P. and L.M.; visualization, M.R., C.D.G., N.R., D.C. and M.D.M.L.; supervision, F.V., G.M.P. and L.M.; project administration, F.V. and L.M. All authors have read and agreed to the published version of the manuscript.

Funding: This research received no external funding.

Institutional Review Board Statement: The study was conducted according to the guidelines of the Declaration of Helsinki. Ethical review and approval were waived for this study, due to the retrospective nature of the analysis.

Informed Consent Statement: Patient consent was waived due to due to the retrospective nature of the analysis.

Data Availability Statement: Data supporting reported results can be found at this link: https://osf.io/k2wh5/?view_only=e59648fbba854840b32ca3988736da6a (accessed on 26 July 2021).

Conflicts of Interest: The authors declare no conflict of interest.

References

1. WHO/Europe. Coronavirus Disease (COVID-19) Outbreak—WHO Announces COVID-19 Outbreak a Pandemic. Available online: https://www.who.int/emergencies/diseases/novel-coronavirus-2019 (accessed on 11 March 2021).
2. Livingston, E.; Bucher, K. Coronavirus Disease 2019 (COVID-19) in Italy. *JAMA* **2020**, *323*, 1335. [CrossRef] [PubMed]
3. Randelli, P.S.; Compagnoni, R. Management of orthopaedic and traumatology patients during the Coronavirus disease (COVID-19) pandemic in northern Italy. *Knee Surg. Sports Traumatol. Arthrosc.* **2020**, *28*, 1683–1689. [CrossRef] [PubMed]
4. Von Elm, E.; Altman, D.G.; Egger, M.; Pocock, S.J.; Gotzsche, P.C.; Vandenbroucke, J.P.; Initiative, S. The Strengthening the Reporting of Observational Studies in Epidemiology (STROBE) statement: Guidelines for reporting of observational studies. *Internist* **2008**, *49*, 688–693. [CrossRef] [PubMed]

5. Afilal, M.; Yalaoui, F.; Dugardin, F.; Amodeo, L.; Laplanche, D.; Blua, P. Forecasting the emergency department patients flow. *J. Med. Syst* **2016**, *40*, 175. [CrossRef] [PubMed]
6. Huang, H.H.; Yen, D.H.; Kao, W.F.; Wang, L.M.; Huang, C.I.; Lee, C.H. Declining emergency department visits and costs during the severe acute respiratory syndrome (SARS) outbreak. *J. Formos. Med. Assoc.* **2006**, *105*, 31–37. [CrossRef]
7. Man, C.Y.; Yeung, R.S.; Chung, J.Y.; Cameron, P.A. Impact of SARS on an emergency department in Hong Kong. *Emerg. Med.* **2003**, *15*, 418–422. [CrossRef] [PubMed]
8. Bhuvaneswari, N.; Prasuna, J.G.; Goel, M.K.; Rasania, S.K. An epidemiological study on home injuries among children of 0-14 years in South Delhi. *Indian J. Public Health* **2018**, *62*, 4–9. [CrossRef] [PubMed]
9. Farrell, S.; Schaeffer, E.K.; Mulpuri, K. Recommendations for the care of pediatric orthopaedic patients during the COVID-19 pandemic. *J. Am. Acad Orthop. Surg.* **2020**, *28*, e477–e486. [CrossRef] [PubMed]
10. Singhal, T. A review of Coronavirus disease-2019 (COVID-19). *Indian J. Pediatr.* **2020**, *87*, 281–286. [CrossRef] [PubMed]
11. Prakash Raju, K.N.J.; Jagdish, S.; Kumar, G.K.; Anandhi, D.; Antony, J. Profile of pediatric trauma among the patients attending emergency department in a tertiary care hospital in South India. *J. Emerg. Trauma Shock* **2020**, *13*, 62–67. [CrossRef] [PubMed]
12. Sephton, B.M.; Mahapatra, P.; Shenouda, M.; Ferran, N.; Deierl, K.; Sinnett, T.; Somashekar, N.; Sarraf, K.M.; Nathwani, D.; Bhattacharya, R. The effect of COVID-19 on a major trauma network. An analysis of mechanism of injury pattern, referral load and operative case-mix. *Injury* **2021**, *52*, 395–401. [CrossRef] [PubMed]
13. Lempesis, V.; Jerrhag, D.; Rosengren, B.E.; Landin, L.; Tiderius, C.J.; Karlsson, M.K. Pediatric distal forearm fracture epidemiology in Malmo, Sweden-Time trends during six decades. *J. Wrist Surg.* **2019**, *8*, 463–469. [CrossRef] [PubMed]
14. Boo, W.H. Exposure to domestic violence during the COVID-19 pandemic: A potent threat to the mental well-being of children. *Malays. J. Med. Sci.* **2021**, *28*, 158–159. [CrossRef] [PubMed]

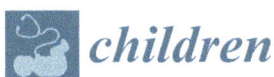

Article

Analysis of Clinical Outcome and Predictors of Mortality in Pediatric Trauma Population: Evidence from a 10 Year Analysis in a Single Center

Ya-Chih Yang [1,2], Tsung-Han Hsieh [3], Chi-Yuan Liu [4,5], Chun-Yu Chang [6,7], Yueh-Tseng Hou [1,2], Po-Chen Lin [1,2], Yu-Long Chen [1,2], Da-Sen Chien [1,2], Giou-Teng Yiang [1,2] and Meng-Yu Wu [1,2,*]

1. Department of Emergency Medicine, Taipei Tzu Chi Hospital, Buddhist Tzu Chi Medical Foundation, New Taipei 231, Taiwan; foxcat721@yahoo.com.tw (Y.-C.Y.); brianann75@gmail.com (Y.-T.H.); taipeitzuchier@gmail.com (P.-C.L.); yulong0129@gmail.com (Y.-L.C.); sam.jan1978@msa.hinet.net (D.-S.C.); gtyiang@gmail.com (G.-T.Y.)
2. Department of Emergency Medicine, School of Medicine, Tzu Chi University, Hualien 970, Taiwan
3. Department of Research, Taipei Tzu Chi Hospital, Buddhist Tzu Chi Medical Foundation, New Taipei 231, Taiwan; tch28047@tzuchi.com.tw
4. Department of Orthopedic Surgery, Taipei Tzu Chi Hospital, Buddhist Tzu Chi Medical Foundation, New Taipei 231, Taiwan; cy.liu@tzuchi.com.tw
5. Department of Orthopedics, School of Medicine, Tzu Chi University, Hualien 970, Taiwan
6. Department of Anesthesiology, Taipei Tzu Chi Hospital, Buddhist Tzu Chi Medical Foundation, New Taipei 231, Taiwan; paulchang1231@gmail.com
7. School of Medicine, Tzu Chi University, Hualien 970, Taiwan
* Correspondence: skyshangrila@gmail.com; Tel.: +886-2-6628-9779; Fax: +886-2-6628-9009

Citation: Yang, Y.-C.; Hsieh, T.-H.; Liu, C.-Y.; Chang, C.-Y.; Hou, Y.-T.; Lin, P.-C.; Chen, Y.-L.; Chien, D.-S.; Yiang, G.-T.; Wu, M.-Y. Analysis of Clinical Outcome and Predictors of Mortality in Pediatric Trauma Population: Evidence from a 10 Year Analysis in a Single Center. *Children* **2021**, *8*, 688. https://doi.org/10.3390/children8080688

Academic Editor: Christiaan J. A. van Bergen

Received: 8 July 2021
Accepted: 8 August 2021
Published: 10 August 2021

Publisher's Note: MDPI stays neutral with regard to jurisdictional claims in published maps and institutional affiliations.

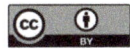

Copyright: © 2021 by the authors. Licensee MDPI, Basel, Switzerland. This article is an open access article distributed under the terms and conditions of the Creative Commons Attribution (CC BY) license (https://creativecommons.org/licenses/by/4.0/).

Abstract: The shock index (SI) is a useful tool for predicting the injury severity and mortality in patients with trauma. However, pediatric physiology differs from that of adults. In the pediatric trauma population, the shock status may be obscured within the normal range of vital signs. Pediatric age-adjusted SI (SIPA) is reported more accurately compared to SI. In our study, we conducted a 10 year retrospective cohort study of pediatric trauma population to evaluate the SI and SIPA in predicting mortality, intensive care unit (ICU) admission, and the need for surgery. This retrospective cohort study included 1265 pediatric trauma patients from January 2009 to June 2019 at the Taipei Tzu Chi Hospital, who had a history of hospitalization. The primary outcome of this investigation was in-hospital mortality, and the secondary outcomes were the length of hospital and ICU stay, operation times, and ICU admission times. The SIPA group can detect changes in vital signs early to reflect shock progression. In the elevated SIPA group, more severe traumatic injuries were identified, including high injury severity score (ISS), revised trauma score (RTS), and new injury severity score (NISS) scores than SI > 0.9. The odds ratio of elevated SIPA and SI (>0.9) to predict ISS ≥ 16 was 3.593 (95% Confidence interval [CI]: 2.175–5.935, $p < 0.001$) and 2.329 (95% CI: 1.454–3.730, $p < 0.001$). SI and SIPA are useful for identifying the compensatory phase of shock in prehospital and hospital settings, especially in corresponding normal to low-normal blood pressure. SIPA is effective in predicting the mortality and severity of traumatic injuries in the pediatric population. However, SI and SIPA were not significant predictors of ICU admission and the need for surgery analysis.

Keywords: shock index; pediatric age-adjusted shock index; trauma; pediatric trauma; mortality

1. Introduction

Despite the advances in medical care, it is observed that ten individuals die due to trauma injuries every minute [1]. Recently, deaths due to trauma have increased and pose a considerable financial burden on health insurance. Based on the current concept of the American College of Surgeons Committee on Trauma (ACS-COT), early accurate prediction of traumatic injury severity could be transferred to higher-level facilities and provide total care for every aspect of the injury. The shock index (SI, the ratio of heart rate to systolic blood pressure) has been reported as a sensitive marker of hemodynamic instability to reflect the shock severity. In previous adult studies, an SI > 0.9 is shown to predict transfusion needs and mortality [2,3]. However, few studies have focused on pediatric populations. The direct application of adult trauma scores to the pediatric population is not suitable [4,5]. In the study by N. Acker et al., [6] the adjusting of SI is promoted by adjusting the age-based pediatric vital signs to provide a higher accuracy than unadjusted SI. This pediatric age-adjusted shock index (SIPA) has been validated in a few studies [6,7]. Other studies have evaluated the role of SI and SIPA in predicting intensive care unit (ICU) admissions. Compared to other symptom scores, SIPA could be calculated by the emergency department or emergency medical services (EMS) without pediatric weight or advanced intervention parameters. In prehospital evaluations, SIPA provided an easy access for emergency medical technicians to predict the traumatic injury severity. However, there is a lack of strong evidence for SIPA in the pediatric population with trauma. Therefore, in our study, we conducted a 10 year retrospective cohort study of pediatric population with trauma to evaluate SI and SIPA in predicting mortality, ICU admission, and operation (OP).

2. Methods

2.1. Study Design and Inclusion Criteria

This was a retrospective cohort study using the Taipei Tzu Chi Hospital trauma database from January 2009 to June 2019 and was approved by the Institutional Review Board of Taipei Tzu Chi Hospital (IRB number: 10-XD-072). The Taipei Tzu Chi Hospital trauma database contains 152 data elements related to trauma patients and hospital information, including detailed patient demographics, prehospital medical conditions, vital signs, in-hospital vital signs, abbreviated injury scale (AIS) score, injury severity score (ISS), and in-hospital and in-emergency department (ED) mortality. We included all pediatric trauma patients aged ≤20 years from January 2009 to June 2019 who visited Taipei Tzu Chi Hospital and had a history of hospitalization. The primary outcome of this investigation was in-hospital mortality, and the secondary outcomes were the length of hospital and ICU stay, OP times, and ICU admission times. The exclusion criteria included (1) patients who were diagnosed with an out-of-hospital cardiac arrest, (2) patients whose clinical outcome or important data were missing, and (3) patients who had no hospitalization. Several trauma scoring systems have been reported to evaluate the trauma severity and predict clinical outcomes. However, there is less evidence to support these findings in the pediatric population. Therefore, we investigated the current trauma score systems in the pediatric population, including the ISS, Glasgow coma scale (GCS), revised trauma score (RTS), SI, National Industrial Security System (NISS), and new trauma and injury severity score (TRISS). A subgroup analysis was also conducted to analyze the traumatic score systems in different age and injury types.

2.2. Shock Index and Pediatric Age-Adjusted Shock Index

The SI, a physiological triage score, was calculated using the recorded heart rate (HR) and systolic blood pressure (SBP) using the following formula: SI = HR/SBP. The SI is a sensitive marker for predicting the shock status, which has been studied in multiple populations, including sepsis, cardiovascular disease, and obstetric population [8]. The normal range for the SI is reported as 0.5–0.7. Some evidence suggests that an SI higher than 0.9 is acceptable to believe hemodynamic instability in patients. Pediatric physiology differs from adults, and the normal range of pediatric vital signs varies with age, which could significantly influence the SI values. Therefore, the SIPA has been proposed to identify and predict hemodynamically unstable children [6]. The cut-off values and normal ranges of SIPA are listed in Table 1.

Table 1. Age-adjusted shock index cutoff value.

Age	Heart Rate	Systolic Blood Pressure	Shock Index Cutoff Value
≤3 years	70–110	90–110	1.2
4–6 years	65–110	90–110	1.2
7–12 years	60–100	100–120	1.0
>12 years	55–90	100–135	0.9

2.3. Statistical Analysis

The demographic details, overall survival, and clinical outcome data were analyzed using the SPSS software (Version 13.0 SPSS Inc, Chicago, IL, USA) for statistical analysis. All continuous variables are reported as the mean, standard deviation (SD), and median. Categorical variables were reported as numbers with percentages. Continuous variables were compared using the independent sample t-test for normally distributed data and the Mann–Whitney U test for non-normally distributed data. The categorical variables were compared using the Pearson chi-squared test or Fisher's exact test. Multivariable logistic regression was used to analyze the clinical outcomes in pediatric trauma patients. The variables with $p < 0.10$, or important variables, were selected for multivariable logistic regression analysis. The area under the receiver operating characteristic curve (AUROC) was used for each outcome to analyze the discrimination of the regression model. All tests were two-sided, and a p value < 0.05 was considered as statistically significant.

3. Results

A total of 1265 patients were identified in the Taipei Tzu Chi Hospital trauma database from January 2009 to June 2019. A detailed flowchart is shown in Figure 1. In the included pediatric trauma population (Table 2), the mean age was 14 years, and 72.1% of the population were boys. The triage distribution of patients was observed to be 55.2% in level II, followed by level III (36.9%). The consciousness level in the emergency department was 91.1% with total alertness (GCS: 15) and severe coma status in 24 patients (1.9%). Of a total of 1265 patients, 760 patients (60.1%) were injured in the street, 268 patients (21.2%) were injured in a public site, and 160 patients (12.6%) were injured at home. The major injury mechanism was traffic accidents (53.1%), followed by the secondary injury mechanism of pediatric trauma. The extremities were the major injury sites, accounting for up to 72.7% of injuries, followed by the head (18.8%) and facial (15.7%) injuries. Fifty-eight pediatric patients were activated by the trauma team. In traumatic score systems, 305 patients presented a high SI, and 171 patients showed an elevated SIPA. Seventy-eight patients had an ISS ≥ 16. In the clinical outcome analysis, the median hospital length of stay (LOS) was 5 days, and 177 patients were admitted to the ICU. Surgical intervention was needed in 867 patients, and 49 patients underwent reoperation. In total, seven patients died during the in-hospital follow-up (Table 3). In the population with a high SI level and elevated SIPA, the blood pressure was significantly lower with respect to the systolic and diastolic blood pressure, associated with higher respiratory and heart rates. These findings reflected an early unstable hemodynamic status. The severe injury population, such as ISS ≥ 16 and high ISS and RTS score, is significant in the abnormal SI and elevated SIPA group. In addition, the high SI level group showed a longer LOS, and the elevated SIPA group had a high mortality rate (Table 4).

All the quantitative variables considered to have potential correlations with the mortality, ICU admission, and the need for surgery showed statistically significant associations, including age, past history, diastolic blood pressure, and the severity of injury (elevated SIPA, ISS, RTS, NISS, and TRISS). To compare the SI value > 0.9 with elevated SIPA, we performed a quantitative assessment of associations by performing an odds ratio (OR) analysis by adjusting for age, past history, diastolic pressure, and severity of injury (ISS ≥ 16). For mortality, the adjusted OR of SI > 0.9 was 2.151 (95% Confidence interval [CI]: 0.322–14.362, p-value: 0.429) and 2.295 in the elevated SIPA group (95% CI: 0.334–15.777, $p = 0.398$). The AUROC was 0.594 in the SI > 0.9 group and 0.648 in the elevated SIPA group. In the prediction of ICU admission, the adjusted OR of SI > 0.9 showed 0.883 (95% CI: 0.560–1.392, $p = 0.591$) and 0.542 in the elevated SIPA group (95% CI: 0.306–0.958, $p = 0.035$). The AUROC was 0.491 in the SI > 0.9 group and 0.471 in the elevated SIPA group. In predicting the need for surgery, the adjusted OR of SI > 0.9 was 1.110 (95% CI: 0.794–1.551, $p = 0.543$) and 1.029 in the elevated SIPA group (95% CI: 0.719–1.473, $p = 0.876$). The AUROC was 0.489 in the SI > 0.9 group and 0.494 in the elevated SIPA group (Figure 2). In the subgroup analysis, home was the major injury site in the population aged ≤8 years. As the age increased, injury at the street increased from 27.1% to 82.3%. In our study, the patients aged between 8 and 12 years had a lower ISS and percentage of ISS ≥ 16 compared to other groups. The mean SI was higher in the age group ≤ 8 years, followed by the 8–12 years group. The young population has up to 70.8% patients with a SI ≥ 0.9; however, only 22.5% of the population was observed to have elevated SIPA. SI was observed to decrease with age, and the percentage of SI ≥ 0.9 is the same. Although the percentage of elevated SIPA also increased with age, the trend was slower than that of SI. In the outcome analysis, the total LOS and the percentage of deaths increased in the high age population (Table 5). In all the patients, the SI of ISS ≥ 16 was significantly higher than the ISS < 16 (mean ± SD: 0.88 ± 0.33 vs. 0.76 ± 0.23). Similar results were observed in the populations of ≤ 8 years, 12–16 years, and 16–20 years. The percentage of SI > 0.9, and elevated SIPA was also significantly higher in the patients with ISS ≥ 16 than in those with ISS < 16 (Figure 3). The total LOS was longer in the severe injury group with ISS ≥ 16; however, the ICU LOS was not significant (Figure 4). Based on the criteria of Acker et al., [6], the patients aged ≤16 years were included for analysis of SIPA and SI > 0.9, predicting the mortality, ICU admission, and the need for surgery. The AUROC curve of elevated SIPA was better than SI > 0.9 in patients aged ≤16 years (AUROC: 0.751 vs. 0.646) (Figure 5).

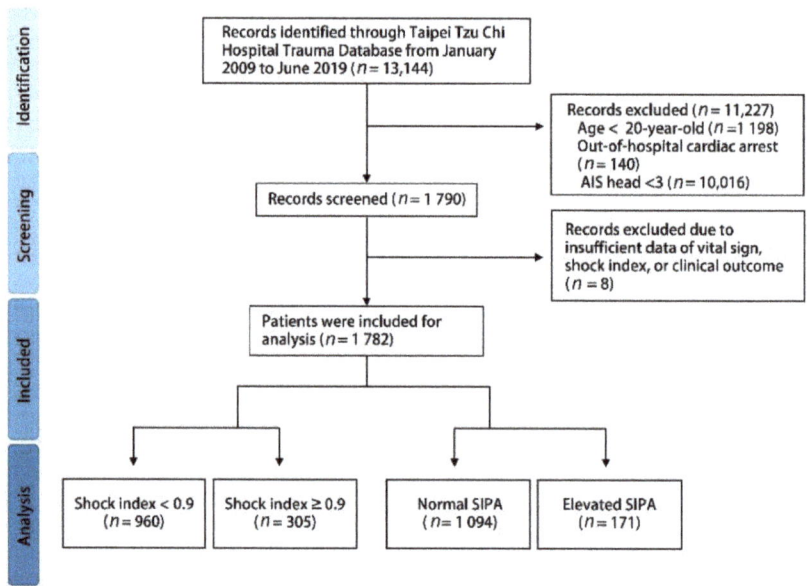

Figure 1. Schematic diagram illustrating the detailed inclusion of pediatric trauma patients.

Table 2. Demographic population of all pediatric trauma patients.

Characteristics	All Pediatric Population N = 1265
Age (years), mean ± SD	14.27 ± 5.51
Male, n (%)	912(72.1%)
Underlying diseases, n (%)	70(5.5%)
Vital sign	
SBP, mean ± SD	126.73 ± 23.48
DBP, mean ± SD	75.33 ± 13.67
RR, mean ± SD	19.17 ± 2.58
HR, mean ± SD	93.56 ± 19.57
Triage	
I	96(7.6%)
II	698(55.2%)
III	467(36.9%)
IV + V	4(0.3%)
Consciousness level	
15	1152(91.1%)
8–15	88(7.0%)
≤8	24(1.9%)
Injury site	
Home	160(12.6%)
Street	760(60.1%)
Public site	268(21.2%)
Others	77(6.1%)
Mechanism	
Motor Vehicle Collision	672(53.1%)
Fall	387(30.6%)
Crushing injury	76(6.0%)
Sharp object	55(4.3%)
Others	75(5.9%)
Injured area	
Head and neck	251(18.8%)
Face	199(15.7%)
Thorax	82(6.5%)
Abdomen	91(7.2%)
Extremity	920(72.7%)
Activation of trauma team	58(4.6%)
Trauma scores	
Shock index	0.77 ± 0.24
Shock index ≥ 0.9	305(24.1%)
SIPA	0.86 ± 0.34
Elevated SIPA	171(13.5%)
ISS, (mean; SD)	6.51 ± 5.80
ISS ≥ 16, (%)	78(6.2%)
RTS, (mean; SD)	7.70 ± 0.63
NISS, (mean; SD)	7.36 ± 6.89
TRISS, (mean; SD)	0.98 ± 0.10
Clinical outcome	
LOS days, (median; IQR)	5.0 (3.0–9.0)
ICU Admission, (%)	177(14.0%)
ICU Readmission, (%)	2(0.2%)
ICU days, (median; IQR)	4.0 (2.0–6.0)
Need for surgery (%)	867(68.5%)
Reoperation (%)	49(3.9%)
Death, (%)	7(0.6%)

SD: standard deviation; IQR: interquartile range; SBP: Systolic blood pressure; DBP: diastolic blood pressure; RR: respiration rate; HR: heart rate; ISS: injury severity score; RTS: revised trauma score; NISS: National Industrial Security System; TRISS: new trauma and injury severity score; LOS days: length of stay days; and ICU: intensive care unit.

Table 3. Demographic population of elevated shock index and age-adjusted pediatric shock index.

Characteristics	SI < 0.9 N = 960	SI ≥ 0.9 N = 305	p-Value	Normal SIPA N = 1094	Elevated SIPA N = 171	p-Value
Age (years), mean ± SD	15.91 ± 4.04	9.09 ± 6.27	<0.001	14.63 ± 5.22	11.97 ± 6.69	<0.001
Male, n (%)	727(75.73%)	185(60.66%)	<0.001	808(73.86%)	104(60.82%)	<0.001
Underlying diseases, n (%)	58(6.04%)	12(3.93%)	0.161	63(5.76%)	7(4.09%)	0.376
Vital sign						
SBP, mean ± SD	133.69 ± 20.63	104.83 ± 17.78	<0.001	130.67 ± 21.64	101.53 ± 18.74	<0.001
DBP, mean ± SD	78.07 ± 12.24	66.70 ± 14.33	<0.001	77.01 ± 12.87	64.54 ± 13.69	<0.001
RR, mean ± SD	18.78 ± 2.0	20.39 ± 3.61	<0.001	19.01 ± 2.23	20.17 ± 4.06	<0.001
HR, mean ± SD	87.19 ± 14.53	113.62 ± 19.85	<0.001	90.05 ± 16.83	116.06 ± 20.90	<0.001
Injury site						
Home	72(7.50%)	88(28.85%)	<0.001	125(11.43%)	35(20.47%)	<0.001
Street	631(65.73%)	129(42.30%)	<0.001	666(60.88%)	94(54.97%)	0.143
Public site	86(8.96%)	29(9.51%)	0.771	104(9.51%)	11(6.43%)	0.194
Others	165(17.19%)	56(18.36%)	0.638	191(17.46%)	30(17.54%)	0.978
ISS, (mean; SD)	6.33 ± 5.28	7.10 ± 7.20	0.084	6.22 ± 5.08	8.39 ± 8.98	0.002
ISS ≥ 16, (%)	46(4.79%)	32(10.49%)	<0.001	52(4.75%)	26(15.20%)	<0.001
RTS, (mean; SD)	7.75 ± 0.52	7.53 ± 0.87	<0.001	7.74 ± 0.55	7.42 ± 0.94	<0.001
NISS, (mean; SD)	7.17 ± 6.32	7.97 ± 8.42	0.126	7.04 ± 6.08	9.40 ± 10.49	0.005
TRISS, (mean; SD)	0.98 ± 0.09	0.97 ± 0.13	0.091	0.98 ± 0.09	0.97 ± 0.12	0.152
LOS days, (median; IQR)	5.0 (3.0–9.0)	3.0 (2.0–7.0)	<0.001	5.0(3.0–9.0)	4.0(2.0–10.0)	0.204
ICU admission, (%)	137(14.27%)	40(13.11%)	0.612	162(14.81%)	15(8.77%)	0.034
ICU readmission, (%)	2(0.21%)	0(0.00%)	1.000	2(0.18%)	0(0.00%)	1.000
ICU days, (median; IQR)	4.0 (3.0–6.0)	3.5 (2.0–6.0)	0.556	4.0(2.0–6.0)	3.0(2.0–5.0)	0.411
Need for surgery (%)	664(69.17%)	203(66.56%)	0.363	753(68.83%)	114(66.67%)	0.571
Reoperation (%)	35(3.65%)	14(4.59%)	0.457	44(4.02%)	5(2.92%)	0.489
Death, (%)	4(0.42%)	3(0.98%)	0.369	4(0.37%)	3(1.75%)	0.056

SD: standard deviation; IQR: interquartile range; SBP: Systolic blood pressure; DBP: diastolic blood pressure; RR: respiration rate; HR: heart rate; ISS: injury severity score; RTS: revised trauma score; NISS: National Industrial Security System; TRISS: new trauma and injury severity score; LOS days: length of stay days; and ICU: intensive care unit.

Table 4. Unadjusted odds ratio for mortality related to in-hospital parameters.

Characteristics	Crude OR of Mortality			Crude OR of ICU Admission			Crude OR of Need for Surgery		
	OR	95% CI	p-Value	OR	95% CI	p-Value	OR	95% CI	p-Value
Age	1.245	0.943–1.644	0.121	1.000	0.971–1.029	0.987	1.022	1.001–1.044	0.040
Male	0.967	0.187–5.008	0.968	1.082	0.756–1.550	0.666	0.928	0.711–1.211	0.584
Underlying diseases, n (%)	13.332	2.925–60.777	<0.001	1.156	0.595–2.246	0.669	0.765	0.464–1.261	0.294
Vital sign									
SBP	0.985	0.953–1.018	0.355	0.999	0.992–1.006	0.716	1.003	0.998–1.009	0.190
DBP	0.937	0.885–0.991	0.023	0.992	0.980–1.003	0.153	1.002	0.993–1.010	0.732
RR	0.850	0.617–1.170	0.319	1.026	0.968–1.088	0.384	1.023	0.976–1.073	0.338
HR	1.006	0.971–1.043	0.726	0.998	0.989–1.006	0.565	1.003	0.997–1.009	0.309
Shock index	7.991	1.033–61.838	0.047	0.853	0.434–1.674	0.644	0.945	0.577–1.545	0.820
Shock index > 0.9	2.375	0.529–10.668	0.259	0.907	0.621–1.324	0.612	0.887	0.674–1.167	0.393
Elevated SIPA	4.867	1.080–21.937	0.039	0.553	0.317–0.964	0.038	0.906	0.643–1.276	0.571
ISS	1.135	1.084–1.189	<0.001	0.996	0.968–1.025	0.785	0.987	0.967–1.006	0.180
ISS ≥ 16	98.833	11.741–831.938	<0.001	0.791	0.388–1.615	0.520	0.719	0.448–1.153	0.171
RTS	0.521	0.395–0.689	<0.001	1.028	0.788–1.341	0.840	1.173	0.980–1.405	0.083
NISS	1.107	1.069–1.145	<0.001	1.002	0.979–1.024	0.896	0.993	0.977–1.010	0.425
TRISS	0.016	0.002–0.106	<0.001	3.741	0.303–46.183	0.304	1.173	0.360–3.823	0.791
Activation of trauma team	56.839	10.778–299.750	<0.001	1.136	0.548–2.355	0.732	0.548	0.322–0.933	0.027
LOS days	1.004	0.972–1.037	0.803	1.035	1.021–1.049	<0.001	0.995	0.986–1.004	0.272

SBP: Systolic blood pressure; DBP: diastolic blood pressure; RR: respiration rate; HR: heart rate; ISS: injury severity score; RTS: revised trauma score; NISS: National Industrial Security System; TRISS: new trauma and injury severity score; and SIPA: pediatric age-adjusted shock index.

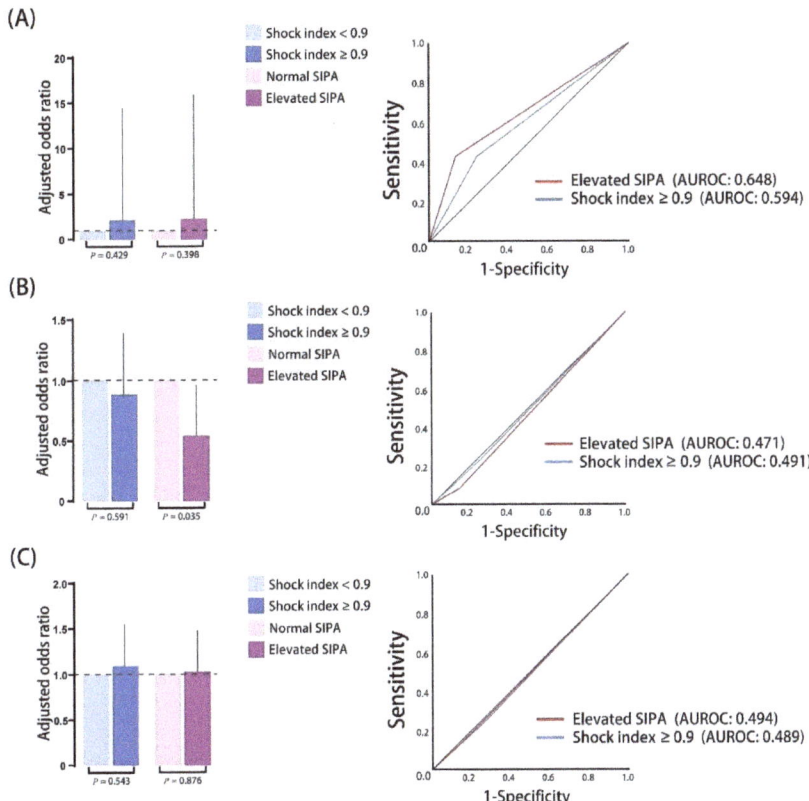

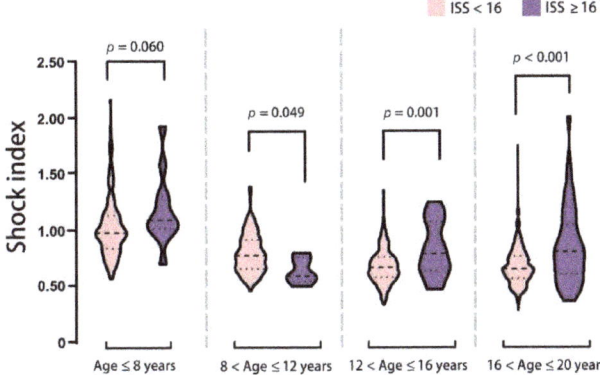

Figure 2. Schematic diagram illustrating the adjusted odds ratio of elevated shock index (SI) > 0.9 and pediatric age-adjusted SI (SIPA) group in (**A**) mortality, (**B**) intensive care unit (ICU) admission, and (**C**) need for surgery with area under the receiver operating characteristic curve (AUROC).

Figure 3. *Cont.*

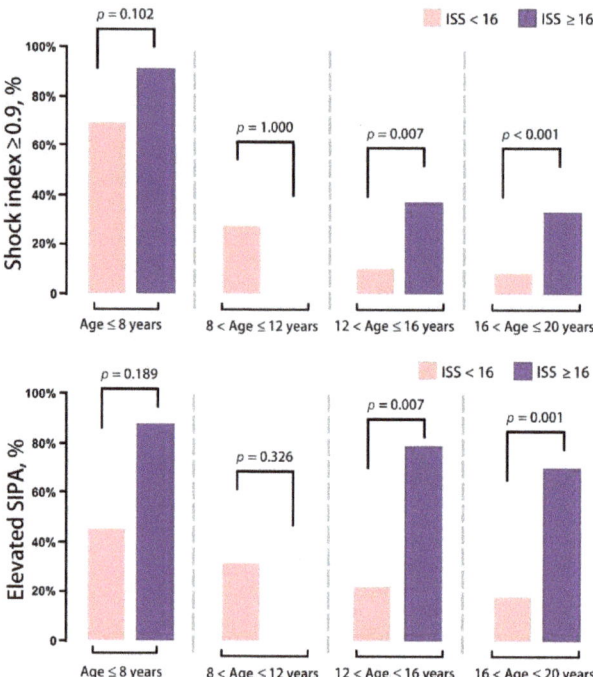

Figure 3. Schematic diagram illustrating the shock index (SI), the percentage of SI ≥ 0.9 and elevated pediatric age-adjusted SI (SIPA) of distribution of high (injury severity score, [ISS] ≥ 16) and low injury (ISS < 16) in different age range.

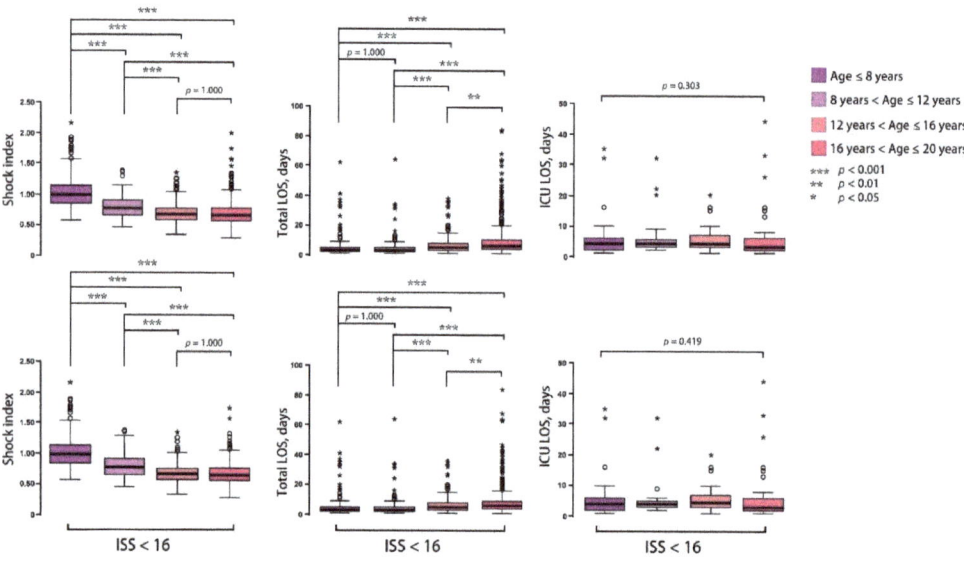

Figure 4. Cont.

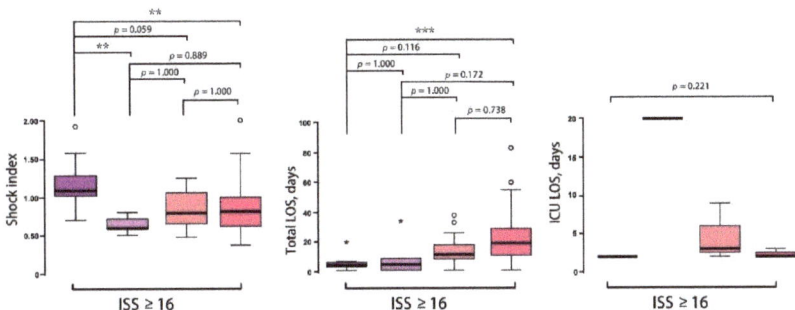

Figure 4. The distribution of shock index, total length of stay (LOS), and intensive care unit (ICU) LOS in different age in high (injury severity score, [ISS] ≥ 16) and low injury (ISS < 16).

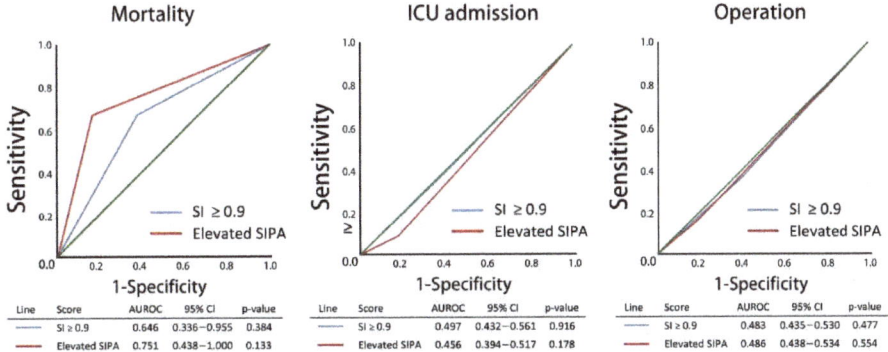

Figure 5. The area under the receiver operating characteristic curve (AUROC) of shock index > 0.9 and elevated pediatric age-adjusted SI (SIPA) predicting mortality, intensive care unit (ICU) admission, and need for surgery in population with age ≤ 16.

Table 5. Subgroup analysis of elevated shock index and age-adjusted pediatric shock index in different age ranges.

Characteristics	Age ≤ 8 year N = 236	8 ≤ Age < 12 year N = 165	12 ≤ Age < 16 year N = 237	16 ≤ Age < 20 year N = 627	p-Value
Age (years), mean ± SD	4.69 ± 2.38	10.65 ± 1.11	14.74 ± 1.16	18.65 ± 1.03	
Male, n (%)	150(36.4%)	113(31.5%)	183(22.9%)	466(25.7%)	0.003
Underlying diseases, n (%)	9(3.8%)	10(6.1%)	13(5.5%)	38(6.1%)	0.624
Vital sign					
SBP, mean ± SD	108.82 ± 19.87	120.5 ± 18.30	131.50 ± 21.56	133.29 ± 22.80	<0.001
DBP, mean ± SD	69.36 ± 15.90	74.52 ± 11.33	75.59 ± 12.35	77.69 ± 13.11	<0.001
RR, mean ± SD	20.78 ± 3.83	18.99 ± 2.05	18.73 ± 1.85	18.76 ± 2.08	<0.001
HR, mean ± SD	109.40 ± 21.23	93.45 ± 15.53	88.93 ± 16.31	89.38 ± 17.91	<0.001
Injury site					
Home	92(39.0%)	28(17.0%)	16(6.8%)	24(3.8%)	<0.001
Street	64(27.1%)	51(30.9%)	129(54.7%)	516(82.3%)	<0.001
Public site	26(11.0%)	25(15.2%)	41(17.4%)	23(3.7%)	<0.001
Others	51(21.6%)	61(37.0%)	50(20.8%)	59(9.4%)	<0.001
ISS, (mean; SD)	5.34 ± 3.40	4.90 ± 2.89	6.70 ± 6.71	7.31 ± 6.54	<0.001
ISS ≥ 16, (%)	12(5.1%)	5(3.0%)	16(6.8%)	45(7.2%)	0.210
RTS, (mean; SD)	7.59 ± 0.83	7.80 ± 0.20	7.70 ± 0.55	7.70 ± 0.64	<0.001
NISS, (mean; SD)	5.88 ± 3.98	5.67 ± 3.39	7.72 ± 8.05	8.24 ± 7.75	<0.001
TRISS, (mean; SD)	0.97 ± 0.15	1.00 ± 0.00	0.98 ± 0.10	0.98 ± 0.09	<0.001
Shock index	1.04 ± 0.27	0.79 ± 0.17	0.69 ± 0.17	0.69 ± 0.19	<0.001
Shock index > 0.9	167(70.8%)	44(26.7%)	29(12.3%)	65(10.4%)	<0.001

Table 5. Cont.

Characteristics	Age ≤ 8 year N = 236	8 ≤ Age < 12 year N = 165	12 ≤ Age < 16 year N = 237	16 ≤ Age < 20 year N = 627	p-Value
Elevated SIPA	53(22.5%)	24(14.5%)	29(12.3%)	65(10.4%)	<0.001
LOS days, (median; IQR)	3(2–5)	3(2–5)	5(3–8)	6(4–11)	<0.001
ICU admission, (%)	33(14.0%)	20(12.1%)	36(15.3%)	88(14.0%)	0.858
ICU readmission, (%)	0(0.0%)	0(0.0%)	0(0.0%)	2(0.3%)	0.564
ICU days, (median; IQR)	4(2–6)	4(3–5.75)	4(3–7)	3(2–6)	0.303
Need for surgery (%)	148(62.7%)	114(69.1%)	165(69.9%)	440(70.2%)	0.200
Reoperation (%)	13(5.5%)	6(3.6%)	10(4.2%)	20(3.2%)	0.461
Death, (%)	0(0.0%)	0(0.0%)	3(1.3%)	4(0.6%)	0.212

SD: standard deviation; IQR: interquartile range; SBP: systolic blood pressure; DBP: diastolic blood pressure; RR: respiration rate; HR: heart rate; ISS: injury severity score; RTS: revised trauma score; NISS: National Industrial Security System; TRISS: new trauma and injury severity score; LOS days: length of stay days; and ICU: intensive care unit.

4. Discussion

An accuracy prediction tool for the shock status is important for physicians and emergency medical technicians to assess the severity of diseases. Several studies have investigated the predictive capability of SI in a population with trauma and compared it with the traditional vital signs, serum biomarkers, and other scoring systems [9]. In the trauma population, the SI has been investigated in hemorrhagic shock for the early recognition of the need for fluid resuscitation. Compared to normal vital signs, SI may be present in the early shock phase, such as the compensatory phase of shock. In the current concept, early resuscitation in the "golden hour" could correct the vicious cycle of hemorrhage injury to prevent an "early death". Therefore, a novel marker to detect hemodynamic instability is effective for early intervention, including activation of the massive transfusion protocol, trauma team, transcatheter arterial embolization (TAE), and resuscitative endovascular balloon occlusion of the aorta (REBOA). In a prospective study by Birkhahn et al. [10], 46 healthy blood donors were included, and 450 mL of blood was removed for 20 min. Although the HR was elevated and SBP was lower, the change in the vital signs was still within the normal range. However, the mean SI was significantly higher. Another retrospective cohort study that analyzed 8111 blunt trauma patients showed that a higher SI was significantly associated with the need for massive transfusion (risk ratio: 8.13, 95% CI: 4.60–14.36) [11]. A similar result was reported by DeMuro et al. [12]. However, in pediatric trauma patients, the SI was not suitable for reflecting hemodynamic instability due to the different physiology of adults. The SIPA by an adjusted normal range of pediatric vital signs has been proposed to predict the outcomes and presented more accurately identified children with shock status. In the study by Acker et al. [6], 543 children with severe blunt injury were included, and the results showed that more severe pediatric trauma patients were identified via elevated SIPA than SI > 0.9, especially in need for transfusion, high-grade liver/spleen laceration, high ISS score, and a high in-hospital mortality rate. Our study showed similar results. The elevated SIPA group can detect changes in vital signs early to reflect shock progression, even if vital signs were within the normal range. An elevated SIPA can signify more severe traumatic injuries, including high ISS, RTS, and NISS scores than SI > 0.9. In our study, the odds ratio of elevated SIPA and SI > 0.9 to predict ISS ≥ 16 was 3.593 (95% CI: 2.175–5.935, $p < 0.001$) and 2.329 (95% CI: 1.454–3.730, $p < 0.001$). These findings suggest that SIPA is more specific than the vital signs or SI alone in predicting the severity of traumatic injury in a pediatric population. In the clinical outcome analysis, an elevated SIPA has a high in-hospital mortality rate. Although SIPA and SI are both effective in predicting the in-hospital mortality, there were no cases of ICU admission and the need for surgery. In previous studies, SIPA was reported to be a better predictor of ICU admission, in-hospital mortality, need for surgery, endotracheal intubation, and blood transfusion [6,7,13]. There are several reasons for this result. First, SIPA is an acute marker which reflected "early death" in the pediatric trauma population. The shock status may be corrected by adequate resuscitation. An initial elevated SIPA is a hint for physicians for an early intervention to prevent shock progression, which may impair the predictive capability of other outcomes in SIPA. In our study, several pediatric trauma patients received early fluid resuscitation to correct abnormal SIPA; additionally, serial follow-up SIPAs were within normal limits. They also did not require other interventions. We believe that a serial elevated SIPA, such as during the first 24 h of admission, is more reliable for predicting ICU admission, in-hospital mortality, and the need for surgery. Second, traumatic injury-induced shock may not only cause hemorrhage. The pediatric airway obstruction caused hypoxia, such as face injury, hemothorax or pneumothorax, may not reflect the shock sign by elevated SIPA. A traumatic brain injury is another important issue that may present with bradycardia, irregular respiration, and widened pulse pressures (Cushing's triad) due to increased intracranial pressure. In our analysis, head and neck injuries accounted for up to 251 patients (18.8%). This may impair the sensitivity of the SIPA to predict the shock status. Finally, pediatric patients are usually irritable and anxious when vital signs are observed. The environmental stress and pain sensations from the traumatic injury stimulate the sympathetic nervous system, leading to tachycardia and hypertension. This may impair the accuracy of the SIPA in predicting the shock status.

This study had several limitations. First, there is an inevitable source of bias in the measurement of the vital signs and triage by different people. In our database, we did not repeat the measurements of vital signs or by the same staff. Second, every patient in the emergency department received different treatment orders, which may have impaired the clinical outcomes, even if the severity of traumatic injury was similar. Third, the serial SIPA or SI was not recorded. In our database, the in-hospital vital signs are only obtained in the emergency department. Therefore, we did not perform SIPA and SI analyses after 24 h or at admission. Finally, this retrospective study did not record the detailed medical history, physical examination, and biomarker analysis, including the injury onset, neurological examination, and serum lactate level.

5. Conclusions

In summary, the SI and SIPA are useful for identifying the compensatory phase of shock in prehospital and hospital settings, especially in corresponding normal to low-normal blood pressure. SIPA is effective for predicting the mortality and severity of traumatic injuries in the pediatric population. However, SI and SIPA were not significant predictors of ICU admission and need for surgery analysis.

Author Contributions: Conceptualization, Y.-C.Y., C.-Y.L., Y.-L.C. and M.-Y.W.; methodology, T.-H.H.; software, T.-H.H. and Y.-L.C.; validation, C.-Y.L., C.-Y.C. and Y.-T.H.; formal analysis, C.-Y.L. and Y.-L.C.; investigation, Y.-C.Y. and Y.-L.C.; resources, C.-Y.L. and G.-T.Y.; data curation, T.-H.H.; writing—original draft preparation, Y.-C.Y., Y.-L.C. and M.-Y.W.; writing—review and editing, Y.-C.Y., Y.-L.C. and M.-Y.W.; visualization, C.-Y.C. and M.-Y.W.; supervision, Y.-T.H.; project administration, P.-C.L., D.-S.C.; funding acquisition, P.-C.L., D.-S.C. and Y.-L.C. All authors have read and agreed to the published version of the manuscript.

Funding: This study was supported by a grant from Taipei Tzu Chi Hospital (TCRD-TPE-110-31, TCRD-TPE-110-34, TCRD-TPE-110-48).

Institutional Review Board Statement: The study was conducted according to the guidelines of the Declaration of Helsinki, and approved by the Institutional Review Board of Taipei Tzu Chi Hospital (IRB number: 10-XD-072).

Informed Consent Statement: Not applicable.

Data Availability Statement: Not applicable.

Conflicts of Interest: The authors declare no conflict of interest.

References

1. World Health Organization. *Injuries and Violence: The Facts 2014*; World Health Organization: Geneva, Switzerland, 2014.
2. Bruijns, S.R.; Guly, H.R.; Bouamra, O.; Lecky, F.; Lee, W.A. The value of traditional vital signs, shock index, and age-based markers in predicting trauma mortality. *J. Trauma Acute Care Surg.* **2013**, *74*, 1432–1437. [CrossRef] [PubMed]
3. Ott, R.; Krämer, R.; Martus, P.; Bussenius-Kammerer, M.; Carbon, R.; Rupprecht, H. Prognostic value of trauma scores in pediatric patients with multiple injuries. *J. Trauma* **2000**, *49*, 729–736. [CrossRef] [PubMed]
4. Eichelberger, M.R.; Gotschall, C.S.; Sacco, W.J.; Bowman, L.M.; Mangubat, E.A.; Lowenstein, A.D. A comparison of the trauma score, the revised trauma score, and the pediatric trauma score. *Ann. Emerg. Med.* **1989**, *18*, 1053–1058. [CrossRef]
5. Nordin, A.; Coleman, A.; Shi, J.; Wheeler, K.; Xiang, H.; Acker, S.; Bensard, D.; Kenney, B. Validation of the age-adjusted shock index using pediatric trauma quality improvement program data. *J. Pediatric Surg.* **2018**, *53*, 130–135. [CrossRef] [PubMed]
6. Acker, S.N.; Ross, J.T.; Partrick, D.A.; Tong, S.; Bensard, D.D. Pediatric specific shock index accurately identifies severely injured children. *J. Pediatric Surg.* **2015**, *50*, 331–334. [CrossRef] [PubMed]
7. Linnaus, M.E.; Notrica, D.M.; Langlais, C.S.; St. Peter, S.D.; Leys, C.M.; Ostlie, D.J.; Maxson, R.T.; Ponsky, T.; Tuggle, D.W.; Eubanks, J.W.; et al. Prospective validation of the shock index pediatric-adjusted (SIPA) in blunt liver and spleen trauma: An ATOMAC+ study. *J. Pediatric Surg.* **2017**, *52*, 340–344. [CrossRef] [PubMed]
8. Koch, E.; Lovett, S.; Nghiem, T.; Riggs, R.A.; Rech, M.A. Shock index in the emergency department: Utility and limitations. *Open Access Emerg. Med. OAEM* **2019**, *11*, 179–199. [CrossRef] [PubMed]
9. Wu, M.-Y.; Chen, Y.-L.; Yiang, G.-T.; Li, C.-J.; Lin, A.S.-C. Clinical Outcome and Management for Geriatric Traumatic Injury: Analysis of 2688 Cases in the Emergency Department of a Teaching Hospital in Taiwan. *J. Clin. Med.* **2018**, *7*, 255. [CrossRef] [PubMed]
10. Birkhahn, R.H.; Gaeta, T.J.; Terry, D.; Bove, J.J.; Tloczkowski, J. Shock index in diagnosing early acute hypovolemia. *Am. J. Emerg. Med.* **2005**, *23*, 323–326. [CrossRef] [PubMed]
11. Vandromme, M.J.; Griffin, R.L.; Kerby, J.D.; McGwin, G., Jr.; Rue, L.W., III; Weinberg, J.A. Identifying Risk for Massive Transfusion in the Relatively Normotensive Patient: Utility of the Prehospital Shock Index. *J. Trauma Acute Care Surg.* **2011**, *70*, 384–390. [CrossRef] [PubMed]
12. DeMuro, J.P.; Simmons, S.; Jax, J.; Gianelli, S.M. Application of the shock index to the prediction of need for hemostasis intervention. *Am. J. Emerg. Med.* **2013**, *31*, 1260–1263. [CrossRef]
13. Acker, S.N.; Bredbeck, B.; Partrick, D.A.; Kulungowski, A.M.; Barnett, C.C.; Bensard, D.D. Shock index, pediatric age-adjusted (SIPA) is more accurate than age-adjusted hypotension for trauma team activation. *Surgery* **2017**, *161*, 803–807. [CrossRef] [PubMed]

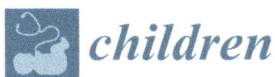

Article

The Etiology and Epidemiology of Pediatric Facial Fractures in North-Western Romania: A 10-Year Retrospective Study

Paul Andrei Țenț [1], Raluca Iulia Juncar [1], Abel Emanuel Moca [1,*], Rahela Tabita Moca [2] and Mihai Juncar [1]

1. Department of Dentistry, Faculty of Medicine and Pharmacy, University of Oradea, 10 Piața 1 Decembrie Street, 410073 Oradea, Romania; tent_andrei@yahoo.com (P.A.Ț.); ralucajuncar@yahoo.ro (R.I.J.); mihaijuncar@gmail.com (M.J.)
2. Doctoral School of Biomedical Sciences, University of Oradea, 1 Universității Street, 410087 Oradea, Romania; rahelamoca@gmail.com
* Correspondence: abelmoca@yahoo.com

Abstract: Pediatric facial fractures are not as common as facial fractures occurring in the adult population. Their therapeutic approach is different because they affect patients with active growth, and have an etiology and epidemiology that vary depending on different cultural, religious and demographic factors. This research aimed to identify the main factors involved in the etiology of pediatric facial fractures, as well as the epidemiology of pediatric facial fractures in a sample of children and adolescents from North-Western Romania. This 10-year retrospective study was performed in a tertiary center for oral and maxillofacial surgery in North-Western Romania. Medical files of patients that were admitted between 1 January 2002 and 31 December 2022 were analyzed. Pediatric patients aged 0 to 18 years were included in this study. The final sample consisted of 142 children and adolescents diagnosed with facial fractures, with this number representing 14.1% of all patients affected by facial fractures. Most frequently, fractures were identified in the 13–18 age group (78.9%, n = 112), which were more often associated with fractures caused by interpersonal violence than caused by road traffic accidents, falls or animal attacks. Boys were more affected (88%, n = 125), and were more frequently associated with fractures caused by interpersonal violence. The most frequently identified etiological factors included interpersonal violence (50%, n = 71), falls (18.3%, n = 26) and road traffic accidents (11.3%, n = 16). In terms of location, the mandible was the most affected facial bone structure (66.2%, n = 94), and patients with mandibular fractures were more frequently associated with fractures caused by interpersonal violence. The incidence of pediatric facial fractures should be lowered because they may interfere with the proper development of the facial skeleton. Establishing measures aimed at preventing interpersonal violence, as well as other causes involved in the etiology of facial fractures is imperative.

Keywords: pediatric facial fractures; etiology; epidemiology; Romania

Citation: Țenț, P.A.; Juncar, R.I.; Moca, A.E.; Moca, R.T.; Juncar, M. The Etiology and Epidemiology of Pediatric Facial Fractures in North-Western Romania: A 10-Year Retrospective Study. *Children* 2022, 9, 932. https://doi.org/10.3390/children9070932

Academic Editor: Christiaan J. A. van Bergen

Received: 14 May 2022
Accepted: 20 June 2022
Published: 21 June 2022

Publisher's Note: MDPI stays neutral with regard to jurisdictional claims in published maps and institutional affiliations.

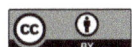

Copyright: © 2022 by the authors. Licensee MDPI, Basel, Switzerland. This article is an open access article distributed under the terms and conditions of the Creative Commons Attribution (CC BY) license (https://creativecommons.org/licenses/by/4.0/).

1. Introduction

Facial trauma can profoundly affect a victim's social life, and have a negative impact on a person's overall quality of life [1]. Facial trauma occurring in adults is the most common diagnosed and treated pathology in maxillofacial surgery services [2], and involves complex treatment, which often requires interdisciplinary collaboration in order to minimize any long-term negative effects [3].

Compared to facial fractures occurring in adult patients, pediatric facial fractures are not as common [4], but their therapeutic approach represents a serious challenge for physicians, especially due to the fact that they occur in actively growing patients [5]. Generally, pediatric facial fractures occurring in children under the age of 5 years do not exceed an incidence rate of 5% [4], but they are more frequent in adolescent patients [5].

Pediatric facial fractures have an etiology that often varies, mostly depending on the age of the child, but the most common causes include fall injuries [6,7], sports accidents [8], motor vehicle accidents [9], or even child abuse [10]. However, the etiology can vary significantly depending on the cultural, religious and demographic background of the patient as well [11]. Age, the presence of intramaxillary teeth, or the topography of lesions influences the treatment of pediatric facial fractures and the choice of a specific therapeutic approach [5,12]. Facial fractures can occur in the frontal bone, the orbita, the nasal bone, the zygomatic bone, the maxilla or the mandible [12]. In the pediatric population, mandibular fractures are among the most common facial fractures, reaching an incidence of up to 50% of all pediatric facial fractures [13]. Their treatment varies from close observation, associated with soft diet and analgesics, to intermaxillary fixation used for short periods of time [13].

Pediatric facial fractures can cause skeletal deformities due to fracture-induced growth defects [13], and should be rapidly and correctly diagnosed and managed, even if the lesions tend to be less severe [14]. Globally, the incidence and etiology of facial fractures vary according to each population studied [2], and this trend is maintained in the pediatric population as well. In the geographic region investigated in this research, the authors did not identify any studies that presented the etiology and epidemiology of pediatric facial fractures. Knowing these aspects is important for preventing and optimally managing facial fractures in a pediatric population [15].

The aim of this research was to identify the main factors involved in the etiology of pediatric facial fractures, as well as the epidemiology of pediatric facial fractures in a sample of children and adolescents from North-Western Romania.

2. Materials and Methods

2.1. Ethical Considerations

The study was approved by the Ethics Committee of the University of Oradea (IRB No. 3402/15.04.2018), and was conducted in accordance with the standards described by the 2008 Declaration of Helsinki and its later amendments. All 18-year-old patients signed an informed consent form at the time of their admission in the medical institution regarding the anonymous use of their medical data for future scientific studies. For minor patients (under the age of 18), the informed consent forms for the anonymous use of patients' medical data were signed by their parents or legal guardians.

2.2. Participants and Data Collection

This ten-year retrospective study was conducted in a tertiary center for oral and maxillofacial surgery from North-Western Romania. All medical files belonging to patients hospitalized in this institution between 1 January 2002 and 31 December 2011 were initially analyzed.

The following inclusion criteria were applied: patients up to 18 years of age, who had at least one facial fracture line at the time of admission, and an acute traumatic episode in the history of the disease; patients for whom the clinical diagnosis was confirmed by a paraclinical examination method (radiographic examination or computed tomographic examination); and patients whose traumatic fractures were treated in the host hospital.

The exclusion criteria were as follows: patients aged 19 years or older, with no facial skeletal fractures, or with pathological bone fractures; and patients for whom the clinical diagnosis was not confirmed by any additional paraclinical examination, who were treated in another hospital, or with incomplete information in the medical records.

The data needed to conduct this research were extracted from patients' medical records. The following variables were analyzed: gender of patients (boys, girls), age of patients (0–6 years, 7–12 years, 13–18 years), living environment of patients (urban, rural), etiology of trauma, location of fracture lines in the facial skeleton (mandible, midface, combined) and the presence of associated lesions in the soft tissues (hematomas, lacerations, abrasions).

All observation sheets were double-checked by the author responsible for data collection and by a member of the team responsible for compiling the statistics. This was performed in order to avoid bias.

2.3. Statistical Analysis

The statistical analysis was performed using IBM SPSS Statistics 26 (IBM, Chicago, IL, USA) and Microsoft Office Excel and Word 2013 (Microsoft, Redmond, WA, USA). All categorical variables were expressed as an absolute or in a percentage form, and were tested using Fisher's Exact Test. Z-tests with Bonferroni corrections were performed in order to detail the results after obtaining the contingency tables.

3. Results

During the 10-year timespan analyzed, a total of 12,645 patients were hospitalized, of which 1569 had facial trauma. After applying the exclusion criteria, 1427 patients were excluded, and 142 patients were included in this study (Figure 1). The age-based exclusion criterion was applied as a final exclusion criteria in order to calculate the total percentage of pediatric patients affected by facial fractures out of the total number of patients (children, adolescents, adults) affected by facial fractures.

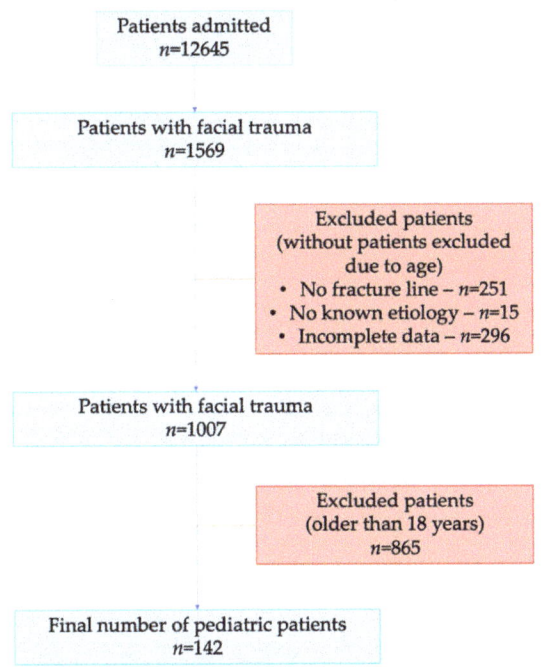

Figure 1. Study flowchart.

The data in Table 1 show the demographic characteristics of the patients investigated. Of the total sample of patients with facial fractures that were admitted during the 10-year timespan, before applying the age-based exclusion criteria (1007 patients), 14.1% ($n = 142$) of the fractures occurred in pediatric patients (with ages between 0 and 18 years). The majority of pediatric patients with fractures were boys (88%, $n = 125$), from urban areas (61.3%, $n = 87$), the most common etiology being interpersonal violence (50%, $n = 71$), followed by fall trauma (18.3%, $n = 26$), and road traffic accidents (11.3%, $n = 16$). Regarding the associated soft tissue lesions, 43.7% ($n = 62$) of children had hematomas, 28.2% ($n = 40$) had lacerations, and 33.1% ($n = 47$) had abrasions. Regarding the location of fractures, 66.2% ($n = 94$) had strictly mandibular fractures, 25.3% ($n = 36$) had only midface fractures, and 8.5% ($n = 12$) had combined fractures (affecting both the midface and the mandible).

Table 1. Distribution of the patients according to the various variables.

Variable	Value
Age (*n*, %)	
>18 years	865 (85.9%)
≤18 years	142 (14.1%)
Age groups (*n*, %)	
0–6 years	8 (5.6%) (0.8% from all facial fractures)
7–12 years	22 (15.5%) (2.2% from all facial fractures)
13–18 years	112 (78.9%) (11.1% from all facial fractures)
Gender (*n*, %)	
Girls	17 (12%)
Boys	125 (88%)
Living environment (*n*, %)	
Rural	55 (38.7%)
Urban	87 (61.3%)
Etiology (*n*, %)	
Interpersonal violence	71 (50%)
Fall	26 (18.3%)
Road traffic accident	16 (11.3%)
Animal attack	15 (10.6%)
Sport accident	10 (7%)
Domestic accident	4 (2.8%)
Fracture line location (*n*, %)	
Mandibular fractures	94 (66.2%)
Midface fractures	36 (25.3%)
Combined fractures	12 (8.5%)
Soft tissue associated lesions (*n*, %)	
Hematomas	62 (43.7%)
Lacerations	40 (28.2%)
Abrasions	47 (33.1%)

n, number; %, percentage.

Data in Figures 2–4 show the distribution of pediatric patients according to the age, gender, living environment and etiology of trauma. Differences between groups were statistically significant according to Fisher's Exact Test, and Z tests with a Bonferroni correction showed that patients aged 0–6 years were more frequently associated with fractures caused by domestic accidents or animal attacks than caused by interpersonal violence, and patients aged 7–12 years were more frequently associated with fractures caused by road traffic accidents, falls or animal attacks than those caused by interpersonal violence. However, patients aged 13–18 years were more frequently associated with fractures caused by interpersonal violence than those caused by road traffic accidents, falls or animal attacks ($p < 0.001$). Regarding the gender of the patients, it was observed that girls were associated more frequently with fractures caused by road traffic accidents than those caused by interpersonal violence, and boys were more frequently associated with fractures caused by interpersonal violence than fractures caused by road traffic accidents ($p = 0.004$). Regarding the living environment of the patients, it was found that children and adolescents from rural areas were more frequently associated with fractures caused by animal attacks than fractures caused by interpersonal violence, road traffic accidents or domestic accidents, and children and adolescents from urban areas were more frequently associated with fractures caused by interpersonal violence, road traffic accidents or domestic accidents than those caused by animal attacks ($p < 0.001$).

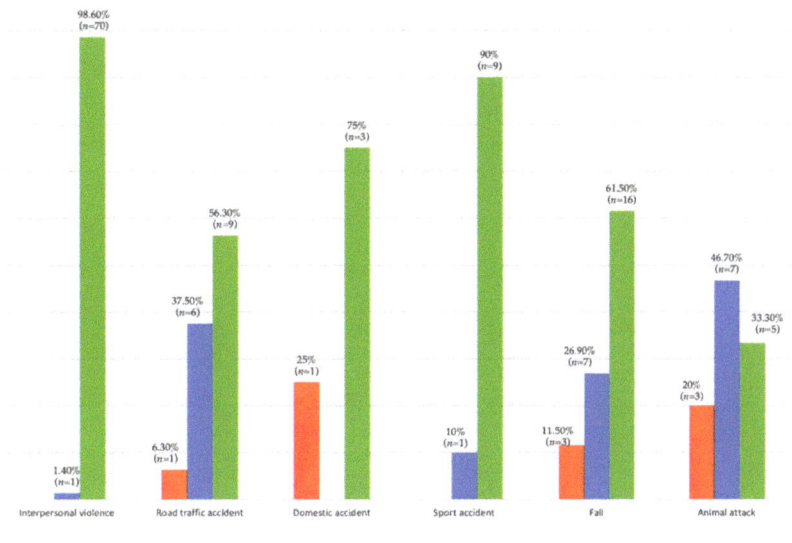

Figure 2. Distribution according to age and etiology.

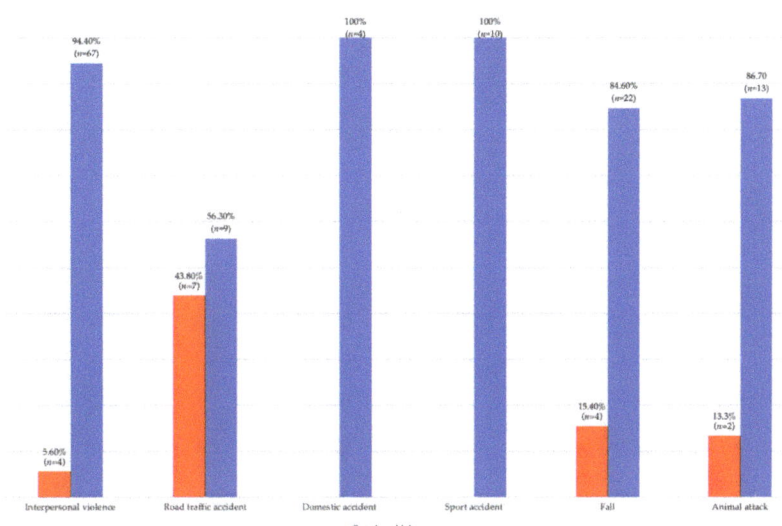

Figure 3. Distribution according to gender and etiology.

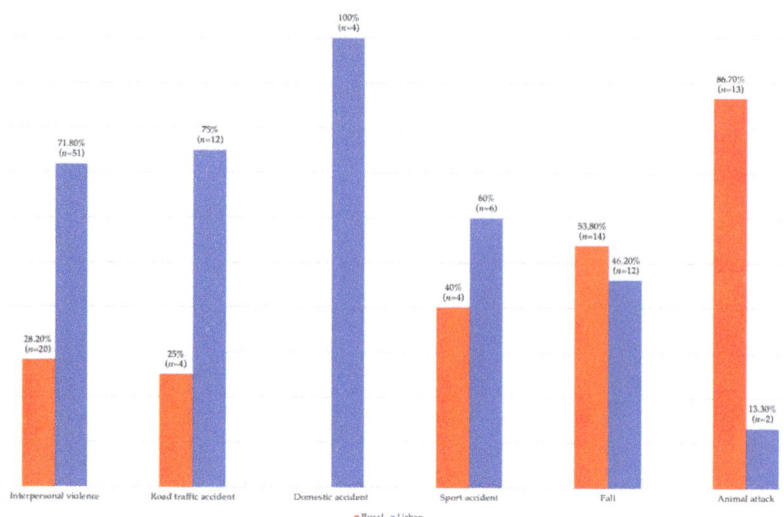

Figure 4. Distribution according to living environment and etiology.

The distribution of pediatric patients related to the location of the fracture line and the etiology of trauma is shown in Figure 5. Differences between groups were statistically significant according to Fisher's Exact Test ($p < 0.001$), and Z tests with a Bonferroni correction showed that children and adolescents with midface fractures were associated more frequently with fractures caused by animal attacks than caused by interpersonal violence, and patients with mandibular fractures were more frequently associated with fractures caused by interpersonal violence than fractures caused by animal attacks. Children and adolescents with combined fractures were associated more frequently with fractures caused by road traffic accidents than those caused by interpersonal violence or falls.

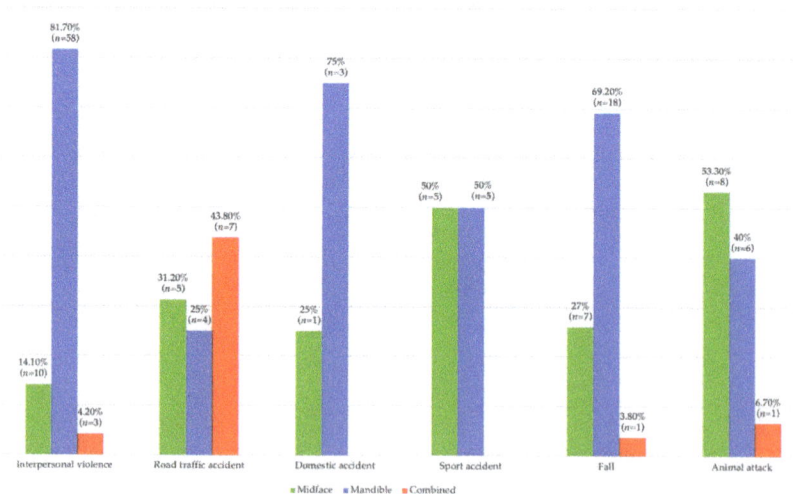

Figure 5. Distribution according to line of fracture and etiology.

Regarding the soft tissues associated lesions, it was observed that children and adolescents without hematomas were more frequently associated with fractures caused by interpersonal violence than fractures caused by road traffic accidents, falls or animal attacks, and patients with hematomas were more frequently associated with fractures caused by road traffic accidents, falls or animal attacks than fractures caused by interpersonal violence ($p < 0.001$). Patients that did not have any lacerations were more frequently associated with fractures caused by interpersonal violence than fractures caused by road traffic accidents, falls or animal attacks, and children with lacerations were more frequently associated with road traffic accidents, falls, animal attacks than those caused by interpersonal violence ($p < 0.001$). Children and adolescents without abrasions were more frequently associated with fractures caused by interpersonal violence than by road traffic accidents, falls or animal attacks, and children with abrasions were more frequently associated with fractures caused by road traffic accidents, falls or animal attacks than those caused by interpersonal violence ($p < 0.001$). The data are detailed in Table 2.

Table 2. Distribution of the pediatric patients according to the presence of soft tissue associated lesions and etiology of trauma.

Etiology		Interpersonal Violence	Road Traffic Accident	Domestic Accident	Sport Accident	Fall	Animal Attack	p *
				Hematomas				
No	n	56	3	2	4	12	3	<0.001
	%	78.9%	18.8%	50%	40%	46.2%	20%	
Yes	n	15	13	2	6	14	12	
	%	21.1%	81.3%	50%	60%	53.8%	80%	
				Lacerations				
No	n	64	7	2	10	13	6	<0.001
	%	90.1%	43.8%	50%	100%	50%	40%	
Yes	n	7	9	2	0	13	9	
	%	9.9%	56.3%	50%	0%	50%	60%	
				Abrasions				
No	n	61	3	2	10	13	6	<0.001
	%	85.9%	18.8%	50%	100%	50%	40%	
Yes	n	10	13	2	0	13	9	
	%	14.1%	81.3%	50%	0%	50%	60%	

n, number; %, percentage; * Fisher's Exact Test.

4. Discussion

Pediatric facial fractures had different etiologies, and their incidence varied according to patients' age, gender and living environment. They are most common in the 13–18 years age group, with interpersonal violence playing a major role in their occurrence. Pediatric facial fractures, although of great importance and with major potential negative effects in the short and long term, do not have a well-characterized epidemiology [16]. They are generally rare, and account for less than 15% of the total number of facial fractures [17]. However, a significant part of the morbidity in the pediatric population is caused by craniofacial fractures [18]. The treatment of facial fractures in children and adolescents differs from the treatment of fractures in adults, considering the fact that pediatric patients have active growth and development [19]. Knowing the etiology and epidemiology of pediatric facial fractures in a specific population is essential for ideal therapeutic management, as well as for successful prevention.

In this research, pediatric facial fractures accounted for 14.1% of all fractures diagnosed for patients admitted in the host institution. The results are consistent with other studies, which reported an incidence of 14.7% [4], 14.6% [20] or 14.1% [21], all of which were below the 15% threshold. A single study was identified that reported an incidence of only 1.01% of facial fractures in the pediatric population under the age of 16 years in India [22], well below the incidence reported in the present study.

Patients were distributed based on age, gender and living environment. The pediatric patients were distributed in three distinct age groups, respectively 0–6 years, 7–12 years and 13–18 years. This distribution was preferred because it comprises three important periods in the development of pediatric patients, namely preschool, school and adolescence [23], but also because it was used in other similar studies [20,23]. The incidence of pediatric facial fractures was influenced by these investigated variables. Thus, the incidence in children under the age of 6 years was 5.6%, a result identical to that obtained by Vyas et al. [4]. Other studies reported a higher incidence in the preschool population [20]. The consensus is, however, that in general, the total number of pediatric patients diagnosed with facial fractures increases with age [4,24].

Regarding the influence of patients' gender on the incidence of pediatric facial fractures, it was observed that the most affected were boys, who, in our study, accounted for 88% (n = 125) of the total number of patients investigated. In general, the literature reports a higher incidence of pediatric fractures in male patients [4,25], which is consistent with our results. In school-age and adolescent patients, the explanation could be correlated with the increased interest in sports, but also with the changing nature of adolescents. In adolescence, the tendency to make risky choices and to have exaggerated emotionally reactions is high [26], thus making adolescent patients prone to various accidents [27]. Studies that report an equally distributed incidence of facial fractures among boys and girls were also identified [28].

The etiology of pediatric facial fractures differs depending on the populations investigated, and involves social, cultural and environmental factors that cause differences between countries [20]. In younger children, most fractures are caused by falls or the practice of various sports [29,30], while in adolescents interpersonal violence is one of the dominant etiological factors responsible for the occurrence of facial fractures [31]. In this study, the main etiological factor in the occurrence of facial fractures was interpersonal violence, which is responsible for 50% of the total number of pediatric facial fractures identified. Additionally, it is important to highlight the fact that out of the total number of cases with fractures caused by interpersonal violence, 98.6% (n = 70) occurred in adolescent patients (13–18 years old). Other etiological factors identified were falls, road traffic accidents, animal attacks, sports accidents and domestic accidents.

Pediatric facial fractures most commonly concern the mandible [16,32,33]. This is due to the prominent position of the mandible in the facial skeleton [34]. In the study conducted on the pediatric population from North-Western Romania, the mandibular fractures were the most frequent facial fractures as well, constituting 66.2% (n = 94) of the total number of fractures diagnosed. Mandibular fractures were the most common fractures caused by interpersonal violence, domestic accidents and falls. Midface fractures are not as common in children and adolescent as mandibular fractures. This is mainly due to the fact that the facial skeleton and paranasal sinuses of children are not fully developed, leading to craniofacial disproportions [35]. In our study, as well, the midface fractures had a much lower incidence than the mandibular fractures, but they were predominant among fractures caused by animal attacks. Combined fractures were the most common facial fractures that occurred in road traffic accidents. This is due to the high kinetic energy developed in accidents [36].

Complications that occur as a result of facial fractures may also affect soft tissues. In this study, we identified hematomas, lacerations and abrasions caused by facial fractures. In contrast to the results of our study where hematomas were the main associated soft tissue lesions (43.7%), Ferreira et al. reported lacerations as the most common soft tissue-associated lesion [36].

It is the authors' belief that this study provides important information regarding the etiology and epidemiology of pediatric facial fractures in a population from North-Western Romania. This information can be used to implement pediatric facial fractures prevention measures, but also to better prepare physicians and nurses for the therapeutic management of facial fractures that occur in children and adolescents.

However, there were some limitations identified in this research. Although the medical institution in which this retrospective study was performed is an oral and maxillofacial surgery hospital, it probably mainly treats the population from North-Western Romania, as it is located in this part of the country; therefore, the etiology and epidemiology of pediatric facial fractures may be different in other regions of the country. At the same time, the study is retrospective, so that data taken from patients' medical records may be incorrectly or incompletely provided at the time of examination and admission of patients. The exact etiology of the trauma could be misreported. Given that the study population was pediatric, the suspicion of domestic abuse must be raised.

5. Conclusions

The incidence of pediatric facial fractures was 14.1%, most of which occurred in patients aged 13–18 years. Boys were the most affected by facial fractures, and the incidence in urban areas was higher than in rural areas. Regarding the causes that led to pediatric facial fractures, it was found that personal violence was responsible for causing half of all pediatric facial fractures. The mandible was the most affected facial bone structure, and the most common soft tissue injuries were hematomas. Overall, all types of fractures require a lower incidence, as they are unwanted events, and in pediatric patients they may interfere with the proper development of the facial skeleton. Measures aimed at preventing interpersonal violence, as well as other causes involved in the etiology of facial fractures are imperative.

Author Contributions: Conceptualization, P.A.T. and M.J.; methodology, P.A.T.; software, R.T.M.; validation, A.E.M. and M.J.; formal analysis, R.I.J.; investigation, P.A.T.; resources, R.I.J. and M.J.; data curation, A.E.M.; writing—original draft preparation, P.A.T.; writing—review and editing, R.I.J. and A.E.M.; visualization, A.E.M.; supervision, M.J.; project administration, A.E.M.; funding acquisition, R.T.M. All authors have read and agreed to the published version of the manuscript.

Funding: This research received no external funding.

Institutional Review Board Statement: The study was conducted in accordance with the Declaration of Helsinki, and approved by the Ethics Committee of the University of Oradea (IRB No. 3402/15.04.2018).

Informed Consent Statement: Informed consent was obtained from all subjects involved in the study.

Data Availability Statement: The data presented in this study are available on request from the corresponding authors. The data are not publicly available due to privacy reasons.

Conflicts of Interest: The authors declare no conflict of interest.

References

1. Manodh, P.; Prabhu Shankar, D.; Pradeep, D.; Santhosh, R.; Murugan, A. Incidence and patterns of maxillofacial trauma-a retrospective analysis of 3611 patients—An update. *Oral Maxillofac. Surg.* **2016**, *20*, 377–383. [CrossRef] [PubMed]
2. Juncar, M.; Tent, P.A.; Juncar, R.I.; Harangus, A.; Mircea, R. An epidemiological analysis of maxillofacial fractures: A 10-year cross-sectional cohort retrospective study of 1007 patients. *BMC Oral Health* **2021**, *21*, 128. [CrossRef] [PubMed]
3. Chukwulebe, S.; Hogrefe, C. The Diagnosis and Management of Facial Bone Fractures. *Emerg. Med. Clin. N. Am.* **2019**, *37*, 137–151. [CrossRef] [PubMed]
4. Vyas, R.M.; Dickinson, B.P.; Wasson, K.L.; Roostaeian, J.; Bradley, J.P. Pediatric facial fractures: Current national incidence, distribution, and health care resource use. *J. Craniofac. Surg.* **2008**, *19*, 339–349. [CrossRef]
5. Boyette, J.R. Facial fractures in children. *Otolaryngol. Clin. N. Am.* **2014**, *47*, 747–761. [CrossRef]
6. Gassner, R.; Tuli, T.; Hächl, O.; Moreira, R.; Ulmer, H. Craniomaxillofacial trauma in children: A review of 3,385 cases with 6060 injuries in 10 years. *J. Oral Maxillofac. Surg.* **2004**, *62*, 399–407. [CrossRef]
7. Nardis Ada, C.; Costa, S.A.; da Silva, R.A.; Kaba, S.C. Patterns of paediatric facial fractures in a hospital of São Paulo, Brazil: A retrospective study of 3 years. *J. Craniomaxillofac. Surg.* **2013**, *41*, 226–229. [CrossRef]
8. Dobitsch, A.A.; Oleck, N.C.; Liu, F.C.; Halsey, J.N.; Hoppe, I.C.; Lee, E.S.; Granick, M.S. Sports-Related Pediatric Facial Trauma: Analysis of Facial Fracture Pattern and Concomitant Injuries. *Surg. J.* **2019**, *5*, e146–e149. [CrossRef]
9. Montovani, J.C.; de Campos, L.M.; Gomes, M.A.; de Moraes, V.R.; Ferreira, F.D.; Nogueira, E.A. Etiology and incidence facial fractures in children and adults. *Braz. J. Otorhinolaryngol.* **2006**, *72*, 235–241. [CrossRef]

10. Berthold, O.; Frericks, B.; John, T.; Clemens, V.; Fegert, J.M.; Moers, A.V. Abuse as a Cause of Childhood Fractures. *Dtsch. Arztebl. Int.* **2018**, *115*, 769–775. [CrossRef]
11. Bakardjiev, A.; Pechalova, P. Maxillofacial fractures in Southern Bulgaria—A retrospective study of 1706 cases. *J. Craniomaxillofac. Surg.* **2007**, *35*, 147–150. [CrossRef]
12. Cole, P.; Kaufman, Y.; Hollier, L.H., Jr. Managing the pediatric facial fracture. *Craniomaxillofac. Trauma Reconstr.* **2009**, *2*, 77–83. [CrossRef] [PubMed]
13. Goth, S.; Sawatari, Y.; Peleg, M. Management of pediatric mandible fractures. *J. Craniofac. Surg.* **2012**, *23*, 47–56. [CrossRef] [PubMed]
14. Hatef, D.A.; Cole, P.D.; Hollier, L.H., Jr. Contemporary management of pediatric facial trauma. *Curr. Opin. Otolaryngol. Head Neck Surg.* **2009**, *17*, 308–314. [CrossRef] [PubMed]
15. Zimmermann, C.E.; Troulis, M.J.; Kaban, L.B. Pediatric facial fractures: Recent advances in prevention, diagnosis and management. *Int. J. Oral Maxillofac. Surg.* **2006**, *35*, 2–13. [CrossRef] [PubMed]
16. Imahara, S.D.; Hopper, R.A.; Wang, J.; Rivara, F.P.; Klein, M.B. Patterns and outcomes of pediatric facial fractures in the United States: A survey of the National Trauma Data Bank. *J. Am. Coll. Surg.* **2008**, *207*, 710–716. [CrossRef]
17. Grunwaldt, L.; Smith, D.M.; Zuckerbraun, N.S.; Naran, S.; Rottgers, S.A.; Bykowski, M.; Kinsella, C.; Cray, J.; Vecchione, L.; Saladino, R.A.; et al. Pediatric facial fractures: Demographics, injury patterns, and associated injuries in 772 consecutive patients. *Plast. Reconstr. Surg.* **2011**, *128*, 1263–1271. [CrossRef] [PubMed]
18. Alcalá-Galiano, A.; Arribas-García, I.J.; Martín-Pérez, M.A.; Romance, A.; Montalvo-Moreno, J.J.; Juncos, J.M. Pediatric facial fractures: Children are not just small adults. *Radiographics* **2008**, *28*, 441–461, quiz 618. [CrossRef]
19. Braun, T.L.; Xue, A.S.; Maricevich, R.S. Differences in the Management of Pediatric Facial Trauma. *Semin. Plast. Surg.* **2017**, *31*, 118–122. [CrossRef]
20. Al-Tairi, N.; Al-Radom, J. Prevalence and Etiology of Pediatric Maxillofacial Fractures in a Group of Yemeni Children and Adolescents. *Open J. Stomatol.* **2021**, *11*, 179–187. [CrossRef]
21. Almahdi, H.M.; Higzi, M.A. Maxillofacial fractures among Sudanese children at Khartoum Dental Teaching Hospital. *BMC Res. Notes* **2016**, *9*, 120. [CrossRef] [PubMed]
22. Ashrafullah; Pandey, R.K.; Mishra, A. The incidence of facial injuries in children in Indian population: A retrospective study. *J. Oral Biol. Craniofac. Res.* **2018**, *8*, 82–85. [CrossRef] [PubMed]
23. Segura-Palleres, I.; Sobrero, F.; Roccia, F.; de Oliveira Gorla, L.F.; Pereira-Filho, V.A.; Gallafassi, D.; Faverani, L.P.; Romeo, I.; Bojino, A.; Copelli, C.; et al. Characteristics and age-related injury patterns of maxillofacial fractures in children and adolescents: A multicentric and prospective study. *Dent. Traumatol.* **2022**, *38*, 213–222. [CrossRef] [PubMed]
24. Ghosh, R.; Gopalkrishnan, K.; Anand, J. Pediatric Facial Fractures: A 10-year Study. *J. Maxillofac. Oral Surg.* **2018**, *17*, 158–163. [CrossRef]
25. Posnick, J.C.; Wells, M.; Pron, G.E. Pediatric facial fractures: Evolving patterns of treatment. *J. Oral Maxillofac. Surg.* **1993**, *51*, 836Y844. [CrossRef]
26. Jaworska, N.; MacQueen, G. Adolescence as a unique developmental period. *J. Psychiatry Neurosci.* **2015**, *40*, 291–293. [CrossRef]
27. Johnson, S.B.; Jones, V.C. Adolescent development and risk of injury: Using developmental science to improve interventions. *Inj. Prev.* **2011**, *17*, 50–54. [CrossRef]
28. Iizuka, T.; Thoren, H.; Annino, D.J.; Hallikainen, D.; Lindqvist, C. Midfacial fractures in pediatric patients. Frequency, characteristics, and causes. *Arch. Otolaryngol. Head Neck Surg.* **1995**, *121*, 1366Y1371. [CrossRef]
29. Haug, R.H.; Foss, J. Maxillofacial injuries in the pediatric patient. *Oral Surg. Oral Med. Oral Pathol. Oral Radiol. Endod.* **2000**, *90*, 126–134. [CrossRef]
30. Mukherjee, C.G.; Mukherjee, U. Maxillofacial trauma in children. *Int. J. Clin. Pediatr. Dent.* **2012**, *5*, 231–236. [CrossRef]
31. Kim, S.H.; Lee, S.H.; Cho, P.D. Analysis of 809 facial bone fractures in a pediatric and adolescent population. *Arch. Plast. Surg.* **2012**, *39*, 606–611. [CrossRef] [PubMed]
32. Shetawi, A.S.; Lim, C.A.; Singh, Y.K.; Portnof, J.E.; Blumberg, S.M. Pediatric maxillofacial trauma: A review of 156 patients. *J. Oral Maxillofacial. Surg.* **2016**, *74*, 1420. [CrossRef] [PubMed]
33. Hong, K.; Jeong, J.; Susson, Y.N.; Abramowicz, S. Patterns of Pediatric Facial Fractures. *Craniomaxillofac. Trauma Reconstr.* **2021**, *14*, 325–329. [CrossRef] [PubMed]
34. Gadicherla, S.; Sasikumar, P.; Gill, S.S.; Bhagania, M.; Kamath, A.T.; Pentapati, K.C. Mandibular Fractures and Associated Factors at a Tertiary Care Hospital. *Arch. Trauma Res.* **2016**, *5*, e30574. [CrossRef]
35. Ferreira, P.; Marques, M.; Pinho, C.; Rodrigues, J.; Reis, J.; Amarante, J. Midfacial fractures in children and adolescents: A review of 492 cases. *Br. J. Oral Maxillofac. Surg.* **2004**, *42*, 501–505. [CrossRef]
36. Hyman, D.A.; Saha, S.; Nayar, H.S.; Doyle, J.F.; Agarwal, S.K.; Chaiet, S.R. Patterns of facial fractures and protective device use in motor vehicle collisions from 2007 to 2012. *JAMA Facial Plast. Surg.* **2016**, *18*, 455–461. [CrossRef]

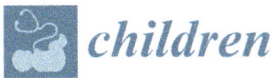

Article

Outcome Analysis of Surgical Timing in Pediatric Orbital Trapdoor Fracture with Different Entrapment Contents: A Retrospective Study

Pei-Ju Hsieh [1] and Han-Tsung Liao [1,2,3,*]

1. Division of Traumatic Plastic Surgery, Department of Plastic and Reconstructive Surgery, Craniofacial Research Center, Chang Gung Memorial Hospital at LinKou, Chang Gung University College of Medicine, Taoyuan City 333, Taiwan; b101103094@tmu.edu.tw
2. College of Medicine, Chang Gung University, Taoyuan City 333, Taiwan
3. Department of Plastic Surgery, Xiamen Chang Gung Hospital, Xiamen 361000, China
* Correspondence: lia01211@gmail.com; Tel.: +886-3-328-1200 (ext. 2946); Fax: +886-3-328-9582

Abstract: Orbital trapdoor fracture occurs more commonly in pediatric patients, and previous studies suggested early intervention for a better outcome. However, there is no consensus on the appropriate timing of emergent intervention due to the insufficient cases reported. In the current retrospective study, we compared the outcomes of patient groups with different time intervals from injury to surgical intervention and entrapment content. Twenty-three patients who underwent surgery for trapdoor fracture between January 2001 and September 2018 at Chang Gung Memorial Hospital were enrolled. There was no significant difference in diplopia and extraocular muscle (EOM) movement recovery rate in patients who underwent surgery within three days and those over three days. However, among the patients with an interval to surgery of over three days, those with muscle entrapment required a longer period of time to recover from EOM movement restriction ($p = 0.03$) and diplopia ($p = 0.03$) than those with soft tissue entrapment. Regardless of time interval to surgery, patients with muscle entrapment took longer time to recover from EOM movement restriction ($p = 0.036$) and diplopia ($p = 0.042$) and had the trend of a worse EOM recovery rate compared to patients with soft tissue entrapment. Hence, we suggested that orbital trapdoor fractures with rectus muscle entrapment should be promptly managed for faster recovery.

Keywords: adolescents; children; pediatric orbital fracture; orbital trapdoor fracture

1. Introduction

Orbital trapdoor fracture occurs more frequently in patient under 18 years old. Due to the inherent elasticity of facial bone, the displaced orbital wall recoils back and traps the soft tissue or rectus muscle, causing extraocular muscle (EOM) movement restriction and diplopia. The injury may also induce oculocardiac reflex by traction on EOM, causing bradycardia, nausea, and syncope [1]. To remove these acute symptoms, releasing the entrapment content is significantly effective. However, not every patient fully recovers from EOM movement restriction and diplopia after the operation. The mechanism remains unclear, but most authors have agreed that the entrapment induces muscle incarceration and causes irreversible muscle fibrosis [2–5].

Previous studies have advocated early intervention to shorten the duration of muscle ischemia [1,6–8]. Moreover, recent studies have also shown that entrapment content significantly influenced the outcome of trapdoor fracture [5,9,10]. However, there is no consensus on the appropriate timing and indication of urgent surgical intervention due to the low incidence of trapdoor fractures and the small sample size.

In our retrospective study, we compared and analyzed the outcome of patient groups with different time intervals from injury to surgical intervention and content of entrapment (muscle versus soft tissue).

Citation: Hsieh, P.-J.; Liao, H.-T. Outcome Analysis of Surgical Timing in Pediatric Orbital Trapdoor Fracture with Different Entrapment Contents: A Retrospective Study. Children 2022, 9, 398. https://doi.org/10.3390/children9030398

Academic Editor: Christiaan J. A. van Bergen

Received: 23 January 2022
Accepted: 7 March 2022
Published: 11 March 2022

Publisher's Note: MDPI stays neutral with regard to jurisdictional claims in published maps and institutional affiliations.

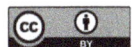

Copyright: © 2022 by the authors. Licensee MDPI, Basel, Switzerland. This article is an open access article distributed under the terms and conditions of the Creative Commons Attribution (CC BY) license (https://creativecommons.org/licenses/by/4.0/).

2. Materials and Methods

2.1. Design and Participants

We recruited patients under 18 with pure orbital wall fractures who underwent surgery at Chang Gung Memorial Hospital, Taiwan, between January 2001 to September 2018.

2.2. Procedures and Measures

A total of 23 patients had orbital trapdoor fractures. Preoperative computed tomography (CT) images and clinical symptoms of restricted EOM movement and diplopia confirmed the trapdoor fracture diagnosis. Patients with incomplete clinical and radiological evidence or a postoperative follow-up duration of fewer than six months were excluded. Cause of fractures, entrapment content, time interval from injury to surgery, the severity of EOM movement restriction and diplopia before and after surgery, and time interval from surgery to full recovery were recorded. Measurements of EOM movement were based on a numeric scale, with 3 representing no limitation and 0 representing no movement in one direction of gaze (Table 1). We evaluated the preoperative EOM movement, and the patient underwent an operation on the same day.

Table 1. The numeric scale for the measurement of EOM movement.

Score	Definition
3	No limitation in one direction of gaze
2	Active movement range > 50% of primary position to the edge of conjunctiva without full motion in one direction of gaze
1	Active movement range < 50% of primary position to the edge of conjunctiva without full motion in one direction of gaze
0	No movement in one direction of gaze

As for surgical intervention, we performed a forced duction test after general anesthesia before incision. The surgery started with a transconjunctival or subciliary approach to the orbital wall. After dissection and exposure of the orbital wall, the entrapped orbital contents were gently released from the fracture site. The fractured wall was patched with MEDPOR (Stryker, Kalamazoo, MI, USA) to prevent recurrent herniation or entrapment. Forced duction tests were performed again at the end of surgery to confirm the complete release of the entrapped tissue. We followed up with the patients every month for over half a year and recorded the latest EOM score and the results of examinations for diplopia. We took the worst preoperative EOM score for analysis regardless of the direction. We then took the postoperative EOM score of the same direction as the preoperative EOM score for comparison.

2.3. Statistical Analysis

Data were analyzed using SPSS V.19.0 (IBM, Portsmouth, UK). The data analysis included descriptive statistics, Fisher's Exact Test, and Mann–Whitney U Test. Significance was established at 0.05. We used Mann–Whitney U Test to analyze the score of EOM movement and time interval from injury to full recovery of both EOM movement restriction and diplopia. Fisher's Exact Test is used for the recovery rate of both EOM movement restriction and diplopia.

3. Results

Of the 23 patients enrolled, the average age was 10.78 years old (SD: 3.57), ranging from 6–18. The male and female ratio was 17:6. The most common cause of injury was falling (30.4%), followed by assault (26.1%), and blunt trauma (21.7%). Among the fracture sites, twenty were at the orbital floor, and three were at the medial orbital wall. As for entrapment content, 12 patients had rectus muscle entrapment, with the rest having pure soft tissue entrapment. The average time interval from injury to operation was 12.95 ± 16.8 days, with 6.0 ± 8.8 and 20.5 ± 20 days in muscle and soft tissue trapdoor fracture, respectively.

The overall recovery rates of EOM movement restriction and diplopia were 87.0% (SD: 33.68%) and 73.91% (SD: 43.91%), respectively. The average time interval to full recovery was 174.47 (SD: 244.91) days for the symptom of EOM movement restrictions and 293.75 (SD: 537.09) days for diplopia (Table 2).

Table 2. Patient Characteristics.

Patient Characteristics (n = 23)	Mean (SD)	
Age (Y)	10.78 (±3.57)	
Gender (M:F)	17:6	
Side (Right: Left)	15:11	
Fracture Site (Orbital Floor: Medial Wall)	20:3	
Entrapment content (Muscle: Soft tissue)	12:11	
Injury Mechanism (n)	Fall: 7	MVA: 3
	Assault: 6	Sports: 2
	Blunt trauma: 5	
Time Interval from Injury to Intervention (Days)	12.95 (±16.84)	
	Muscle: 6.03 (±8.79)	
	Soft Tissue: 20.50 (±19.99)	
Pre-OP EOM movement Score	0.90 (±1.07)	
	Muscle: 0.25 (±0.60)	
	Soft Tissue: 1.59 (±1.04)	
Post-OP EOM movement Score	2.80 (±0.64)	
Improvement in EOM movement restriction	1.9 (±1.1)	
Full Recovery Rate of EOM movement restriction	87.0% (±33.68%)	
Pre-OP Diplopia (percentage)	87.0% (±33.68%)	
Post-OP Diplopia (percentage)	26.09% (±43.91%)	
Full Recovery Rate of Diplopia	73.91% (±43.91%)	
Interval to full recovery of EOM movement restriction (Days)	174.47 (±244.91)	
Interval to full recovery of Diplopia (Days)	293.75 (±537.09)	

Pre-OP means preoperative; Post-OP means postoperative; EOM means extraocular muscle.

We initially divided the patients into two groups—surgical intervention within three days (Early) and over three days (Late). There was no significant difference between the two groups in preoperative EOM movement, diplopia, postoperative symptoms, and recovery time (Table 3). We then stratified the patient group with surgical time interval by entrapment content. There was no significant difference between the muscle and soft tissue entrapment group which performed surgery within three days in post-op EOM movement, EOM movement full recovery rate, persistent diplopia rate, and interval to full recovery of EOM movement and diplopia. Patients with muscle entrapment showed worse preoperative EOM movement than those with soft tissue entrapment at surgical timing of more than three days (p = 0.026). There was no significant difference in the recovery rate in EOM movement restriction and diplopia between the two types of entrapment content, but the subgroup with muscle entrapment took significantly longer to recover from both EOM movement restriction (p = 0.030) and diplopia (p = 0.030) at surgical timing of more than three days (Table 4).

Furthermore, we divided the patients by their entrapment content—rectus muscle versus pure soft tissue. The patients with muscle entrapment had more serious preoperative EOM movement restriction (p = 0.002) and needed a longer time for EOM movement (p = 0.036) and diplopia (p = 0.042) recovery, significantly. (Table 5) We also divided each group into early and late surgical interventions. Although the trends of worse recovery rate and longer recovery time from EOM movement restriction and diplopia were found, there were no significant differences between subgroups in both types of entrapment content (Table 6).

Table 3. Comparison of functional outcome by time interval to surgical intervention.

Time Interval (Days)	Pre-OP EOM Movement	Pre-OP Diplopia	Post-OP EOM Movement	EOM Movement Full Recovery Rate	Interval to Full EOM Movement Recovery	Persistent Diplopia	Interval to Diplopia Recovery
≤3 Days (n = 7)	0.21 ± 0.36	71.43 ± 45.18%	2.86 ± 0.36	85.71 ± 34.99%	84.07 ± 54.68	14.29% ± 34.99%	91.06 ± 51.80
>3 Days (n = 16)	1.19 ± 1.18	93.75 ± 24.21%	2.81 ± 0.73	87.50 ± 33.07%	214.01 ± 291.70	31.25% ± 46.35%	382.42 ± 643.04
p-Value	p = 0.082	p = 0.209	p = 0.585	p = 1.000	p = 0.624	p = 0.621	p = 0.535

Pre-OP means preoperative; Post-OP means postoperative; EOM means extraocular muscle.

Table 4. Comparison of functional outcome by surgical time interval and subgroups of entrapment contents.

Entrapment Content		Pre-OP EOM Movement	Pre-OP Diplopia	Post-OP EOM Movement	EOM Movement Full Recovery Rate	Interval to Full EOM Movement Recovery	Persistent Diplopia	Interval to Diplopia Recovery
≤3 Day (n = 7)	Muscle (n = 6):	0.17 ± 0.37	83.33 ± 37.27%	2.83 ± 0.37	83.33 ± 37.27%	96.46 ± 49.13	83.33 ± 37.27%	104.62 ± 42.94
	Soft Tissue (n = 1):	0.50	100.00%	3.00	100.00%	9.72	0.00%	9.72
	p-Value	p = 0.334	p = 0.286	p = 0.683	p = 1.000	p = 0.699	p = 1.000	p = 0.699
>3 Day (n = 16)	Muscle (n = 6):	0.33 ± 0.75	83.33 ± 37.27%	2.50 ± 1.12	66.67 ± 47.14%	399.51 ± 358.18	50.00 ± 50.00%	751.26 ± 832.75
	Soft Tissue (n = 10):	1.70 ± 1.03	90.91 ± 0.29%	3.00	100.00%	102.72 ± 132.78	20.00 ± 40.00%	161.11 ± 271.22
	p-Value	p = 0.026	p = 0.375	p = 0.197	p = 0.125	p = 0.030	p = 0.299	p = 0.030

Table 5. Comparison of functional outcome by entrapment contents.

Entrapment Content	Pre-OP EOM Movement	Pre-OP Diplopia	Post-OP EOM Movement	EOM Movement Full Recovery Rate	Interval to Full EOM Movement Recovery	Persistent Diplopia	Interval to Diplopia Recovery
Muscle (n = 12)	0.25 ± 0.60	83.33 ± 37.27%	2.67 ± 0.85	75.00 ± 43.30%	247.99 ± 297.17	66.67 ± 47.14%	541.78 ± 742.00
Soft Tissue (n = 11)	1.59 ± 1.04	90.91 ± 28.75%	3.0	100.00%	94.26 ± 129.39	81.82 ± 38.57%	147.35 ± 262.23
p-Value	p = 0.002	p = 1.000	p = 0.166	p = 0.217	p = 0.036	p = 0.640	p = 0.042

Table 6. Comparison of functional outcome by entrapment contains and subgroup of surgical timing interval.

Time Interval (Days)		Pre-OP EOM Movement	Pre-OP Diplopia	Post-OP EOM Movement	EOM Movement Full Recovery Rate	Interval to Full EOM Movement Recovery	Persistent Diplopia	Interval to Diplopia Recovery
Muscle (n = 12)	≤3 Days (n = 6):	0.17 ± 0.37	83.33 ± 37.27%	2.83 ± 0.37	83.33 ± 37.27%	96.46 ± 49.13	83.33 ± 37.27%	104.62 ± 42.94
	>3 Days (n = 6):	0.33 ± 0.75	83.33 ± 37.27%	2.50 ± 1.12	66.67 ± 47.14%	399.51 ± 358.18	50.00 ± 50.00%	751.26 ± 832.75
	p-Value	$p = 0.902$	$p = 1.000$	$p = 0.902$	$p = 1.000$	$p = 0.078$	$p = 0.545$	$p = 0.078$
Soft Tissue (n = 11)	≤3 Days (n = 1):	0.50	100.00%	3.00	100.00%	9.72	0.00%	9.72
	>3 Days (n = 10):	1.70 ± 1.03	90.91 ± 0.29%	3.00	100.00%	102.72 ± 132.78	20.00 ± 40.00%	161.11 ± 271.22
	p-Value	$p = 0.336$	$p = 0.091$	-	-	$p = 0.527$	$p = 1.000$	$p = 0.343$

4. Discussion

Due to the inherited elasticity of bone, pediatric patients encountering a blunt injury have a higher rate of trapdoor fractures than blowout fractures. The displaced bone would transiently snap back to its original position and impinge on the herniated tissue, causing the lower portion of extraocular tissue to be incarcerated. The incidence of entrapment in pure orbital wall fracture in pediatric patients was approximately 5.8% [5], and the age of patients ranged from 6–16 years old [2,11].

With a longer duration of incarceration, there is a higher rate of persistent diplopia. The exact mechanisms of persistent diplopia are still under debate, but it is mostly accepted that the trapped tissue would undergo ischemia and result in irreversible fibrosis and scarring [3,4]. Therefore, early surgical intervention for pediatric trapdoor fracture should be encouraged to better recover from EOM movement restriction and diplopia. As opposed to the traditional management of a 2-week waiting period of observation for a common blowout fracture, Jordan et al. [12] presented a case series and found that patients with intervention over two weeks had no full recovery of EOM movement restriction. In a retrospective study presented by Grant et al. [6], 19 patients with trapdoor fracture were enrolled and segregated into two groups by the overall means of time interval to intervention—5 days. They found a negative correlation between time interval and degree of EOM movement after releasing the entrapped content in the late intervention group (>5 days). Neinstein et al. [7] analyzed their participants retrospectively; the mean of time to surgery in the patients with full return of EOM function was 6.4 days compared with 14.2 days in those with residual diplopia. Yoon et al. [8] conducted a study in which patients were divided into three groups by intervention at 0–5 days, 5–14 days, and over 14 days. In the first month after surgery, early intervention within five days resulted in the greatest reduction of EOM movement limitation. Yang et al. [10] investigated patients with shorter surgical intervention and segregated them into three groups by surgical timing of fewer than 24 h, 24–72 h, and over 72 h. The authors found no significant differences in recovery rate and interval to full recovery between the three groups. For general trapdoor fracture, surgical timing within 3–7 days seems to bring a better recovery rate and shorter interval to full recovery.

Recent studies have mentioned that the entrapped content and type of fracture may affect the initial severity of diplopia and EOM movement restriction as well as the postoperatively outcomes. In the study by Gerbino et al. [2], they analyzed the outcome of patients with different extents of fracture bone displacement. With intervention performed within 24 h, in patients with minor bone fragment displaced, the tissue was trapped more tightly and had a higher incidence of residual diplopia. As for entrapment content, patients with rectus muscle tended to have more severe preoperative EOM movement restriction. Su et al. [9] performed a study on patients with delayed surgical intervention. They divided the patients by entrapment content and stratified them by their severity of preoperative EOM movement limitation. While the extent of initial EOM movement restriction did not affect the recovery rate and time interval to full recovery, the patient subgroup with rectus muscle entrapment took a significantly longer time to full recovery. Besides surgical timing, other factors that affected the preoperative symptoms of trapdoor fracture were proved to have some influences on the outcome [6,10]. Therefore, surgical timing could be adjusted according to the patient's extent of injury and entrapment contents. Our study also demonstrated that muscle entrapment leads to delayed recovery of EOM movements and diplopia.

Early diagnosis of trapdoor fracture may be decisive for the outcome for pediatric patients. According to previous studies, indications to surgical intervention should not rely on merely radiographic evidence of entrapment [1,2,8,13]. Contents of entrapment would occasionally be too subtle to be recognized in CT images, and the concordance rate to operative findings was reported to be 50% in the pediatric population [9,13]. Thin-sliced CT images and missing rectus signs were recommended for entrapment content discovery. Yet, correlation to severe clinical evidence is considered a critical indication of surgery [13,14].

Since children may be difficult to approach during an emergency due to the inability to describe their discomfort and poor cooperation, physical examination plays a significant role in diagnosis. External clinical signs such as ecchymosis, edema, and enophthalmos are relatively minimal in children compared to adults. Instead, EOM movement restriction could indicate a high possibility of muscle entrapment even without radiographic findings. Moreover, muscle entrapment may also bring oculocardiac reflex (OCR), which is more commonly seen in children and adolescents [15]. Arrhythmia caused by OCR may put pediatric patients in danger but could be easily relieved by releasing the injured rectus muscle. Kim et al. [1] found a strong association between nausea and vomiting and extraocular muscle entrapment. In other words, severe OCR should be considered a sign of muscle entrapment and taken as one of the indications for immediate surgery [16–18]. Compared to pure soft tissue entrapment, muscle entrapment with delayed intervention would need a longer time to recover and higher risks for persistent diplopia and fatal complications. Therefore, even though the exact cut-off timing for intervention is still under debate, the urgency of an operation could be considered according to the symptom severity.

Limitations of this study include its retrospective nature and relatively small sample size. The number of participants in the early intervention group was insufficient for statistical validity as our institute is classified as a tertiary medical center and our patients are mostly composed of referral from other local hospitals which leads to delayed visit and management. Furthermore, most of the recruited patients with pure soft tissue entrapment in this study visited our hospital more than three days after injury because they were unaware of the severity due to mild diplopia or EOM movement restriction. Moreover, some children did not receive surgery because of mild symptoms and signs. However, the surgical timing still remains vital as previous studies have recommended that patients with soft tissue entrapment should be treated as having muscle entrapment when they present restriction in EOM [9].

5. Conclusions

In conclusion, we recommend early intervention for patients with rectus muscle entrapment and severe symptoms of trapdoor fracture. Although an appropriate timing remained unknown, our study showed that patients with muscle entrapment would have a shorter interval to full recovery if receiving surgical intervention within three days. Although the recovery rate is not related to either surgical timing or entrapment content, early intervention should be conducted to lower the risks of potentially fatal complications, improve the outcomes, and enhance faster recovery.

Author Contributions: Conceptualization, H.-T.L.; methodology, H.-T.L.; formal analysis, P.-J.H.; investigation, P.-J.H.; data curation, H.-T.L. and P.-J.H.; writing—original draft preparation, P.-J.H.; writing—review and editing, H.-T.L.; supervision, H.-T.L.; project administration, H.-T.L. All authors have read and agreed to the published version of the manuscript.

Funding: This research received no external funding.

Institutional Review Board Statement: The study was conducted according to the guidelines of the Declaration of Helsinki and approved by the Institutional Review Board of Chang Gung Memorial Hospital (protocol code 202102062B0 Date: 20 December 2021).

Informed Consent Statement: Informed consent was obtained from all subjects involved in the study.

Data Availability Statement: The data that support the findings of this study are available on request from the corresponding author. The data are not publicly available due to privacy and ethical restrictions.

Conflicts of Interest: The authors declare no conflict of interest.

References

1. Kim, J.; Lee, H.; Chi, M.; Park, M.; Lee, J.; Baek, S. Endoscope-Assisted Repair of Pediatric Trapdoor Fractures of the Orbital Floor: Characterization and Management. *J. Craniofacial Surg.* **2010**, *21*, 101–105. [CrossRef] [PubMed]
2. Gerbino, G.; Roccia, F.; Bianchi, F.A.; Zavattero, E. Surgical Management of Orbital Trapdoor Fracture in a Pediatric Population. *J. Oral Maxillofac. Surg.* **2010**, *68*, 1310–1316. [CrossRef] [PubMed]
3. Iliff, N.; Manson, P.N.; Katz, J.; Rever, L.; Yaremchuk, M. Mechanisms of Extraocular Muscle Injury in Orbital Fractures. *Plast. Reconstr. Surg.* **1999**, *103*, 787–799. [CrossRef] [PubMed]
4. Smith, B.; Lisman, R.D.; Simonton, J.; della Rocca, R. Volkmann's Contracture of the Extraocular Muscles Following Blowout Fracture. *Plast. Reconstr. Surg.* **1984**, *74*, 200–216. [CrossRef] [PubMed]
5. Sugamata, A.; Yoshizawa, N.; Shimanaka, K. Timing of Operation for Blowout Fractures with Extraocular Muscle Entrapment. *J. Plast. Surg. Hand Surg.* **2013**, *47*, 454–457. [CrossRef] [PubMed]
6. Grant, H.J., 3rd; Patrinely, J.R.; Weiss, A.H.; Kierney, P.C.; Gruss, J.S. Trapdoor Fracture of the Orbit in a Pediatric Population. *Plast. Reconstr. Surg.* **2002**, *109*, 482–489, discussion 90–95. [CrossRef] [PubMed]
7. Neinstein, M.R.; Phillips, J.H.; Forrest, C.R. Pediatric Orbital Floor Trapdoor Fractures: Outcomes and Ct-Based Morphologic Assessment of the Inferior Rectus Muscle. *J. Plast. Reconstr. Aesthet. Surg.* **2012**, *65*, 869–874. [CrossRef] [PubMed]
8. Yoon, C.K.; Seo, M.S.; Park, Y.G. Orbital Trapdoor Fracture in Children. *J. Korean Med. Sci.* **2003**, *18*, 881–885. [CrossRef] [PubMed]
9. Su, Q.Y.; Shen, B.X.; Lin, M.; Fan, X. Delayed Surgical Treatment of Orbital Trapdoor Fracture in Paediatric Patients. *Br. J. Ophthalmol.* **2019**, *103*, 523–526. [CrossRef] [PubMed]
10. Yang, W.J.; Woo, J.E.; An, H.J. Surgical Outcomes of Orbital Trapdoor Fracture in Children and Adolescents. *J. Craniomaxillofac. Surg.* **2015**, *43*, 444–447. [CrossRef] [PubMed]
11. Criden, R.M.; Ellis, F.J. Linear Nondisplaced Orbital Fractures with Muscle Entrapment. *J. Am. Assoc. Pediatr. Ophthalmol. Strabismus* **2007**, *11*, 142–147. [CrossRef] [PubMed]
12. Jordan, R.D.; Allen, L.H.; White, J.; Harvey, J.; Pashby, R.; Esmaeli, B. Intervention within Days for Some Orbital Floor Fractures: The White-Eyed Blowout. *Ophthalmic Plast. Reconstr. Surg.* **1998**, *14*, 379–390. [CrossRef] [PubMed]
13. Alinasab, B.; Qureshi, A.R.; Stjärne, P. Prospective Study on Ocular Motility Limitation Due to Orbital Muscle Entrapment or Impingement Associated with Orbital Wall Fracture. *Injury* **2017**, *48*, 1408–1416. [CrossRef] [PubMed]
14. Parbhu, C.K.; Galler, K.E.; Li, C.; Mawn, L.A. Underestimation of Soft Tissue Entrapment by Computed Tomography in Orbital Floor Fractures in the Pediatric Population. *Ophthalmology* **2008**, *115*, 1620–1625. [CrossRef] [PubMed]
15. Sires, S.B.; Stanley, R.B., Jr.; Levine, L.M. Oculocardiac Reflex Caused by Orbital Floor Trapdoor Fracture: An Indication for Urgent Repair. *Arch. Ophthalmol.* **1998**, *116*, 955–956. [PubMed]
16. Firriolo, M.J.; Ontiveros, N.C.; Pike, C.M.; Taghinia, A.H.; Rogers-Vizena, C.R.; Ganor, O.; Greene, A.K.; Meara, J.G.; Labow, B.I. Pediatric Orbital Floor Fractures: Clinical and Radiological Predictors of Tissue Entrapment and the Effect of Operative Timing on Ocular Outcomes. *J. Craniofac. Surg.* **2017**, *28*, 1966–1971. [CrossRef] [PubMed]
17. Mehmood, N.; Hasan, A. Oculocardiac Reflex: An Underrecognized but Important Association with Orbital Trap Door Fractures. *Pediatr. Emerg. Care* **2021**, *37*, e1731–e1732. [CrossRef]
18. Tarbet, C.; Siegal, N.; Tarbet, K. White-Eyed Blowout Fracture with Muscle Entrapment Misdiagnosed as Increased Intracranial Pressure: An Important Clinical Lesson. *Am. J. Emerg. Med.* **2021**, *48*, 375.e1–375.e3. [CrossRef] [PubMed]

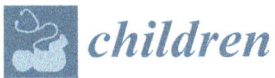

Review

Pediatric Clavicle Fractures and Congenital Pseudarthrosis Unraveled

Lisa van der Water [1,*], Arno A. Macken [1], Denise Eygendaal [1,2] and Christiaan J. A. van Bergen [1]

1. Depeartment of Orthopedic Surgery, Amphia Hospital, 4818 CK Breda, The Netherlands; arnomacken@gmail.com (A.A.M.); denise@eygendaal.nl (D.E.); CvanBergen@amphia.nl (C.J.A.v.B.)
2. Department of Orthopaedics and Sports Medicine, Erasmus University Medical Center Rotterdam, 3015 GD Rotterdam, The Netherlands
* Correspondence: lisa.vanderwater@gmail.com

Abstract: Clavicle fractures are commonly seen in the pediatric and adolescent populations. In contrast, congenital pseudarthrosis of the clavicle is rare. Although both conditions may present with similar signs and symptoms, especially in the very young, clear differences exist. Clavicle fractures are often caused by trauma and are tender on palpation, while pseudarthrosis often presents with a painless protuberance on the clavicle, which becomes more prominent as the child grows. Its presence may only become apparent after trauma, as it is usually asymptomatic. The diagnosis is confirmed on plain radiography, which shows typical features to distinguish both entities. Both clavicle fractures and congenital pseudarthrosis are generally treated conservatively with a high success rate. Operative treatment for a fracture can be indicated in the case of an open fracture, severely displaced fracture, floating shoulder, neurovascular complications or polytrauma. Congenital pseudarthrosis requires operative treatment if the patient experiences progressive pain, functional limitation and late-onset thoracic outlet symptoms, but most operations are performed due to esthetic complaints.

Keywords: clavicle; fracture; pseudarthrosis; pediatric; children; treatment; diagnosis

1. Introduction

Clavicle fractures frequently occur in the pediatric and adolescent populations [1]. Diagnosis and treatment of these fractures are generally straightforward but can be particularly challenging in select cases. Therefore, it is important to have a thorough understanding of the underlying principles. Furthermore, a pediatric clavicle fracture should be differentiated from congenital pseudarthrosis, which may have a similar presentation (especially in neonates) but may require a different treatment approach. Congenital pseudarthrosis of the clavicle is characterized by a failure in the fusion of the medial and lateral ossification centers of the clavicle [2]. This article aims to provide an overview of the diagnosis, treatment and complications of pediatric clavicle fractures and congenital pseudarthrosis based on the most recent literature.

2. Epidemiology

Clavicle fractures account for 10–15% of all pediatric fractures [1]. The majority of patients with a clavicle fracture are male (91.2%), and most clavicle fractures are seen between the ages of 10 and 19 years (incidence rate of 91.7 per 100,000) [1,3]. Fractures on the left side (58%) and on the non-dominant side (56%) are slightly more common [4]. Most clavicle fractures occur in the middle section of the bone, accounting for 70% to 95% of all pediatric clavicle fractures [1,5,6]. Displaced fractures of the clavicle are relatively common, ranging from 28% to 67% of all clavicle fractures in children and adolescents [1,4,6,7].

Clavicle fractures occur most frequently as a result of sports (66%), horseplay (12%), riding a bike (6%), a fall (6%) or another type of accident (3%) [4]. However, clavicle fractures may also occur during childbirth, particularly in the case of shoulder dystocia [8,9].

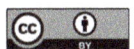

Although less than 4% of all children are born with this fracture, it is the most common fracture during childbirth, accounting for almost a third of all birth traumas [8–10].

On the other hand, congenital pseudarthrosis of the clavicle is a rare condition, and currently, available evidence relies on case reports (approximately 200 in total), with no studies reporting the incidence [2]. Congenital pseudarthrosis occurs more frequently in females and most commonly on the right side [2,6]. Isolated left clavicle pseudarthrosis occurs in less than 10%, and in most cases, presents in combination with dextrocardia or situs inversus [2]. Bilateral pseudarthrosis has been reported in about 10% of cases, often in combination with a high subclavian artery and cervical ribs or vertical upper ribs [2].

Congenital pseudarthrosis is often associated with abnormalities of ossification during the embryonic stage and is associated with genetic syndromes like Ehlers-Danlos, Al-Awadi/Ras-Rothschild, Kabuki and Prader-Willi [2].

2.1. Anatomy

Development of Clavicle

The clavicle develops from two ossification centers that are initially connected by pre-cartilage surrounded by perichondrium [2]. Physiological ossification of the clavicle occurs during the fourth week of gestation, and the two ossification centers fuse near the seventh week [2]. The epiphysis of the medial part of the clavicle does not ossify until the age of 20, and the lateral epiphysis does not ossify until the age of 25 years [1].

2.2. Trauma Mechanism

Most fractures are caused by blunt trauma to the shoulder or upper arm (60%), trauma to the clavicle or chest (24%) or a fall on an outstretched arm (11%) [4].

Concomitant fractures are rare in children and occur mostly in high-energy accidents involving sports or motorized vehicles [1,11]. The most common concomitant fractures are those of the ribs, spine, extremities and facial bones [1]. However, other concomitant injuries such as brachial plexopathy, compression of the subclavian vein and other neurovascular injuries are more common [1,7].

Another important trauma mechanism of clavicle fracture is peri-natal injury. Birth fractures are associated with shoulder dystocia and difficult delivery [8]. Risk factors for clavicle fractures are similar to risk factors related to a difficult delivery and shoulder dystocia, namely: instrumented delivery, macrosomia, post-term delivery, procedural induction of labor, prolonged labor, advanced maternal age, multiparity and excessive weight gain during the pregnancy [8]. Peri-natal clavicle fractures are often seen in combination with a fractured humerus, brachial plexus injury and injuries to the phrenic and recurrent laryngeal nerves [8]. In rare cases, an iatrogenic clavicle fracture is unavoidable to ensure successful delivery.

2.3. Classification of Fractures

The Allman classification divides clavicle fractures into three groups: type 1 fractures are located in the middle third of the clavicle, type 2 fractures are located in the part lateral to the coracoclavicular ligament, and type 3 fractures are located in the medial third (Figure 1) [11,12].

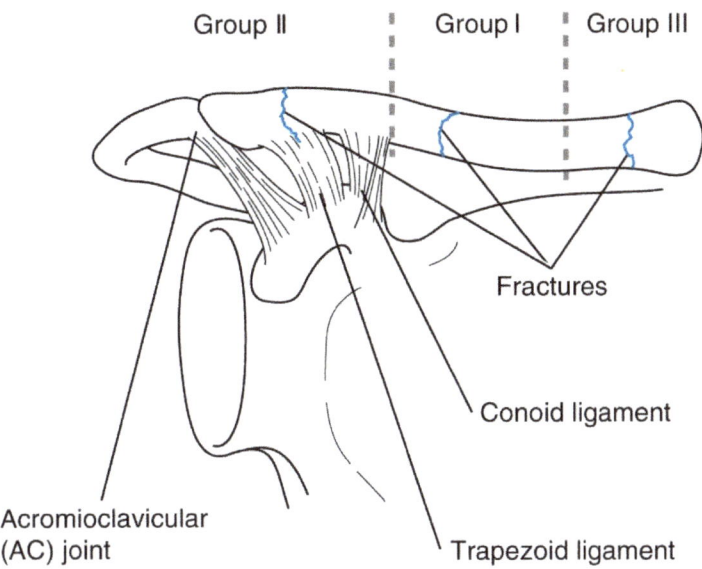

Figure 1. The Allman classification for clavicle fractures [13].

2.4. Development of Pseudarthrosis

Pseudarthrosis of the clavicle is characterized by the incomplete or absent union of the two ossification centers [2]. Although the exact cause of pseudarthrosis is unknown, several theories have been developed as to why the fusion of the two ossification centers fails [2]. One theory is that the excessive pressure from the pulsing subclavian artery during the development of the clavicle causes non-union of the ossification centers, especially if cervical ribs are present, which add to the increased pressure [2]. Another theory is that the non-union is caused by an altered intrauterine position of the fetus and cranial localization of the right subclavian artery [2]. Additionally, rare case reports [14–18] of family members with pseudarthrosis suggest inheritance to attribute to the development of pseudarthrosis, although there is a lack of conclusive evidence to support this hypothesis.

2.5. Classification of Pseudarthrosis

Kite proposed a classification system for congenital pseudarthrosis of the clavicle based on the differences in anatomy, clinical representation and pathology [2,19].

Type I includes patients who have clavicular non-union at birth, caused by hypoplasia of the distal fragment [2,19]. Pressure on the protuberance is painful, and radiographs show a larger medial fragment than lateral fragment with clear spacing between them [2,19]. For this type, the distance between the fragments and their positioning should be assessed before surgery is considered [2,19].

Type II includes patients with congenital bone deficiency who have a physiologically formed clavicle at birth which is more fragile and prone to fractures [2,19]. For this type, surgery could be considered after a fracture has occurred [2,19].

3. Diagnosis

3.1. Clavicle Fracture

Clavicle fractures are often the result of trauma and can present as a deformity or open fracture, although visible deformity may also be absent [4,20,21]. The fracture is tender on palpation, and movement of the shoulder is labored, painful and sometimes limited [2,20]. Plain radiographs usually confirm the clinical suspicion of a fracture, yet a recent study found that it is not necessary for proper diagnosis and treatment [22]. Several studies have demonstrated ultrasound to be reliable for diagnosis of clavicle fractures both in neonates and older children [23–25]. One study of 58 patients found a sensitivity of 89.7% and specificity of 89.5% [25]. Ultrasound has the advantage of reducing radiation exposure but is dependent on the experience of the operator.

3.2. Pseudarthrosis

Pseudarthrosis of the clavicle often presents as a painless protuberance on the clavicle, most commonly in the middle third or lateral third of the bone [2]. In addition, during the first days after birth, a hypermobile segment can be seen [2]. The protuberance usually becomes larger and more evident as the child grows (Figure 2), sometimes causing atrophy of the overlying skin [2]. Furthermore, pseudarthrosis of the clavicle is often associated with a change in the alignment of the shoulder and a winged scapula [26–28]. This can cause a limited range of motion in all three planes, but especially when lifting the arm above the head [26–28]. Apart from appearance, pseudarthrosis is usually asymptomatic. However, some patients do experience pain, discomfort or functional limitations, such as late-onset thoracic outlet syndrome [2]. Although it is logical to expect the altered biomechanics to lead to a long-term impairment of the shoulder, we found no studies reporting long-term outcomes. This may be due to the low incidence of pseudo-arthrosis of the clavicle.

To confirm the diagnosis, plain radiographs need to show a clear separation between two fragments of the clavicle [2]. The fragments often have a characteristic shape towards the end facing the defect. Generally, one of the fragments appears as an "elephant's foot" shape (the fragment is wider at the end compared to the shaft) and the other shows a "pencil point" shape (the fragment is increasingly thin towards the end) (Figure 2) [2]. The medullary canal is closed and sclerotic, but no bone callus is formed [2]. The medial fragment is often positioned superior to the lateral fragment due to muscle forces and the weight of the arm [2].

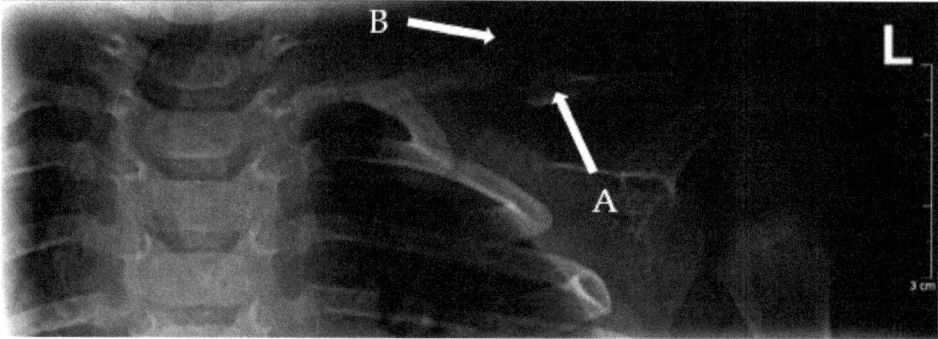

Figure 2. Left-sided pseudo-arthrosis (Type I) of the clavicle showing an elephant's foot (A) and pencil point sign (B).

3.3. Differential Diagnosis

A congenital pseudarthrosis should be differentiated from a clavicle fracture. The latter is tender on palpation and is associated with a trauma or traumatic birth [2]. Old clavicle fractures can present with callus formation, which can help distinguish the difference between old and new fractures [2]. In general, pseudarthrosis is a painless protuberance (Figure 3) on the clavicle without callus formation [2]. Furthermore, several other diagnoses can have a similar presentation and should be considered in the differential diagnosis. This includes cleidocranial dysplasia, which is characterized by the absence or hypoplasia of the clavicle (usually bilateral) and presents with an increased anterior position of the shoulder but is otherwise asymptomatic [2,29]. In addition, cleidocranial dysplasia is associated with overall increased range of motion of the joints and several specific facial features (late ossification of the fontanelle, wide and protruding forehead and excess teeth) [29]. Another is neurofibromatosis, which can also cause dysplasia of the clavicle and may appear similar to a fracture or pseudarthrosis. Most of these patients have hyperpigmented "coffee stains" on their skin, pathognomonic for neurofibromatosis [2,30].

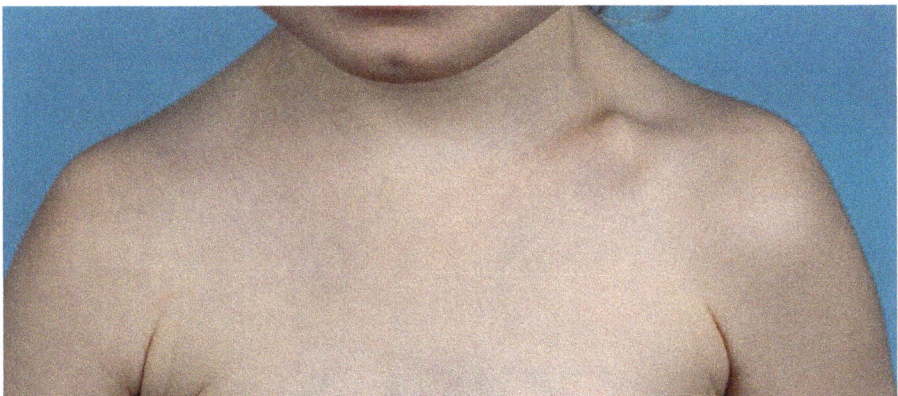

Figure 3. Congenital pseudo-arthrosis patient with an imminent protuberance on the left clavicle.

4. Treatment and Complications
4.1. Clavicle Fracture
4.1.1. Non-Operative Treatment

Non-operative treatment is indicated for all fractures without displacement or other complicating factors [1,21]. The majority of clavicle fractures are treated conservatively (Figure 4b), even with significant shortening and total displacement, because children have the ability to reconstitute fracture shortening and displacement that would need surgery in adults [6,21,31–36]. To immobilize the fracture, a supportive sling, collar 'n' cuff or figure-of-eight bandage is prescribed for several weeks [6,21,31]. The exact length of immobilization is dependent on the severity of the fracture, the age of the child and the amount of pain [6,21,31]. The children are also instructed to avoid high-risk activities [6].

Outcomes of non-operative treatment are generally satisfactory in children and adolescents [37–39]. Most patients prefer the cosmetic outcome of conservative treatment [37]. However, in adolescents, conservative treatment may lead to longer functional recovery and longer time until a stable union is achieved, compared to younger children [40,41]. Non-union and mal-union are rare in children but occur slightly more frequently in the non-operative group [6,40,41].

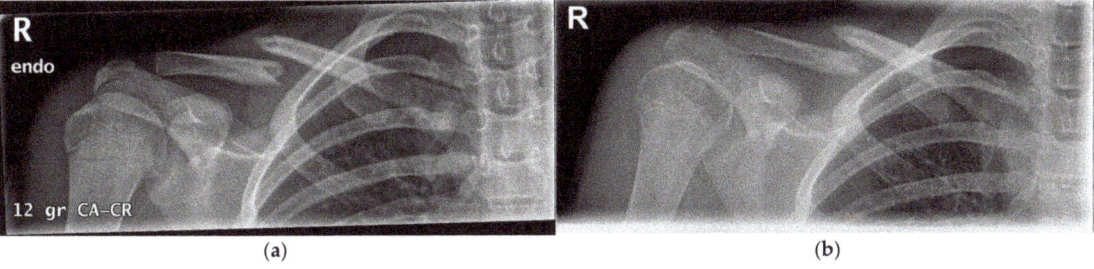

Figure 4. (a) Right clavicle fracture (Group I) with extreme displacement. (b) After 5 weeks of conservative treatment, early callus formation is visible.

4.1.2. Operative Treatment

A small percentage of fractures require primary surgical fixation (1.6%) [6]. Fixation is indicated in the case of an open fracture, imminent open fracture, neurovascular injury, symptomatic non-union, symptomatic malunion, floating shoulder or polytrauma [1,6,34,35,42]. Relative indications for operative treatment are significantly displaced fractures (>100% of shaft width) (Figures 4a, 5a and 6a), severe comminution and significantly shortened fractures (> 15–20 mm absolute or > 14% relative shortening) [1,6,34,35,42–49].

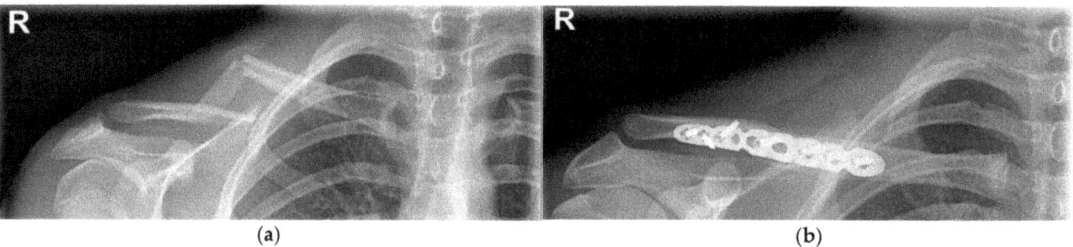

Figure 5. (a) Segmental right clavicle fracture (Group I), with extreme displacement. (b) Surgical fixation using the plate-and-screw method.

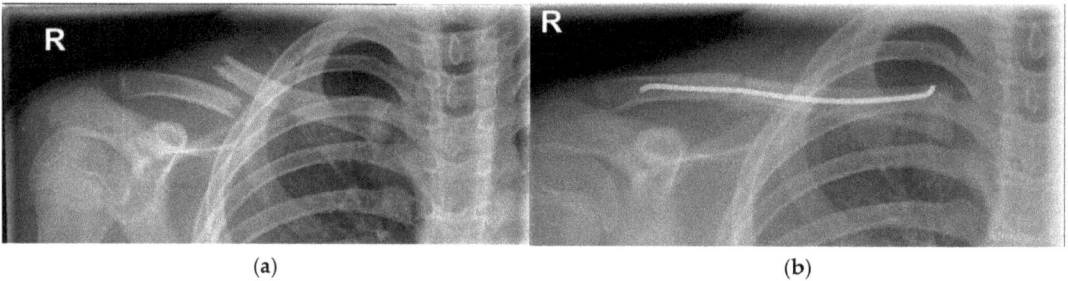

Figure 6. (a) Right clavicle fracture (Group I) with extreme displacement. (b) Surgical fixation with an intramedullary wire.

The indication for surgery for fractures with significant shortening is actively discussed in the literature. Some studies have shown beneficial effects of surgery in children with a significantly shortened clavicle fracture, such as a lower incidence of mal-union and non-union [27,34,42,43,45–51]. However, other studies found no significant difference in outcome compared to the conservative treatment for shortened fractures [35,36,48,52]. This ambiguity is partially caused by the different methods of measuring clavicle shortening: end-to-end, cortex-to-corresponding cortex and relative shortening compared to the uninjured side [4]. Different methods may result in different cut-off values for the amount of shortening [4]. Therefore, an exact cut-off value for the amount of shortening that would be an indication for surgery cannot be concluded from the literature. In children and adolescents, clavicle shortening should be expressed in percentage shortening relative to the uninjured clavicle [4,34]. Until further consensus is reached, the choice of treatment for fracture shortening should be based on additional complicating factors, age, years of growth remaining, potential for remodeling and level of functional demand [34,42,51].

Several internal fixation methods can be used, such as plate and screw fixation (Figure 5b), screw-only fixation and intramedullary fixation (Figure 6b) [6]. Plate and screw fixation is the most commonly used technique [6]. Plate fixation has advantages over the other techniques: it provides strong fixation and compression of the small fractured fragments [44]. However, it requires an open exposure with corresponding soft tissue damage and risk of infection [44]. To reduce the size of the incision, other techniques such as the minimally invasive plate osteosynthesis (MIPO) technique, screw fixation only or intramedullary nail fixation can be used [44].

Outcomes after surgical treatment are generally satisfactory, yet not (significantly) superior to non-operative treatment [37–39]. There is an incongruence in the literature regarding the superiority of surgical treatment or non-operative treatment in children and adolescents. Some studies report superior outcomes in adolescents after surgery compared to non-operative treatment [40,41]. However, other studies report no clear difference in outcomes between operative and non-operative treatment in children or adolescents [6,38,39,44]. Possible advantages of surgery for adolescents are shorter recovery time, fewer cases of mal-union and non-union and shorter time to achieve union [40–44,47,49,51]. However, conservative treatment comes with a lower risk of complications and remains the preferred treatment in the far majority of pediatric patients.

4.1.3. Revision Surgery

Revision surgery is required in the case of a refracture and non-union due to failed osteosynthesis [1,5,44]. Non-union is rare and occurs almost exclusively in patients with complete fracture displacements and refractures [5,6]. The incidence of non-union increases with increased age [6]. This may be related to skeletal maturity and more forceful trauma, which increases the chance of completely displaced fractures and concomitant injuries [6].

Bone-grafting is often used in the case of non-union, but is increasingly difficult with increased displacement [53]. Kubiak and Slongo reported that in a study of 15 patients that underwent wire or nail fixation, all patients had to undergo revision surgery [54]. Furthermore, Luo et al. reported that out of 23 patients who were surgically treated (19 with a plate and 4 with an intramedullary nail), 5 (21.7%) experienced complications (refracture, prominence of the implant and non-union due to implant failure), of whom 4 needed a revision surgery [5]. Additionally, many patients prefer to have the hardware removed due to discomfort or esthetic complaints [5].

4.1.4. Return to Sports

Before returning to sports, the child should have a full range of motion, normal shoulder strength, bony healing and no tenderness on palpation [43,55]. Operative treatment could allow athletes to return to sports faster than a conservative treatment, especially for significantly displaced or shortened fractures [56–58]. On the contrary, in some cases, the hardware (i.e., plate, screws, pin) is removed before returning to sports, which can cause a delay [43].

On average, the time to return to sports is similar for operative and non-operative treatment because it depends on individual characteristics such as age, type and severity of the fracture and the nature of their sport [43,55,56,58].

Patients can return to non-contact sports six weeks after injury in most cases [43]. Athletes can resume contact and collision sports when solid bony union occurs, which is usually after 2–4 months [43].

4.2. Congenital Pseudarthrosis

4.2.1. Non-Operative Treatment

The majority of patients are treated conservatively (i.e., observation only, no interventions), especially if they experience minimal symptoms and do not have esthetic complaints due to the protuberance [2,7].

Outcomes after non-operative treatment are generally excellent; most patients do not experience any pain, discomfort or limited range of motion [59].

4.2.2. Operative Treatment

Indications for surgical treatment are progressive pain, functional limitation and late-onset thoracic outlet syndrome [2]. However, most operations are performed for cosmetic reasons [2]. It is recommended to perform surgery between the ages of 2 to 6 years [14,60,61].

Surgery is considered in Kite type I patients, where the fragments are less than 1 cm apart [2,19]. A displacement greater than 1 cm has a much higher incidence of non-consolidation and complications after surgery [2,19].

Several surgical treatment options are used: resection of the focus of the pseudarthrosis with the option of using a bone graft, osteosynthesis or both [2]. For stabilization, different techniques are used: an intramedullary Kirschner-wire, plate and screws, screws only, a Steinmann intramedullary pin or external fixation [2,19]. Above the age of 8 years, a bone graft is needed to achieve full consolidation [2]. The most commonly used donor site for bone grafting is the iliac crest, but the tibia, ribs and vascularized fibular grafts can also be used [2].

Post-operative treatment includes immobilization with a Velpeau sling or Desault bandage for four to six weeks [2,62].

Outcomes after surgical treatment are generally successful but appear most successful in cases with minimum or no fragment displacement and an intact periosteum and with the use of a bone graft [2].

Complications are very rare but do occur. Scar tissue may become hypertrophic, painful or form a keloid [2]. Furthermore, one case of a clavicle fracture through one of the screw holes (after the removal of the plate and screws) and one case of neuropraxia of the brachial plexus have been reported [63,64]. The most common complication is non-union, which is often an indication for revision surgery [63].

5. Conclusions

Clavicle fractures and congenital pseudarthrosis can be difficult to differentiate on first inspection, specifically immediately after birth. Even though pseudarthrosis of the clavicle is rare, with only a few hundred cases reported in the literature [65], it should be included in the differential diagnosis of a neonatal clavicle fracture, as undetected pseudarthrosis can cause problems at a later age. However, there are several diagnostic differences between clavicle fractures and congenital pseudarthrosis of the clavicle that can help distinguish them. Clavicle fractures are often a result of trauma, are suddenly tender on palpation and cause labored, painful or limited movement of the shoulder. Cases of congenital pseudarthrosis of the clavicle often present with a painless protuberance on the clavicle, which can become larger over time. In most cases, it is asymptomatic.

Both clavicle fractures and pseudarthrosis can be treated operatively or non-operatively, both with great success rate and patient satisfaction. Most patients with either are treated conservatively. Possible surgical indications for a clavicle fracture include an open fracture, significantly displaced fracture, shortened fracture or complications caused by the fracture. The majority of operations are successful and lasting. However, in some cases, revision surgery is required for non-union. For congenital pseudarthrosis, surgical treatment is considered in cases of progressive pain, functional limitation and late-onset thoracic outlet syndrome. However, most surgeries for congenital pseudarthrosis of the clavicle are performed because of cosmetic reasons.

In conclusion, this article provides a comprehensive, evidence-based overview of pediatric clavicle fractures and congenital pseudarthrosis. Some important issues remain open for discussion, including clear indications for surgical treatment. Most of the current knowledge is based on case studies, underpowered studies or adult-based studies. Therefore, future high-level studies in the pediatric population will need to contribute to our knowledge on these challenging pathologies.

Author Contributions: Conceptualization, L.v.d.W. and C.J.A.v.B.; writing—original draft preparation, L.v.d.W.; writing—review and editing, A.A.M., D.E. and C.J.A.v.B.; visualization, L.v.d.W. and C.J.A.v.B.; supervision, C.J.A.v.B.; project administration, L.v.d.W. and C.J.A.v.B. All authors have read and agreed to the published version of the manuscript.

Funding: This research received no external funding.

Informed Consent Statement: Not applicable.

Acknowledgments: The authors would like to thank J.M. De Groot, for revising and improving the overall quality of the English language of this article.

Conflicts of Interest: The authors declare no conflict of interest.

References

1. van der Meijden, O.A.; Gaskill, T.R.; Millett, P.J. Treatment of clavicle fractures: Current concepts review. *J. Shoulder Elb. Surg.* **2012**, *21*, 423–429. [CrossRef]
2. de Figueiredo, M.J.P.S.S.; Dos Reis Braga, S.; Akkari, M.; Prado, J.C.L.; Santili, C. Congenital pseudarthrosis of the clavicle. *Rev. Bras. Ortop.* **2012**, *47*, 21–26. [CrossRef]
3. van Tassel, D.; Owens, B.D.; Pointer, L.; Moriatis Wolf, J. Incidence of clavicle fractures in sports: Analysis of the NEISS Database. *Int J. Sports Med.* **2014**, *35*, 83–86. [CrossRef] [PubMed]
4. Ellis, H.B.; Li, Y.; Bae, D.S.; Kalish, L.A.; Wilson, P.L.; Pennock, A.T.; Nepple, J.J.; Willimon, S.C.; Spence, D.D.; Pandya, N.K.; et al. Descriptive Epidemiology of Adolescent Clavicle Fractures: Results From the FACTS (Function after Adolescent Clavicle Trauma and Surgery) Prospective, Multicenter Cohort Study. *Orthop J. Sports Med.* **2020**, *8*. [CrossRef] [PubMed]
5. Luo, T.D.; Ashraf, A.; Larson, A.N.; Stans, A.A.; Shaughnessy, W.J.; McIntosh, A.L. Complications in the treatment of adolescent clavicle fractures. *Orthopedics* **2015**, *38*, e287–e291. [CrossRef] [PubMed]
6. Hughes, K.; Kimpton, J.; Wei, R.; Williamson, M.; Yeo, A.; Arnander, M.; Gelfer, Y. Clavicle fracture nonunion in the paediatric population: A systematic review of the literature. *J. Child. Orthop.* **2018**, *12*, 2–8. [CrossRef]
7. O'Neill, B.J.; Molloy, A.P.; Curtin, W. Conservative Management of Paediatric Clavicle Fractures. *Int. J. Pediatr.* **2011**, *2011*, 172571. [CrossRef]
8. Yenigül, A.E.; Yenigül, N.N.; Başer, E.; Özelçi, R. A retrospective analysis of risk factors for clavicle fractures in newborns with shoulder dystocia and brachial plexus injury: A single-center experience. *Acta Orthop. Traumatol. Turc.* **2020**, *54*, 609–613. [CrossRef]
9. Beall, M.H.; Ross, M.G. Clavicle fracture in labor: Risk factors and associated morbidities. *J. Perinatol.* **2001**, *21*, 513–515. [CrossRef]
10. Linder, N.; Linder, I.; Fridman, E.; Kouadio, F.; Lubin, D.; Merlob, P.; Yogev, Y.; Melamed, N. Birth trauma-risk factors and short-term neonatal outcome. *J. Matern. Neonatal Med.* **2013**, *26*, 1491–1495. [CrossRef]
11. O'Neill, B.J.; Hirpara, K.M.; O'Briain, D.; McGarr, C.; Kaar, T.K. Clavicle fractures: A comparison of five classification systems and their relationship to treatment outcomes. *Int. Orthop.* **2011**, *35*, 909–914. [CrossRef]
12. Allman, F.L. Fractures and ligamentous injuries of the clavicle and its articulation. *J. Bone Jt. Surg. Am.* **1967**, *49*, 774–784. [CrossRef]
13. Trumble, T.E.; Cornwall, R.; Budoff, J.E. *Core Knowledge in Orthopaedics—Hand, Elbow, and Shoulder*, 1st ed.; Mosby: Philadelphia, PA, USA, 2006; ISBN 9780323027694.
14. Alldred, A.J. Congenital pseudarthrosis of the clavicle. *J. Bone Jt. Surg. Br.* **1963**, *45*, 312–319. [CrossRef]
15. Price, B.D.; Price, C.T. Familial congenital pseudoarthrosis of the clavicle: Case report and literature review. *Iowa Orthop. J.* **1996**, *16*, 153–156.
16. Toledo, L.C.; MacEwen, G.D. Severe complication of surgical treatment of con-genital pseudarthrosis of the clavicle. *Clin. Orthop. Relat. Res.* **1979**, *139*, 64–67.
17. Shim, J.S.; Chang, M.J. Congenital pseudarthrosis of the clavicle—Report of 4 cases treated with surgical methods. *J. Korean Orthop. Assoc.* **2008**, *43*, 396–399. [CrossRef]
18. Persiani, P.; Molayem, I.; Villani, C.; Cadilhac, C.; Glorion, C. Surgical treatment of congenital pseudarthrosis of the clavicle: A report on 17 cases. *Acta Orthop. Belg.* **2008**, *74*, 161–166. [PubMed]
19. Kite, J.H. Congenital pseudarthrosis of the clavicle. *South. Med. J.* **1968**, *61*, 703–710. [CrossRef] [PubMed]
20. Ray, P.; King, I.C.; Thomas, P.S.W. Vacuum phenomenon in the shoulder of a child. *BMJ Case Rep.* **2019**, *12*, e226724. [CrossRef]
21. Kihlström, C.; Möller, M.; Lönn, K.; Wolf, O. Clavicle fractures: Epidemiology, classification and treatment of 2 422 fractures in the Swedish Fracture Register; an observational study. *BMC Musculoskelet. Disord.* **2017**, *18*, 82. [CrossRef]
22. Lirette, M.P.; Bailey, B.; Grant, S.; Jackson, M.; Leonard, P. Can paediatric emergency clinicians identify and manage clavicle fractures without radiographs in the emergency department? A prospective study. *BMJ Paediatr. Open* **2018**, *2*, e000304. [CrossRef] [PubMed]
23. Katz, R.; Landman, J.; Dulitzky, F.; Bar-Ziv, J. Fracture of the clavicle in the newborn. An ultrasound diagnosis. *J. Ultrasound Med.* **1988**, *7*, 21–23. [CrossRef] [PubMed]
24. Kayser, R.; Mahlfeld, K.; Heyde, C.; Grasshoff, H. Ultrasonographic imaging of fractures of the clavicle in newborn infants. *J. Bone Jt. Surg. Br.* **2003**, *85*, 115–116. [CrossRef] [PubMed]
25. Chien, M.; Bulloch, B.; Garcia-Filion, P.; Youssfi, M.; Shrader, M.W.; Segal, L.S. Bedside ultrasound in the diagnosis of pediatric clavicle fractures. *Pediatr. Emerg. Care* **2011**, *27*, 1038–1041. [CrossRef]

26. Hillen, R.J.; Burger, B.J.; Pöll, R.G.; van Dijk, C.N.; Veeger, D. The effect of experimental shortening of the clavicle on shoulder kinematics. *Clin. Biomech.* **2012**, *27*, 777–781. [CrossRef] [PubMed]
27. Matsumura, N.; Ikegami, H.; Nakamichi, N.; Nakamura, T.; Nagura, T.; Imanishi, N.; Aiso, S.; Toyama, Y. Effect of shortening deformity of the clavicle on scapular kinematics: A cadaveric study. *Am. J. Sports Med.* **2010**, *38*, 1000–1006. [CrossRef]
28. Matsumura, N.; Nakamichi, N.; Ikegami, H.; Nagura, T.; Imanishi, N.; Aiso, S.; Toyama, Y. The function of the clavicle on scapular motion: A cadaveric study. *J. Shoulder Elb. Surg.* **2013**, *22*, 333–339. [CrossRef] [PubMed]
29. Beals, R.K.; Sauser, D.D. Nontraumatic disorders of the clavicle. *J. Am. Acad Orthop. Surg.* **2006**, *14*, 205–214. [CrossRef]
30. Korf, B.R. Neurofibromatosis. *Handb. Clin. Neurol.* **2013**, *111*, 333–340. [CrossRef]
31. Andersen, K.; Jensen, P.O.; Lauritzen, J. Treatment of clavicular fractures. Figure-of-eight bandage versus a simple sling. *Acta Orthop. Scand.* **1987**, *58*, 71–74. [CrossRef]
32. Randsborg, P.H.; Fuglesang, H.F.; Røtterud, J.H.; Hammer, O.L.; Sivertsen, E.A. Long-term patient-reported outcome after fractures of the clavicle in patients aged 10 to 18 years. *J. Pediatr. Orthop.* **2014**, *34*, 393–399. [CrossRef]
33. Schulz, J.; Moor, M.; Roocroft, J.; Bastrom, T.P.; Pennock, A.T. Functional and radiographic outcomes of nonoperative treatment of displaced adolescent clavicle fractures. *J. Bone Jt. Surg. Am.* **2013**, *95*, 1159–1165. [CrossRef] [PubMed]
34. Leal-Oliva, A.; Mora-Ríos, F.G.; Mejía-Rohenes, C.; López-Marmnolejo, A.; Acevedo-Cabrera, M.J. Acortamiento relativo de clavícula en fracturas pediátricas: Su importancia en la decisión del tratamiento conservador [Relative clavicle shortening in pediatric fractures: Its importance when selecting conservative treatment]. *Acta Ortop. Mex.* **2014**, *28*, 82–87. [PubMed]
35. Swarup, I.; Maheshwer, B.; Orr, S.; Kehoe, C.; Zhang, Y.; Dodwell, E. Intermediate-Term Outcomes Following Operative and Nonoperative Management of Midshaft Clavicle Fractures in Children and Adolescents: Internal Fixation May Improve Outcomes. *JB JS Open Access* **2021**, *6*, e20.00036. [CrossRef] [PubMed]
36. McGraw, M.A.; Mehlman, C.T.; Lindsell, C.J.; Kirby, C.L. Postnatal growth of the clavicle: Birth to 18 years of age. *J. Pediatr. Orthop.* **2009**, *29*, 937–943. [CrossRef] [PubMed]
37. Riiser, M.O.; Molund, M. Long-term Functional Outcomes and Complications in Operative Versus Nonoperative Treatment for Displaced Midshaft Clavicle Fractures in Adolescents: A Retrospective Comparative Study. *J. Pediatr. Orthop.* **2021**, *41*, 279–283. [CrossRef]
38. Scott, M.L.; Baldwin, K.D.; Mistovich, R.J. Operative Versus Nonoperative Treatment of Pediatric and Adolescent Clavicular Fractures. *JBJS Rev.* **2019**, *7*, e5. [CrossRef] [PubMed]
39. Mukhtar, I.A.; Yaghmour, K.M.; Ahmed, A.F.; Ibrahim, T. Flexible intramedullary nailing versus nonoperative treatment for paediatric displaced midshaft clavicle fractures. *J. Child. Orthop.* **2018**, *12*, 104–110. [CrossRef] [PubMed]
40. McIntosh, A.L. Surgical treatment of adolescent Clavicle Fractures: Results and complications. *J. Pediatr. Orthop.* **2016**, *36* (Suppl. 1), S41–S43. [CrossRef] [PubMed]
41. Song, M.H.; Yun, Y.H.; Kang, K.; Hyun, M.J.; Choi, S. Nonoperative versus operative treatment for displaced midshaft clavicle fractures in adolescents: A comparative study. *J. Pediatr. Orthop. Part B* **2019**, *28*, 45–50. [CrossRef] [PubMed]
42. Fanter, N.J.; Kenny, R.M.; Baker, C.L., III; Baker, C.L., Jr. Surgical treatment of clavicle fractures in the adolescent athlete. *Sports Health* **2015**, *7*, 137–141. [CrossRef] [PubMed]
43. Pecci, M.; Kreher, J.B. Clavicle fractures. *Am. Fam. Physician* **2008**, *77*, 65–70.
44. Kim, H.Y.; Yang, D.S.; Bae, J.H.; Cha, Y.H.; Lee, K.W.; Choy, W.S. Clinical and Radiological Outcomes after Various Treatments of Midshaft Clavicle Fractures in Adolescents. *Clin. Orthop. Surg.* **2020**, *12*, 396–403. [CrossRef] [PubMed]
45. Lazarides, S.; Zafiropoulos, G. Conservative treatment of fractures at the middle third of the clavicle: The relevance of shortening and clinical outcome. *J. Shoulder Elb. Surg.* **2006**, *15*, 191–194. [CrossRef] [PubMed]
46. Hill, J.M.; McGuire, M.H.; Crosby, L.A. Closed treatment of displaced middle-third fractures of the clavicle gives poor results. *J. Bone Jt. Surg. Br.* **1997**, *79*, 537–539. [CrossRef]
47. Herzog, M.M.; Whitesell, R.C.; Mac, L.M.; Jackson, M.L.; Culotta, B.A.; Axelrod, J.R.; Busch, M.T.; Willimon, S.C. Functional outcomes following non-operative versus operative treatment of clavicle fractures in adolescents. *J. Child. Orthop.* **2017**, *11*, 310–317. [CrossRef]
48. Bae, D.S.; Shah, A.S.; Kalish, L.A.; Kwon, J.Y.; Waters, P.M. Shoulder motion, strength, and functional outcomes in children with established malunion of the clavicle. *J. Pediatr. Orthop.* **2013**, *33*, 544–550. [CrossRef] [PubMed]
49. Vander Have, K.L.; Perdue, A.M.; Caird, M.S.; Farley, F.A. Operative versus nonoperative treatment of midshaft clavicle fractures in adolescents. *J. Pediatr. Orthop.* **2010**, *30*, 307–312. [CrossRef]
50. Ledger, M.; Leeks, N.; Ackland, T.; Wang, A. Short malunions of the clavicle: An anatomic and functional study. *J. Shoulder Elb. Surg.* **2005**, *14*, 349–354. [CrossRef]
51. Pandya, N.K.; Namdari, S.; Hosalkar, H.S. Displaced clavicle fractures in adolescents: Facts, controversies, and current trends. *J. Am. Acad. Orthop. Surg.* **2012**, *20*, 498–505. [CrossRef]
52. Parry, J.A.; Van Straaten, M.; Luo, T.D.; Simon, A.L.; Ashraf, A.; Kaufman, K.; Larson, A.N.; Shaughnessy, W.J. Is There a Deficit After Nonoperative Versus Operative Treatment of Shortened Midshaft Clavicular Fractures in Adolescents? *J. Pediatr. Orthop.* **2017**, *37*, 227–233. [CrossRef] [PubMed]
53. Pennock, A.T.; Edmonds, E.W.; Bae, D.S.; Kocher, M.S.; Li, Y.; Farley, F.A.; Ellis, H.B.; Wilson, P.L.; Nepple, J.; Gordon, J.E.; et al. Adolescent clavicle nonunions: Potential risk factors and surgical management. *J. Shoulder Elb. Surg.* **2018**, *27*, 29–35. [CrossRef] [PubMed]

54. Kubiak, R.; Slongo, T. Operative treatment of clavicle fractures in children: A review of 21 years. *J. Pediatr. Orthop.* **2002**, *22*, 736–739. [CrossRef] [PubMed]
55. Housner, J.A.; Kuhn, J.E. Clavicle fractures: Individualizing treatment for fracture type. *Physician Sportsmed.* **2003**, *31*, 30–36. [CrossRef]
56. Burnier, M.; Barlow, J.D.; Sanchez-Sotelo, J. Shoulder and Elbow Fractures in Athletes. *Curr Rev. Musculoskelet. Med.* **2019**, *12*, 13–23. [CrossRef]
57. Hoogervorst, P.; van Schie, P.; van den Bekerom, M.P. Midshaft clavicle fractures: Current concepts. *EFORT Open Rev.* **2018**, *3*, 374–380. [CrossRef]
58. Souza, N.A.S.M.; Belangero, P.S.; Figueiredo, E.A.; Pochini, A.C.; Andreoli, C.V.; Ejnisman, B. Displaced midshaft clavicle fracture in athletes—should we operate? *Rev. Bras. Ortop.* **2018**, *53*, 171–175. [CrossRef]
59. Odorizzi, M.; FitzGerald, M.; Gonzalez, J.; Giunchi, D.; Hamitaga, F.; De Rosa, V. Posttraumatic Pseudoarthrosis of a Clavicle Fracture in an 11-Year-Old Girl: A Case Report and Analysis. *Case Rep. Orthop.* **2020**, *2020*, 4069431. [CrossRef]
60. Owen, R. Congenital pseudarthrosis of the clavicle. *J. Bone Jt. Surg. Br.* **1970**, *52*, 644–652. [CrossRef]
61. Sakellarides, H. Pseudarthrosis of the clavicle. *J. Bone Jt. Surg* **1961**, *43*, 130. [CrossRef]
62. Da Costa, J.C. *Modern Surgery*, 4th ed.; W.B. Saunders: Philadelphia, PA, USA, 1903; Chapter 34 Bandages; p. 11.
63. Dzupa, V.; Bartonicek, J.; Zidka, M. Fracture of the clavicle after surgical treatment for congenital pseudarthrosis. *Med. Sci. Monit.* **2004**, *10*, CS1–CS4. [PubMed]
64. Padua, R.; Romanini, E.; Conti, C.; Padua, L.; Serra, F. Bilateral congenital pseudarthrosis of the clavicle report of a case with clinical, radiological and neurophysiological evaluation. *Acta Orthop. Belg.* **1999**, *65*, 372–375. [PubMed]
65. Di Gennaro, G.L.; Cravino, M.; Martinelli, A.; Berardi, E.; Rao, A.; Stilli, S.; Trisolino, G. Congenital pseudarthrosis of the clavicle: A report on 27 cases. *J. Shoulder Elb. Surg.* **2017**, *26*, e65–e70. [CrossRef] [PubMed]

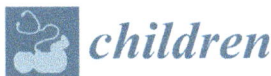

Article

Plate Fixation for Irreducible Proximal Humeral Fractures in Children and Adolescents—A Single-Center Case Series of Six Patients

Florian Freislederer [1,*], Susanne Bensler [2], Thomas Specht [1], Olaf Magerkurth [3] and Karim Eid [1,*]

1 Department of Orthopaedics and Traumatology, Kantonsspital Baden (KSB), Im Ergel 1, 5404 Baden, Switzerland; thomas.specht@ksb.ch
2 Unit for Musculoskeletal Radiology, Department of Radiology, Kantonsspital Baden (KSB), Im Ergel 1, 5404 Baden, Switzerland; susanne.bensler@ksb.ch
3 Unit for Pediatric Radiology, Department of Radiology, Kantonsspital Baden (KSB), Im Ergel 1, 5404 Baden, Switzerland; olaf.magerkurth@ksb.ch
* Correspondence: freislederer.florian@gmail.com (F.F.); karim.eid@ksb.ch (K.E.)

Abstract: Background: Recommended treatment for severely displaced proximal humeral fractures in children is the closed reduction and percutaneous fixation by K-wires or intramedullary nailing. Methods: From January 2016 to January 2017 6, 21 children/adolescents (range 8 to 16 years) with proximal humeral fractures were treated surgically for severe displacement. In these six patients, several attempts of closed reduction were unsuccessful, and an open reduction was performed. The humeral head was fixed with a 3.5 mm T-plate without affecting the growth plate. Plate removal was performed at a mean interval of 132 days after initial surgery. Two years after initial surgery, the clinical outcome was assessed by the Constant–Murley score and QuickDASH score (including sport/music and work) and the shoulder joint was evaluated with a standardized sonographic examination for the rotator cuff and the conjoint tendon. Results: In all six patients, dorsal displacement of the fracture was irreducible due to the interposition of tendinous or osseous structures. Intraoperatively, the interposed structures were the long biceps tendon in two, periosteal tissue in two, a bony fragment in one, and the long biceps tendon together with the conjoint tendon in one case. At mean follow-up of 26 months (range 22 months to 29 months), patients showed very good clinical results with an excellent mean Constant–Murley score of 97.5 (range 91 to 100) and mean QuickDASH score (including sport/music and work) of 5.5 (range 0–20.8). An X-ray follow-up 6 weeks after surgery demonstrated early consolidation and correct alignment in all patients. A sonographic evaluation at 2 years post injury showed that the biceps and the conjoined tendon were intact in all patients. Conclusions: If a proximal humeral fracture is not reducible by closed means, a tissue entrapment (most likely biceps tendon) should be considered. Treatment with an open reduction and plate fixation yields very good clinical and radiological results and preserves interposed structures as the biceps and conjoint tendon.

Keywords: humerus fracture; proximal humeral fracture; children; plate fixation; ORIF; tissue entrapment; biceps

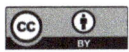

1. Introduction

Proximal humeral fractures in children and adolescents are rare injuries, representing less than 5% of all pediatric fractures with a peek incidence between the age of 11 and 15 years [1–3]. These fractures can be physeal or metaphyseal. Metaphyseal fractures account for about 70% of the cases [4]. The muscle attachments of the rotator cuff proximally, and of the deltoid, as well as of the pectoralis major distally, are responsible for the specific fracture pattern.

Muscular tension displaces the proximal fragment in varus and posteromedially, whereas the distal fragment moves anteriorly and in adduction (Figure 1A,B).

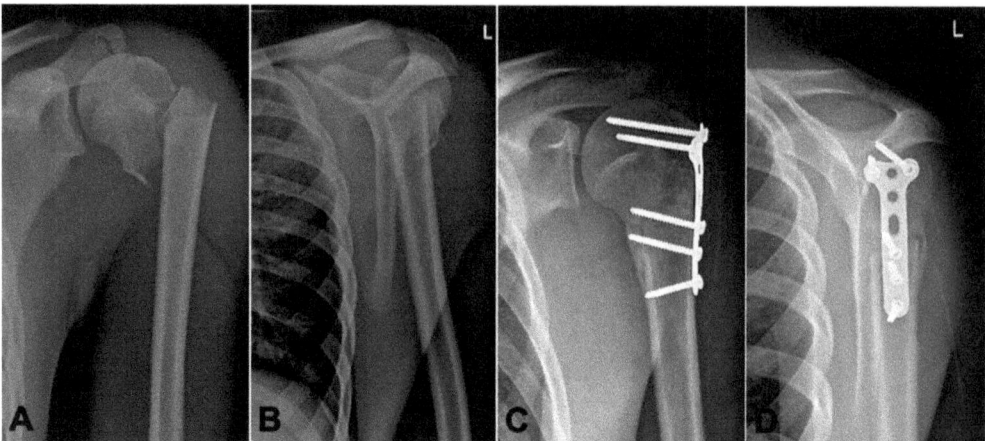

Figure 1. Radiographic shoulder views (Pat. N° 4) (ap/Neer). (**A,B**): Dorsally displaced humeral head. (**C,D**): 10 weeks after open reduction and plate fixation.

Another explanation for the anterior displacement of the distal fragment might be the thinner and weaker anterior periosteum [5].

Neer and Horwitz classified proximal humeral fractures in children in four grades according to the severity of displacement (I: <5 mm; II: <1/3 shaft width; III: <2/3 shaft width; IV: >2/3 shaft width) [2].

Most fractures of the proximal humerus in the skeletally immature are not or only minimally displaced and can be treated conservatively [4,6,7].

The management of severely displaced proximal humeral fractures in children is still controversial [3]. Most of the displaced proximal humeral fractures (Neer and Horwitz ≥ III) are treated by closed reduction and intramedullary nailing or by percutaneous fixation with K-wires [2,8,9]. Due to the high remodeling potential, moderate malalignment after closed reduction is acceptable. In addition, since around 80% of the longitudinal growth of the humerus results from the proximal physis, any mechanical interference with the growth plate by implant materials is usually avoided [10,11].

However, insufficient alignment after closed reduction may require open reduction and stable fixation which has already been described 40 years ago by Weber with an excellent clinical outcome [4,12–14].

In our institution, closed reduction and pin fixation are routinely performed to address displaced pediatric proximal humerus fractures. If secondary displacement is observed or primary reduction is not satisfactory, presumably due to tissue entrapment, open reduction and internal fixation are performed.

The aim of the study is to assess clinical and radiological results after an open reduction, plate fixation and plate removal of irreducible displaced proximal humeral fractures in older children and to evaluate the functional integrity of the tissue—mainly the long head of the biceps tendon—interposed in the irreducible fracture.

2. Material and Methods

Between January 2016 and January 2017, 21 skeletally immature patients with proximal humeral fractures were treated at the authors institute (level 1 trauma hospital). Six of these patients (29%) were treated by open reduction and internal fixation. All of these six patients were included in the study.

The inclusion criteria were: available standard x-rays in anteroposterior (AP) and Neer view preoperatively and 6 weeks postoperatively, severely displaced humeral fracture (Neer–Horwitz III/IV), not reducible by closed means, open physis and hardware removal performed. After 2 years, patients were prospectively assessed with a clinical and sonographic examination. Informed consent was obtained from the patient's or her/his legal representative.

Approval by the Ethical committee Nordwestschweiz Nr. 2018-01405 was obtained.

2.1. Surgical Technique

All of the operative procedures were carried out under general anesthesia. The patients were positioned in beach chair position. An initial attempt of closed reduction was conducted in all patients. This was performed by gentle longitudinal traction with abduction and external rotation of the arm. An image intensifier was used to monitor reduction. If closed reduction failed, the surgeon proceeded with open reduction by means of an anterior deltopectoral approach. Entrapped tissue or periosteum were gently freed. Once reduction was achieved, a 3.5 mm T-plate was contoured on the anterolateral part of the proximal humerus and temporary K-wires were inserted through the plate holes to hold the reduction. Under image intensifier, attention was drawn not to injure the physeal plate by the drill or the screws. After confirming anatomical reduction, the K-wires were then replaced with conventional cortical screws.

Surgical wounds were closed with absorbable VICRYL (Ethicon, Raritan, NJ, USA; Johnson & Johnson, New Brunswick, NJ, USA) sutures. Skin was closed using absorbable MONOCRYL (Ethicon, Raritan, NJ, USA; Johnson & Johnson, New Brunswick, NJ, USA) sutures.

Postoperatively, a brace (type Gilchrist) was applied for 2 weeks. For the first 6 weeks, range of motion was limited to 90° abduction and flexion. For the first 2 weeks, only passive mobilization out of the brace was allowed, followed by actively assisted movements.

2.2. Clinical Assessment

Patient outcome was assessed by clinical and sonographic evaluation. The clinical examination was carried out by a single independent observer and sonography by a single radiologist specifically trained in musculoskeletal imaging. The Constant–Murley score and QuickDASH (Disability of the Arm, Shoulder and Hand) score (including sport and music/work modules) were used for objective assessment [15,16]. The Constant–Murley score is a 100-point shoulder score, which assesses the range of motion of the treated shoulder joint. Forward flexion, extension, abduction, and low (arm in adduction) and high (arm in 90° of abduction) external and internal rotation were measured using the standardized neutral-zero method in degrees. A goniometer was used for the measurement. The abduction strength was measured using a spring balance (Macro-Line 80020, Fa. Pesola), which was attached distally on the forearm adjacent to the wrist with the method described and validated by Bankes et al. [17]. Strength was measured with the arm in 90 degrees abduction, full extension of the elbow, and the palm of the hand in pronation. The patient was asked to maintain this position for five seconds. This procedure was repeated three times, with at least a one-minute time interval. The average in kilograms (kg) was noted. The same procedure was performed with the contralateral arm. The measurement should be pain free. If pain was present or the patient was unable to abduct above 90°, the score equaled zero. The strength score was calculated from the highest score of the three attempts. The score corresponds to the force in kilogram.

We also performed this procedure with the contralateral arm to obtain the individual Constant score as described by Fialka et al. [15]. For interpretation, the results of the Constant–Murley score were divided into four subscales: excellent 90–100; satisfactory 80–89; unsatisfactory 70–79; failure > 70. The QuickDASH outcome measure was a 100-point shoulder score. It measured a 30-item (+4 sports/music, +4 work) questionnaire of physical and social function with symptoms in any or all joints in the upper extremity. The lower the DASH score, the better the outcome.

In addition, medical records were reviewed. All patients had a normal shoulder function and no previous operations on the affected side. Radiological evaluation included standard anteroposterior and Neer view of the shoulder. Follow-up radiographs were carried out six weeks and between two and three months postoperatively. Subsequently, hardware removal was performed.

2.3. Ultrasound Imaging

All patients were scanned in a sitting position with a relaxed arm hanging freely on the side. For the examination, a GE LOGIQ E9 ultrasound system (GE Healthcare; Chicago, IL, USA) with a linear transducer with a bandwidth of 6–15 MHz was used.

The tendons of the subscapularis, supraspinatus and infraspinatus tendon were examined along their long and short axis.

The subscapularis tendon was examined with the arm externally rotated and the elbow fixed at the iliac crest. For the evaluation of the supraspinatus tendon, the patient's arm was placed posteriorly, with the palmar side of the hand on the superior aspect of the iliac wing with the elbow flexed and directed posteriorly. To examine the infraspinatus tendon, the arm was placed anteriorly with the hand on the opposite shoulder.

The long head of the biceps tendon was examined along the long and short axis with the arm placed in slight internal rotation. The integrity of the conjoint tendon was examined also in both planes with the arm placed in external rotation.

3. Results

There were five boys and one girl with a mean age of 14 years (8–16 years). At the time of injury, mostly accidents during physical activities which caused an isolated injury to the proximal humerus, all fractures were proximal metaphyseal fractures. Five patients had a Neer–Horwitz Grade III fracture and one had a Grade IV (patient N° 4, see Table 1) completely displaced fracture of the proximal humerus (Figure 1A,B). In these six patients, a closed reduction was attempted; in five patients, an immediate conversion to open surgery with open reduction and internal plate fixation was necessary.

Table 1. Outcome with 2-year follow-up after open reduction, internal plate fixation and early (mean 4 months postoperative) plate removal.

Case N°	Age	Sex	Reduction Method	Constant Score	QuickDASH Score				Subjective Outcome
					Total	Disability	Sport/Music	Work	
1	12 years	M	Closed/Open [1]	98	0	0			Satisfied
2	14 years	F	Open	91	11.25	5	6.25	0	Very satisfied
3	14 years	M	Open	100	0	0	0		Very satisfied
4	14 years	M	Open	95	20.8	8.3	12.5	0	Very satisfied
5	16 years	M	Open	97	10	10			Very satisfied
6	8 years	M	Open	100	1	1	0		Very satisfied

[1] secondary open reduction due to dislocation after closed reduction and percutaneous pinning (see also Figure 2).

The first patient (N° 1, Table 1, Figure 2) from this series was initially treated with a closed reduction and percutaneous pinning; due to secondary displacement, an open reduction and internal fixation was necessary.

For this patient, it was apparent that a closed reduction was impossible due to the interposition of soft tissue at the fracture site. Tissue entrapment was intraoperatively observed in all of the six cases (the long biceps tendon in two cases (Pat. N° 1 and 5), periosteal tissue in two cases (Pat. N° 3 and 6), a bony fragment in one case (Pat. N° 4), and both the long biceps tendon as well as the conjoint tendon in one case (Pat. N° 4)) (Figure 3).

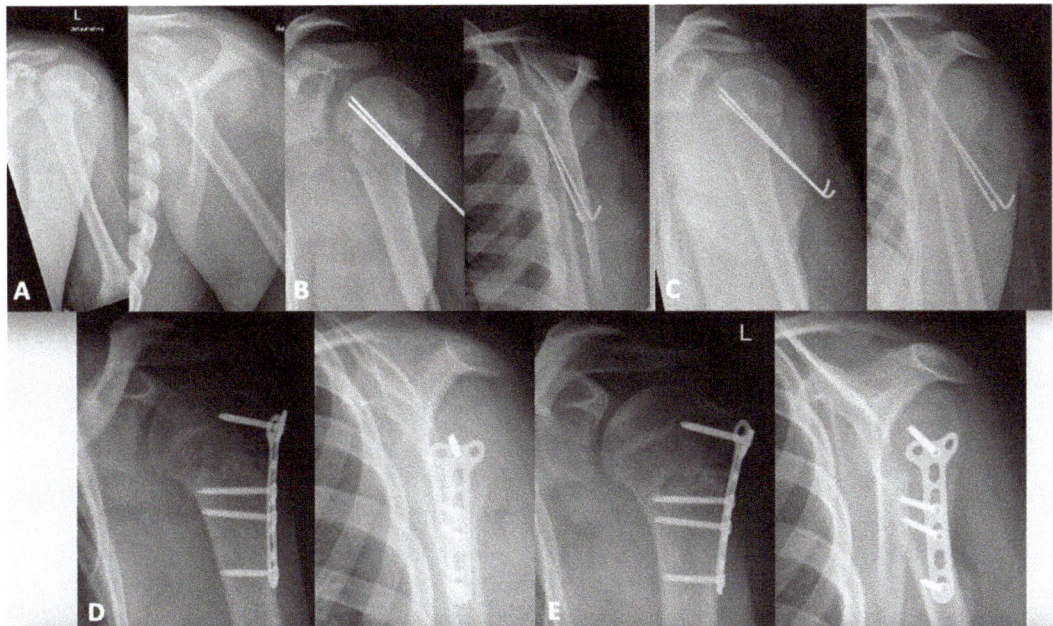

Figure 2. Chronologic radiographic images of Pat. N° 1. (**A**) Initial images after trauma with a posteriorly displaced proximal humeral fracture. (**B**) After closed reduction and transepiphyseal fixation. (**C**) X-ray 1 day after surgery shows posterior displacement in the Neer view (right side). (**D**) Open reduction and T-plate fixation. (**E**) X-ray follow-up 10 weeks after open reduction and plate-fixation with anatomical reduction and fracture healing.

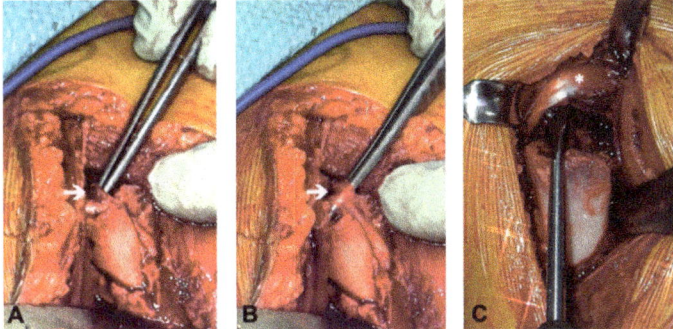

Figure 3. Intraoperative findings. (**A**) Entrapment of the long biceps tendon (white arrow) in the fracture gap (Pat. N° 1, see also Figure 2); (**B**) freed long biceps tendon (Pat. N° 1, see also Figure 2); (**C**) freed conjoint tendons (white asterisk) (Pat. N° 4, see also Figure 1).

The scheduled removal of the hardware was performed in all six patients. The implants were removed under general anesthesia as a day case procedure without difficulty at a mean time of 4.4 months after surgery (range 3–5.3 months).

The mean follow-up was 26 months (range: 22 months to 29 months) after fracture fixation. The Constant–Murley Shoulder and QuickDASH (including sport and music/work modules) scores are presented in (Table 1). The Constant–Murley score at the final follow-up was 97.5 (range 91 to 100) and the mean overall QuickDASH score (including sport and music/work) was 5.5 (range 0–20.8). Analyzing the subtypes of the QuickDASH score, we found a score of 3 for disability (range 0–10), 3.125 for sport and music (range 0–12.5) and 0 for work.

All fractures showed advanced radiological healing at the 10–12 weeks follow-up (Figure 1C,D). Postoperatively, there was no loss of reduction, residual deformity or screw migration.

A sonographic examination of the shoulder two years postoperatively showed normal rotator cuff, long head of biceps and conjoint tendon (Figure 4).

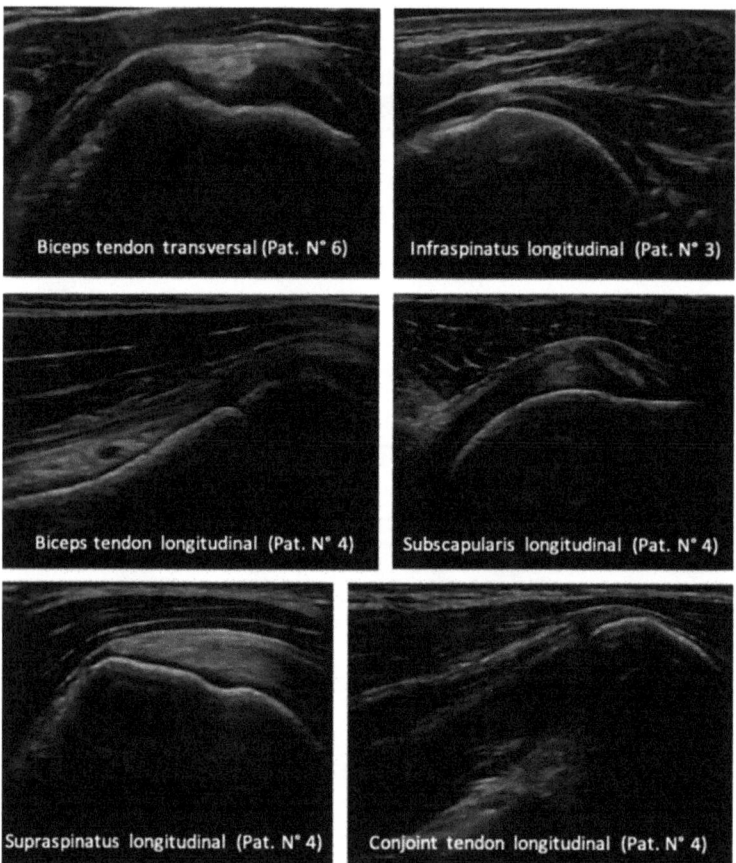

Figure 4. Sonographic scans 2 years postoperatively of the soft tissue surrounding the shoulder joint.

No major complication was observed related to primary surgery or plate removal. None of the patients presented with vascular or neurological complications. All patients showed a rather apparent skin scar, known to appear frequently in this location [4]. Three out of six patients reported the scar to be esthetically disturbing. Two patients described a feeling of irritation at the operative scar, which they attributed to the plate irritation. This resolved completely after plate removal. At the 2-year follow-up, five patients were very satisfied and one was satisfied with the outcome.

4. Discussion

Recommended treatment for severely displaced proximal humeral fractures in children is closed reduction and percutaneous fixation by K-wires or intramedullary nailing [4,5,18]. We presented a series of six patients treated by an open reduction and plate fixation, in which either secondary displacement occurred, or closed reduction was unsatisfactory.

Two years postoperatively, we were able to demonstrate excellent shoulder function and preserved anatomical integrity of the entrapped tissues, namely, the biceps and conjoint tendon. To the best of our knowledge, this is the first report on the integrity of the interposed structures. It might well be questioned, whether these structures would have been intact, if a closed reduction had been accepted.

The first patient of this series (Figure 2) was initially treated with a closed reduction and percutaneous pinning. Due to secondary displacement, a revision with an open reduction and internal fixation was necessary caused by a biceps entrapment. Subsequently, we treated unreducible fractures by an open reduction and internal plate fixation and found tissue entrapment to be present in all cases.

All fractures healed completely, and functional scores were excellent at a 2 year follow-up with symmetrical shoulder movement (Figure 5). The obstacle to reduction was, in most cases, the entrapped biceps tendon. In one case, the entrapped conjoint tendons inhibited reduction and in one other case periosteal tissue.

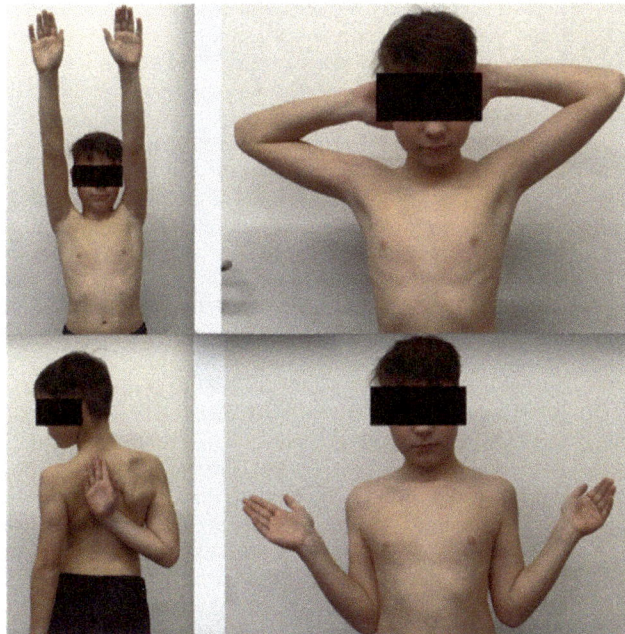

Figure 5. Range of motion after plate fixation of a proximal humerus fracture on the right site (Patient N° 6).

Dobbs et al. examined a subgroup of older adolescents and mentioned patients with irreducible fractures due to tissue entrapment which needed an open reduction [11].

The entrapment of the long head of the biceps tendon or periosteum was mentioned earlier but has not been identified as a major cause for irreducible fractures [4,5,11]. Lucas et al. did not find entrapment of the tendon of the long head of the biceps in the fracture site in four patients, which were assessed by magnetic resonance imaging.

In contrast, Bahrs et al. described open reduction in Neer III and IV fractures in 17 of their 31 patients. They found that in nine of these patients, the biceps tendon was entrapped in the fracture site. They concluded that a failed closed reduction should be interpreted as a possible soft tissue entrapment (most likely biceps tendon) and that these cases should be addressed with an open reduction and the removal of the entrapped structures [14].

Performing an open reduction, we could liberate the tissue interposed in the fracture side and achieve an anatomical reduction. To achieve a stable fixation of our reduction without crossing the physeal plate, we decided to use a T-plate fixation.

The use of a plate for an internal fixation after an open reduction has rarely been considered. In the aforementioned study of Bahrs et al., twelve patients were treated with a K-wire or screw fixation, and a plate fixation was used only in five patients. As early as 42 years ago, Weber et al. described treatment of severely displaced or irreducible infratubercular proximal humerus fractures by an open reduction and plate fixation without complications and symmetrical function of the shoulders.

In contrast to the generally preferred use of k-wires, a plate fixation avoids direct injury to the physis if screws are placed with the use of an image intensifier. If planned hardware removal is performed 3–6 months after initial surgery, tethering of the epiphyseal plate is not to be anticipated [14]. The drawback of the plate fixation, however, is the necessity of its removal at 3 months.

A plate fixation provides a stable fixation of the reduced fracture. Anatomical fracture healing is of upmost importance in adolescents (>12 years), where the remodeling capacity is limited [19]. In the present study, the average age of patients was 13 years. There is only limited data on the outcome of adolescent patients with this fractures [11].

In contrast to the plate fixation, any wire or elastic nail in metaphyseal and epiphyseal fractures will pass the epiphyseal plate and damage it to a certain degree. Excellent outcomes without limb shortening or axial deviation of the proximal humerus after K-wire or intramedullary nailing are reported [4,6,8]. Nevertheless, a physeal arrest and progressive deformity can be a potential risk of any crossing stabilization [20]. Peterson et al. reported on physeal injury in physeal fractures at three different sites (proximal humerus, distal humerus, distal femur) and recorded 100% premature closure in the three cases in which a K-wire internal fixation had passed the physis [21]. Intramedullary retrograde stabilization with ESIN has been recommended as the standard fixation method for proximal humeral fractures in children and adolescents, but this technique has some major drawbacks, such as nail penetration into the joint cavity, humeral head perforation, physeal damage due to multiple perforation and the displacement of the proximal fragment by pushing with the ESIN tips [4]. Zivanovic et al. observed complications in 5 of 16 patients: 2 humeral head perforations, 10° of residual varus deformation in 2 patients and difficulties in nail extraction in one patient. Similar complications were reported by other authors [8,22].

Our study has its limitations. First, the number of patients treated was small and general treatment recommendations could not be deducted. We did not have a control group that would demonstrate any superiority compared to other treatment strategies.

Second, due to the ethical restrictions, the study lacked a late radiographic follow-up at two years. However, as clinical results were excellent and ultrasound did not show any deformity of the tuberosities or the humeral head, it seems reasonable to state, that the growth plate was not subjected to any injury or tethering.

A drawback of our proposed treatment is the requirement of a second surgery.

We do agree with the generally accepted age and deformity-based decision making [4,5,18,23], but want to emphasize that tissue entrapment, which inhibits closed reduction, is very likely in Neer III and IV fractures, and may be underestimated in the literature so far.

5. Conclusions

If a proximal humeral fracture is not reducible by closed means, a tissue entrapment (most likely biceps tendon and conjoined tendon) has to be considered as an obstacle to the reduction. An open reduction and plate fixation not only yield excellent clinical results, but allow the functional and anatomical integrity of the entrapped tendons.

Author Contributions: Conceptualization, F.F., T.S. and K.E.; methodology, F.F., T.S., S.B., O.M. and K.E.; validation, F.F. and K.E. investigation, F.F. and S.B.; data curation, F.F.; writing—original draft preparation, F.F. and S.B.; writing—review and editing, F.F. and K.E.; visualization, F.F.; supervision, K.E.; All authors have read and agreed to the published version of the manuscript.

Funding: This research received no external funding.

Institutional Review Board Statement: The study was conducted according to the guidelines of the Declaration of Helsinki, and approved by the Institutional Review Board (or Ethics Committee) of Ethical committee Nordwestschweiz Nr. 2018-01405, 05. September 2018.

Informed Consent Statement: Informed consent was obtained from all subjects involved in the study.

Data Availability Statement: The data presented in this study are stored and openly available in the secretary bureau of the Department of Orthopaedics and Traumatology, Kantonsspital Baden, Im Ergel 1, 5404 Baden, Switzerland.

Conflicts of Interest: The authors declare no conflict of interest.

References

1. Landin, L.A. Epidemiology of children's fractures. *J. Pediatr. Orthop.* **1997**, *6*, 79–83. [CrossRef]
2. Neer. Fractures of the proximal humeral epiphyseal plate. *Clin. Orthop. Relat. Res.* **1965**, *41*, 24–31.
3. Shrader, M.W. Proximal humerus and humeral shaft fractures in children. *Hand Clin.* **2007**, *23*, 431–435. [CrossRef] [PubMed]
4. Lefevre, Y.; Journeau, P.; Angelliaume, A.; Bouty, A.; Dobremez, E. Proximal humerus fractures in children and adolescents. *Orthop. Traumatol. Surg. Res.* **2014**, *100*, S149–S156. [CrossRef]
5. Bishop, J.Y.; Flatow, E.L. Pediatr. Shoulder Trauma. *Clin. Orthop. Relat. Res.* **2005**, *432*, 41–48. [CrossRef] [PubMed]
6. Rajan, R.A.; Hawkins, K.J.; Metcalfe, J.; Konstantoulakis, C.; Jones, S.; Fernandes, J. Elastic stable intramedullary nailing for displaced proximal humeral fractures in older children. *J. Child. Orthop.* **2008**, *2*, 15–19. [CrossRef]
7. Kinderchirurgie, D.G.F. Leilinien der deutschen Gesellschaft für Kinderchirurgie—Proximale Humerusfraktur beim Kind. *Awmf. Online* **2016**, *4*, 1–5.
8. Fernandez, F.F.; Eberhardt, O.; Langendorfer, M.; Wirth, T. Treatment of severely displaced proximal humeral fractures in children with retrograde elastic stable intramedullary nailing. *Injury* **2008**, *39*, 1453–1459. [CrossRef] [PubMed]
9. Chee, Y. Treatment of severely displaced proximal humeral fractures in children with elastic stable intramedullary nailing. *J. Pediatr. Orthop.* **2006**, *15*, 45–50. [CrossRef] [PubMed]
10. Dameron, J.R. Fractures Involving the Proximal Humeral Epiphyseal Plate. *J. Bone Jt. Surg.* **1969**, *51*, 289–297. [CrossRef]
11. Dobbs, M.B. Severely Displaced Proximal Humeral Epiphyseal Fractures. *J. Pediatr. Orthop.* **2003**, *23*, 208–215. [CrossRef] [PubMed]
12. Pandya, N.K.; Behrends, D.; Hosalkar, H.S. Open reduction of proximal humerus fractures in the adolescent population. *J. Child. Orthop.* **2012**, *6*, 111–118. [CrossRef]
13. Schwendenwein, E.; Hajdu, S.; Gaebler, C.; Stengg, K.; Vecsei, V. Displaced fractures of the proximal humerus in children require open/closed reduction and internal fixation. *Eur. J. Pediatr. Surg.* **2004**, *14*, 51–55. [CrossRef]
14. Bahrs, C.; Zipplies, S.; Ochs, B.G.; Rether, J.; Oehm, J.; Eingartner, C.; Rolauffs, B.; Weise, K. Proximal Humeral Fractures in Children and Adolescents. *J. Pediatr. Orthop.* **2009**, *29*, 238–242. [CrossRef] [PubMed]
15. Fialka, C.; Oberleitner, G.; Stampfl, P.; Brannath, W.; Hexel, M.; Vécsei, V. Modification of the Constant-Murley shoulder score-introduction of the individual relative Constant score Individual shoulder assessment. *Int. J. Care Inj.* **2005**, *36*, 1159–1165. [CrossRef]
16. Quatman-Yates, C.C.; Gupta, R.; Paterno, M.V.; Schmitt, L.C.; Quatman, C.E.; Ittenbach, R.F. Internal Consistency and Validity of the QuickDASH Instrument for Upper Extremity Injuries in Older Children. *J. Pediatr. Orthop.* **2013**, *33*, 838–842. [CrossRef]
17. Bankes, M.J.K.; Crossman, E.; Emery, R.J. A standard method of shoulder strength measurement for the Constant score with a spring balance. *J. Shoulder Elb. Surg.* **1998**, *7*, 116–121. [CrossRef]
18. Pahlavan, S.; Baldwin, K.D.; Pandya, N.K.; Namdari, S.; Hosalkar, H. Proximal humerus fractures in the Pediatr. population: A systematic review. *J. Child. Orthop.* **2011**, *5*, 187–194. [CrossRef]
19. Binder, H.; Schurz, M.; Aldrian, S.; Fialka, C.; Vecsei, V. Physeal injuries of the proximal humerus: Long-term results in seventy two patients. *Int. Orthop.* **2011**, *35*, 1497–1502. [CrossRef] [PubMed]
20. Boyden. Partial premature closure of distal radial physis associated with Kirschner wire fixation. *Orthopedics* **1991**, *14*, 585–588. [CrossRef]
21. Peterson, H.A. *Physeal Injury Other Than Fracture*; Springer: Berlin, Heidelberg, 2011.
22. Kelly, D.M. Flexible Intramedullary Nailing of Pediatr. Humeral Fractures: Indications, Techniques, and Tips. *J. Pediatr. Orthop.* **2016**, *36*, 49–55. [CrossRef] [PubMed]
23. Beaty, J.H. Fractures of the proximal humerus and shaft in children. *Instr. Course Lect.* **1992**, *41*, 369–372.

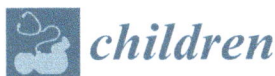

Article

Diagnosis and Treatment for Pediatric Supracondylar Humerus Fractures with Brachial Artery Injuries

Tu Ngoc Vu [1,2,3], Son Hong Duy Phung [1,3,*], Long Hoang Vo [4] and Uoc Huu Nguyen [1,3,*]

1. Department of Surgery, Hanoi Medical University, Hanoi 100000, Vietnam; vungoctu@hmu.edu.vn
2. Department of Cardiovascular and Thoracic Surgery, Hanoi Medical University Hospital, Hanoi 100000, Vietnam
3. Department of Cardiovascular and Thoracic Surgery, Viet Duc University Hospital, Hanoi 100000, Vietnam
4. Institute for Preventive Medicine and Public Health, Hanoi Medical University, Hanoi 100000, Vietnam; vohoanglonghmu@gmail.com
* Correspondence: hongsony81@yahoo.com (S.H.D.P.); uocdhyhn101@yahoo.com.vn (U.H.N.)

Citation: Vu, T.N.; Phung, S.H.D.; Vo, L.H.; Nguyen, U.H. Diagnosis and Treatment for Pediatric Supracondylar Humerus Fractures with Brachial Artery Injuries. *Children* **2021**, *8*, 933. https://doi.org/10.3390/children8100933

Academic Editor: Christiaan J. A. van Bergen

Received: 5 September 2021
Accepted: 11 October 2021
Published: 18 October 2021

Publisher's Note: MDPI stays neutral with regard to jurisdictional claims in published maps and institutional affiliations.

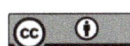

Copyright: © 2021 by the authors. Licensee MDPI, Basel, Switzerland. This article is an open access article distributed under the terms and conditions of the Creative Commons Attribution (CC BY) license (https://creativecommons.org/licenses/by/4.0/).

Abstract: (1) Background: This study aims to describe the clinical and paraclinical characteristics of and the diagnostic approach to brachial artery injuries in pediatric supracondylar humerus fractures, as well as to evaluate intraoperative vascular anatomical lesions and early postoperative results. (2) Methods: A retrospective, hospital-based analysis of medical records at Viet Duc University Hospital (Vietnam), using a sample of children under 16 years who met the diagnostic criteria for supracondylar humerus fractures with brachial artery injuries between January 2016 and December 2020, was performed. A total of 50 patients were included in the analysis. (3) Results: Out of 50 pediatric patients, 36 patients were male (72%) and the mean age was 5.85 years (range, 1.5–14 years). Before treatment, there were 46 patients with severely displaced fractures which were classified as Gartland type III (92%). Following casting, the percentage of those with severely displaced fractures was reduced significantly to 12%, while there were no patients with Gartland type III fractures after percutaneous pinning. Doppler sonography failed to assess vascular lesions at the fracture site before and after casting in most patients. Two-thirds of surgical cases had only vasospasm, without physical damage to the vessel wall or intravascular thrombosis. Preoperative Doppler spectrum analysis was not consistent with the severity of intraoperative brachial artery injury. Out of 24 patients with vasospasm, we performed vascular blockade using papaverin in 11 cases and intraoperative balloon angioplasty of the brachial artery using the Fogarty catheter in 13 cases. Brachial artery graft was performed with 12 patients who had anatomical damage to the vascular wall. A complication of embolism occurred in one patient immediately after surgery, and two patients had superficial infections. One month following surgery, 2 out of 36 patients had a temporary loss of sensation in the area of incision. (4) Conclusions: Most pediatric patients did not present with symptoms of critical limb ischemia similar to those associated with lower extremity vascular injuries. The diagnosis and treatment of pediatric supracondylar humerus fractures with vascular injury is difficult and time-consuming, especially in cases of transverse fractures.

Keywords: supracondylar humerus fracture; vascular injury; brachial artery injuries

1. Introduction

Supracondylar fractures of the humerus are the most prevalent kind of fractures, accounting for approximately 60% of all elbow fractures and 3–7% of pediatric fractures [1,2]. They are most common in young children between 5 and 10 years of age. More than 95% of these fractures are extension fractures, which may result in a variety of neurological and vascular complications. About 10% to 20% of displaced supracondylar fractures present alterations in vascular status [3,4]. An absent radial pulse was observed in 7% to 12% of all fractures and up to 19% in displaced fractures. Brachial artery injuries are often a consequence of stretching, entrapping or disrupting the neurovascular structures on the proximal fragment, as well as, though less frequently, of reduction maneuvers or immobilization of the elbow in the hyperflexion position [5,6].

The diagnosis and morphology of the anatomical lesion as well as the surgical treatment of this form of injury in children are markedly different from the extremity arterial injuries which are more common in adults. Through treating this pathology at our institution, we identified the following key concerns. Firstly, most brachial artery injuries in children do not have obvious symptoms of ischemia. Therefore, the implementation of intensive diagnostic procedures, as well as emergency surgery which is similar to that performed in cases of adult vascular trauma, can increase the risk of complications and consume unnecessary medical and social resources. Secondly, the application of Doppler ultrasound and multislice computed tomography angiography (CT-A) in children is not easy, especially for those who are not yet of school age. Anesthesia must be used in order to ensure the safety and effectiveness of these methods. As a result, the duration of the evaluation is prolonged and the pediatric patient may have to undergo anesthesia several times during the course of treatment, thereby increasing the risk of complications from anesthesia. Thirdly, once the vessel wall is opened for examination, the potential for endothelium lesion damage leads to actual occlusion of the artery because of the small diameter of the pediatric brachial artery. Once the vessel wall is opened for examination, the potential for endothelium lesion damage leads to actual occlusion of the artery because of the small diameter of the pediatric brachial artery. If the lesion is long, there is no alternative solution with artificial vessels or saphenous veins, as in adults. In addition, intervention on brachial arteries in pediatric patients has potential risks for adverse outcomes, such as vasodilation or vasoconstriction [7,8], large and bad scars [7,9] and osteomyelitis [10].

To better inform practice so as to minimize the duration of treatment and avoid the unnecessary consumption of medical resources, while ensuring that pediatric patients receive effective treatment for their injuries and avoid more complicated vascular complications, is the ultimate goal of this research. Our aims were to describe the clinical and paraclinical characteristics and the diagnostic approach to brachial artery injuries in pediatric supracondylar humerus fractures, and to evaluate intraoperative vascular anatomical lesions and early postoperative results.

2. Methods

2.1. Patients

This study was retrospectively performed using medical records at Viet Duc University Hospital, one of the oldest and largest surgical public hospitals in Vietnam, in the period from January 2016 to December 2020. We examined the data of patients who were under 16 years of age, had a diagnosis of traumatic arterial injury in the upper extremity and underwent treatment at our institution. Diagnostic criteria for supracondylar humerus fractures with brachial artery injuries included radiographs showing supracondylar humerus fractures and loss of the ulnar/radial pulse. We excluded those patients who had experienced previous elbow fracture(s) that caused limited movement and deformity.

2.2. Data Collection

Clinical parameters: age (years), age group (<3 years/3–<13 years/≥13 years), gender (male/female), injured side in the upper extremity (right/left), mechanism of injury (high energy trauma/other), types of bone fractures (closed fracture/open fracture), time interval between the beginning of trauma and arrival to the first health facility (hours), time interval between the beginning of trauma and arrival to the operating room (hours) and clinical symptoms.

Paraclinical parameters:
a. X-ray: Gartland classification of fractures (type 1/type 2/type 3);
b. Doppler sonography: vascular lesions at fracture site (thrombosis/crush injury/vasoconstriction), Doppler waveforms (monophasic flow/biphasic flow/triphasic flow) and flow velocity under the fracture site (m/s);

c. Multislice CT-A for vascular injuries: short lesion, <5 mm/long lesion, ≥5 mm. Multislice CT-A was indicated for those with ischemic symptoms after unsuccesful conservative fracture treatment using casts.

Treatment:
a. Conservative fracture treatment using casts;
b. Vascular trauma treatment: intraoperative vascular blockade using papaverine/ intraoperative balloon angioplasty of the brachial artery using the Fogarty catheter/ Brachial artery graft by great saphenous vein;
c. Early result and one-month reexamination were based on clinical assessment, elbow radiograph and Doppler sonography; handling complications included bone displacement and embolism.

2.3. Data Analysis

Data were sorted, cleaned, coded and entered into Epidata 3.1. Then, a software program (SPSS, version 23.0; IBM, Armonk, NY, USA) was used for all statistical analyses. Descriptive statistics, such as frequency, percentage, mean, standard deviation and interquartile range, were used to summarize preoperative, intraoperative and postoperative parameters.

3. Results

Among 50 pediatric patients, 36 patients were male (72%) and the mean age was 5.85 years (range, 1.5–14 years). The mean time interval between the beginning of trauma and arrival to the first health facility was 12 h (range, 1–120 h), and the mean time interval between the beginning of trauma and arrival to the operating room was 52.8 h (range, 4–168 h). Injuries were commonly the result of high energy trauma ($n = 49, 98\%$). 31 patients injured their left arm (62.0%), while 19 injured their right arm (38.0%). Most patients were diagnosed with Gartland type III fractures ($n = 46, 92\%$), the rest with Gartland type II fractures ($n = 4, 8\%$). Pink hand was present in 49 patients with supracondylar fractures (98%), and purple hand in only 1 case (2%) (Table 1).

Table 1. Clinical characteristics at admission.

Characteristic	Patient ($N = 50$)
Gender, no. (%)	
Male	36 (72.0)
Female	14 (28.0)
Age, years	
Mean (years)	5.85
Min–Max (years)	1.5–14
Time interval between the beginning of trauma and arrival to the first health facility (hours)	
Mean (hours)	12
Min–Max (hours)	1–120
Time interval between the beginning of trauma and arrival to the operating room (hours)	
Mean (hours)	52.8
Min–Max (hours)	4–168
Mechanism of injury, no. (%)	
High energy trauma	49 (98.0%)
Other *	1 (2.0%)
Injured side, no. (%)	
Right arm	19 (38.0%)
Left arm	31 (62.0%)

Table 1. *Cont.*

Characteristic	Patient (N = 50)
Gartland classification of fractures, no. (%)	
Type II	4 (8.0%)
Type III	46 (92.0%)
Types of bone fractures, no. (%)	
Closed fracture	49 (98.0%)
Open fracture	1 (2.0%)
Ischemia in the upper extremities, no. (%)	
Cold limb	11 (22.0%)
Warm limb	39 (78.0%)
Skin color in hand, no. (%)	
Pink hand	49 (98.0%)
Purple hand	1 (2.0%)

* This involved the arm being rammed into by a buffalo.

Figure 1 indicates changes of the Gartland classification of supracondylar humerus fractures following casting and percutaneous pinning. Before treatment, there were 46 patients with severely displaced fractures; these were classified as Gartland type III (92%). Following casting, the percentage of those with severely displaced fractures decreased significantly to 12%, while there were no patients with Gartland type III fractures after pinning.

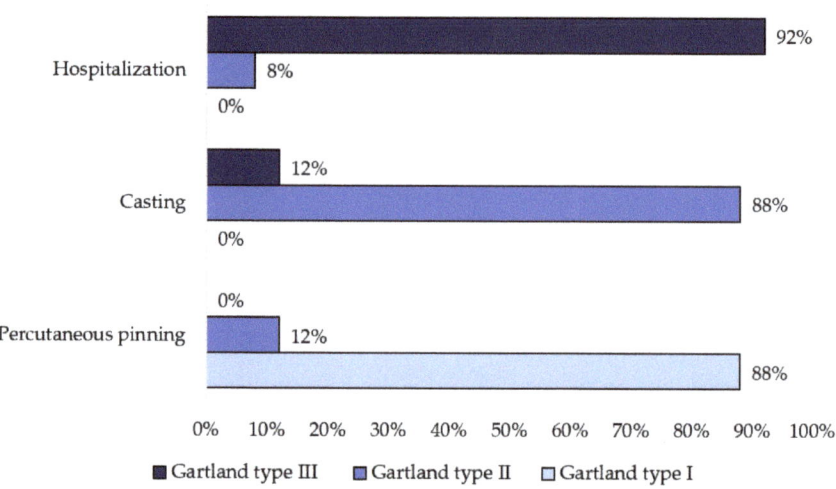

Figure 1. Changes of the Gartland classification of supracondylar humerus fractures after casting and after pinning.

Doppler sonography failed to assess vascular lesions at the fracture site before and after casting in most patients (Table 2).

Out of 50 patients, all cases were firstly treated by casting, from them, 14 cases were successfully treated with a cast. Other 36 cases were indicated for surgery. As was shown in Table 3, all pediatric patients in the age group of 13 years or over intraoperatively had found vessel injury. Most lesions having length of ≥5 mm were indicated for surgery, while lesions < 5 mm were treated conservatively.

Table 2. Brachial artery injuries and flow velocity around the fracture site with Doppler sonography classification, before and after casting.

	Before Cast (N = 50)	After Cast (N = 50)
Brachial artery injuries, no. (%)		
No assessment	43 (86%)	45 (90%)
Thrombosis	1 (2%)	0 (0%)
Contusion	2 (4%)	3 (6%)
Vasospasm	4 (8%)	2 (4%)
Flow velocity under the fracture site (m/s), mean (SD)	16 (8.5)	18.2 (9.7)
Doppler waveforms		
Monophasic flow	22 (44%)	25 (50%)
Biphasic flow	28 (56%)	21 (42%)
Triphasic flow	0 (0%)	4 (8%)

Table 3. Frequency of treatment methods with age group and length of lesions on multislice CT-A.

	Surgical Treatment (N = 36)	Conservative Treatment (N = 14)
Age group (yrs), Frequency (%)		
<3 years	2 (5.56)	1 (7.14)
3–<13 years	32 (88.89)	13 (92.86)
≥13 years	2 (5.56)	0 (0.00)
Patient age, mean (SD)	6.28 (2.87)	4.75 (2.06)
	Surgical Treatment (N = 21)	**Conservative Treatment (N = 7)**
Length of lesions on multislice CT-A		
Lesions < 5 mm	1 (16.7%)	5 (83.3%)
Lesions ≥ 5 mm	20 (90.9%)	2 (9.1%)

Two-thirds of surgical cases had only vasospasm without vessel wall contusion or intravascular thrombosis (n = 24, 66.7%) (Figure 2).

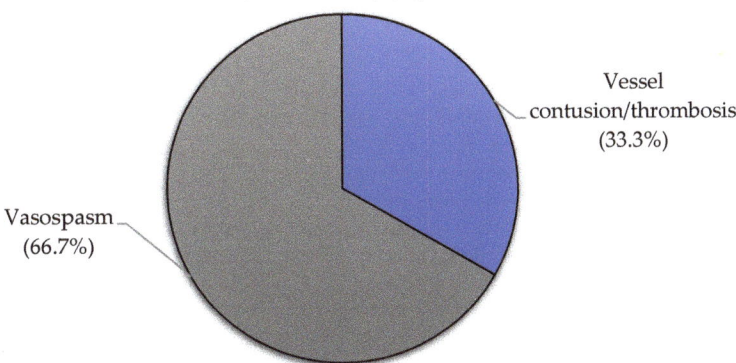

Figure 2. Intraoperative blood vessel injury in pediatric patients undergoing surgical treatment.

No patients under 3 years of age had anatomical damage of the vessel wall, while there were two patients over 13 years of age who were diagnosed with vessel wall contusion. Of the cases with long-segment lesions on multislice CT-A (≥5 mm) that were operated on, only one-third of the lesions were actually vascular contusion. Preoperative Doppler spectrum analysis was not consistent with the severity of intraoperative brachial artery injury. Out of 24 patients with vasospasm, we performed intraoperative vascular blockade using papaverin in 11 patients and intraoperative balloon angioplasty of the brachial artery using the Fogarty catheter in 13 patients. A brachial artery graft using great saphenous vein was performed in 12 patients with vascular wall contusion (Table 4).

Table 4. Association of intraoperative vascular injury with age group, lesions on multislice CT, preoperative Doppler spectrum analysis and brachial artery graft in pediatric patients undergoing surgical treatment.

	Vasospasm	Vascular Contusion/Thrombosis
Age group (years), no. (%)		
<3 years	2 (100%)	0 (0%)
3–<13 years	22 (68.8%)	10 (31.2%)
≥13 years	0 (0%)	2 (100%)
Length of lesions on multislice CT-A, no. (%)		
Lesions < 5 mm	1 (6.7)	0 (0.0)
Lesions ≥ 5 mm	14 (93.3)	7 (100.0)
Doppler waveforms, no. (%)		
Monophasic flow	17 (71.4)	7 (58.3)
Biphasic flow	7 (28.6)	5 (41.7)
Brachial artery graft, no. (%)		
Blockade	11 (100%)	0 (0%)
Angioplasty	13 (100%)	0 (0%)
Anastomosis end-to-end or using graft	0 (0%)	12 (100%)

As shown in Table 5, we recorded a complication of embolism occurring in one patient immediately after surgery and superficial infections in two patients. One month following surgery, 2 out of 36 patients experienced a temporary loss of sensation around an incision.

Table 5. Postoperative results and one-month re-examination ($N = 36$).

Postoperative Results	Patient
Embolism immediately after surgery, no. (%)	1 (2.8)
Superficial infection immediately after surgery, no. (%)	2 (5.5)
Temporary loss of sensation around an incision one month after surgery, no. (%)	2 (5.5)

4. Discussion

4.1. Clinical Condition

Non-dominant hand injuries occur more frequently in pediatric insupracondylar humerus fractures. The incidence of fractures in men and women is almost equal [11,12]. Most fractures occurred in male children. The most common age is around 5–6 years old. This is the age when children are preparing or starting school and their awareness is still immature; it is difficult for them to control their movements and body postures, yet they are eager to learn and explore the world around them. 62% of children had fractures in the left hand, which is mostly non-dominant and less flexible compared to the right hand. Most were closed fractures due to high energy trauma, only a single case admitted to the hospital being an open fracture, caused by a buffalo ramming into the arm. The injury is mainly due to falling against the hand and the grounding distance is not too large, so all patients were in a stable condition when they were admitted to hospital.

Most of the patients had type III fractures based on the Gartland classification (92%). This is consistent with injury to the brachial artery in supracondylar humerus fractures, where the artery is trapped in the fracture. According to Pham Quang Tri [13], six out of eight patients with supracondylar humerus fractures with vascular injury had Gartland type III displacement. Most of the children who came to the hospital did not have obvious symptoms of ischemia. Only a few children showed cold extremities (22%) and cyanosis (2%), while none of them showed signs of ischemia or of severe or irreversible limb bleeding, which is common in adult limb vascular trauma. In our study, time intervals between the beginning of trauma and arrival at the first health facility, as well as arrival to the operating room, were much longer than the ideal time (6 h after the accident) to restore circulation after acute extremity embolism in adults. The prolonged time of hospital admission and delaying surgery in children could be explain by several reasons. First, the ischemia of the injury hand is not severe and it don't influence on their condition. Second, diagnostic imaging procedures such as Doppler ultrasound, X-ray, and multislide CT-A, and casting procedure take more time among small children compared to among adults. Finally, the treatment algorism for this injury is casting firstly, after that, if the pulse is restored, we will keep stop on conservative treatment. If the pulse is not restored, we send to multislide CT-A and consider to surgery.

4.2. Preoperative Imaging

In the study of Phan Quang Tri [13], among 102 cases of supracondylar fractures that were treated with born reposition and percutaneous pinning under C-arm control. There were 8 cases of brachial artery injury, accounting for 7.48% in general and 57.2% of cases with complications. Because the clinical signs and symptoms of ischemia are not clear and difficult to find out in small children, especially those who are not yet of school age. Diagnostic imaging plays an important role in decision between surgical and conservative treatments. Most of the children being at school age, with little or no sense of cooperation, vascular imaging diagnostic procedures are very difficult to perform with high quality. The performance of vascular diagnostic tests requires anesthesia, leading to difficulties in deploying human resources and equipment, as well as carrying an increased risk of adverse consequences.

Because it is performed in emergency conditions with a lack of patient's cooperation, cast, edema, and hematoma, only a very small number (<10%) of Doppler ultrasound analyses can directly evaluate the blood vessels at the level of the fracture, including the vessel wall and lumen. That information is quite needed for verify diagnosis of upper extremity vascular injury. In our study, more than half of the pediatric patients undergo a multislice CT-A of the upper extremity, whereas in adult patients these lesions are very rare to require this diagnostic procedure. Multislice CT-A enables an assessment of the perfusion status of the entire vascular system of the upper extremity but does not accurately assess the damage to the vessel wall and lumen in children. We found that all cases with length of lesion of the brachial artery on CT-A less than 5 mm did not necessarily require surgery. In addition, all study patients who had the lesions longer than 5 mm were indicated to surgery, but in only half of them can find out the vascular contusion intraoperatively. Therefore, multislice CT-A may be useful mainly in the decision of conservative therapy, i.e., those with short lesions (less than 5 mm) (Figure 3).

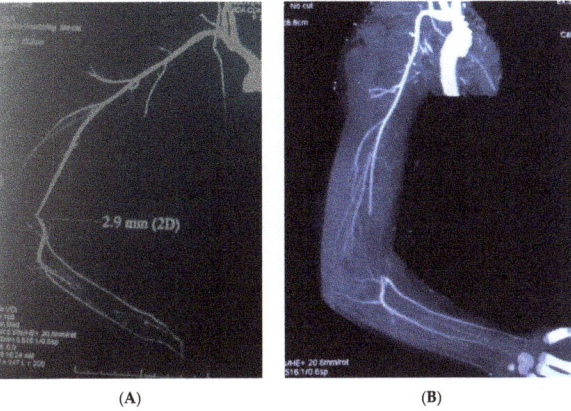

Figure 3. Brachial artery injuries in multislice CT-A. (**A**) Lesions < 5 mm. (**B**) Lesions ≥ 5 mm.

4.3. Efficacy of Vascular Rehabilitation after Treatment

For conventional closed supracondylar fractures of the humerus, treatment is achieved mainly by reposition of fractured born and cast or pinning. In cases with vascular injury, the good born reposition may enable to decompress blood vessels and restore blood flow. However, even with perfect born reposition, surgical treatment is still needed to treat the vascular injury in case having really anatomical damage to the vascular wall.

Among the techniques for achieving and maintaining born reposition, pinning is the most effective method, but it is also the most invasive and time-consuming, and is associated with risk of complications. By contrast, casts present the simplest and least invasive technique; they may not gave perfect reposition but could decompress vessel and restore blood flow. In this study, when patients were mainly diagnosed with type III displaced supracondylar fractures of the humerus before treatment (92%), this figure decreased significantly after cast to 12% and 0% after pinning (Figure 4).

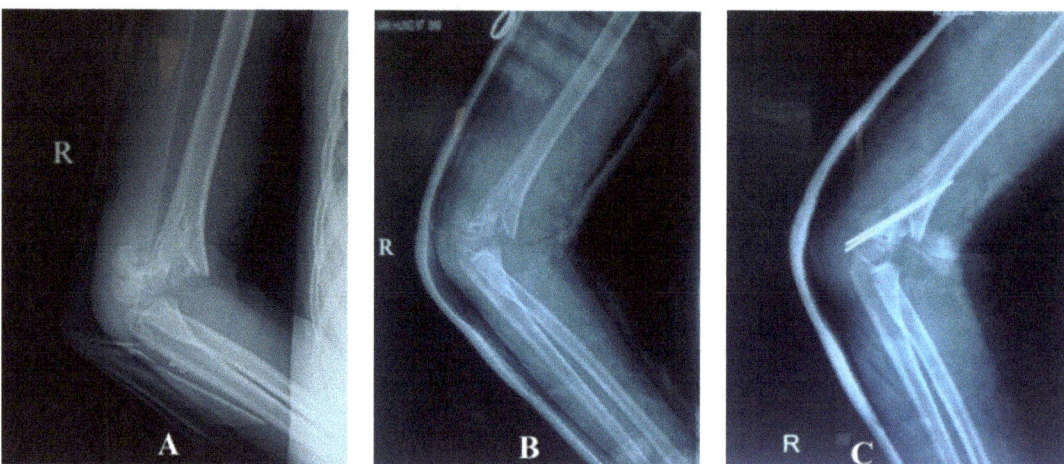

Figure 4. X-rays of supracondylar fractures of the humerus. (**A**) Before reposition—Gartland type III. (**B**) After reposition—Gartland type II. (**C**) After operative pinning—Gartland type II.

4.4. Vascular Injury, Surgical Management and Related Factors

Regarding the cases of conservative treatment when born reposition and cast was applied but the radial pulse was still not found, if Doppler ultrasound analysis showed reduced blood flow and there were long-length of lesions on a multislice CT-A, patients were indicated for surgery with born reposition, pinning and re revascularization.

Intraoperatively found that, two-thirds of surgical cases had vasospasm without anatomical damage of the vessel wall or intravascular thrombosis. In most cases, following born reposition and cast, the blood vessels have been released from the fracture and only a few are still stuck in the fracture. All cases of surgery fractured born was reposited and fixed by pinning with K-wire from the lateral side. In cases with vasospasm. Blood flow will be restored by extra-vessel papaverine blockage or balloon dilatation of the brachial artery using a Fogarty catheter or cutting damaged artery and performing anastomosis end-to-end or replace it by great saphenous graft, while a brachial artery had wall damage (Figure 5).

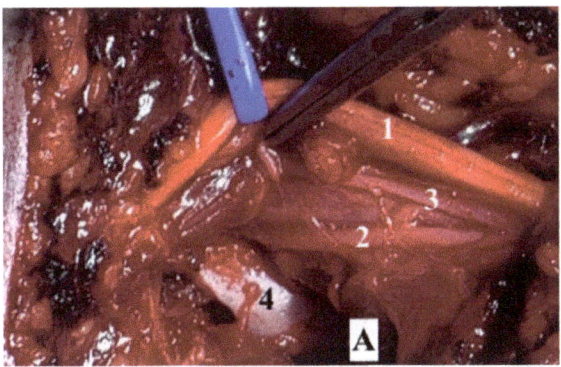 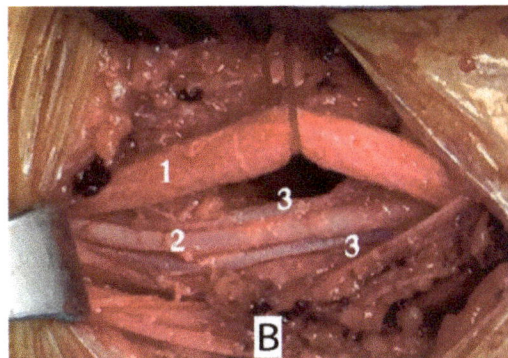

Figure 5. (**A**) Arterial entrapment in the fracture socket. (**B**) Freeing the artery from the fracture socket. (**1**: median nerve; **2**: brachial artery; **3**: brachial vein; **4**: fracture location.)

With vasospasm, there were several cases of short spasm which is not dilated after the pinning and blocking using papaverin. This opens the blood flow very weakly but without damage to the vessel wall and thrombosis of the lumen. This explains why on a multislice CT-A there can be seen a loss of the long brachial artery but no damage to the vessel wall during surgery. Therefore, if Doppler ultrasound accurately assesses the status of contusion in the transverse fracture and non-thrombotic lumen, angioplasty will most likely not need to be performed. This leads to a real vascular injury and the risk of a serious vascular complication, especially where a specialist in vascular surgery is not available (Figure 6).

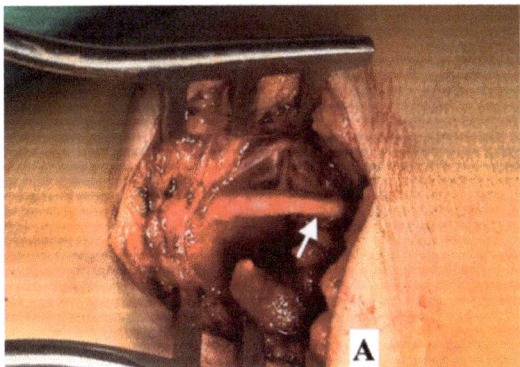 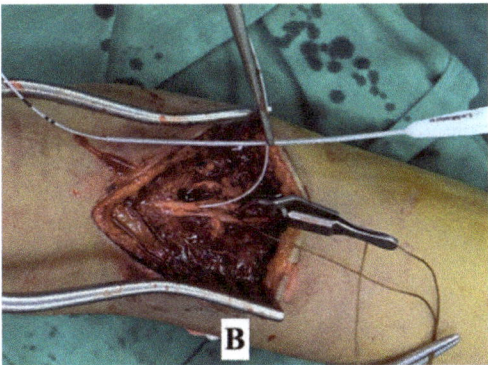

Figure 6. Vasospasm of brachial artery and its surgical management. (**A**) Vasospasm. (**B**) Balloon dilatation of the brachial ar-tery using the Fogarty catheter.

Comparing intraoperative finding of vascular lesions with the age group of the patient, we found that patients under 3 years of age only had vasospasm, while those over 13 years of age only had vascular contusion. This can be explained by ossification in the humerus bone. The ossification centers begin to fuse together at age 3 years and the ossification process completes by the age of 13 [14]. Therefore, in children less than 3 years of age, the bone structure is almost entirely cartilage which is not capable of causing damage to the vessel wall, while since the bone structure in children over 13 years old is almost adult, the pathology of vascular trauma is similar to that of an adult with typical vessel contusion and thrombosis. In the study, direct anastomosis end-to-end was performed when the lesions were short (less than 1 cm). In addition, the choice of grafting with saphenous vein is very difficult because of the very small size of vessel in children. However, in older children with sufficiently large vein size, the artery bypass grafting can be used if the damage to the vessel wall is long, which avoids missing the injury with postoperative embolism as a result. We documented the case of a patient who suffered a thrombosis immediately after direct anastomosis end-to-end surgery and who was then re-operated on using grafting with saphenous vein. The cause of complication may be not completely removement of the damaged segment, short length and tension of vessel, may also be due to the failed technique or the inadequate anticoagulation (Figure 7).

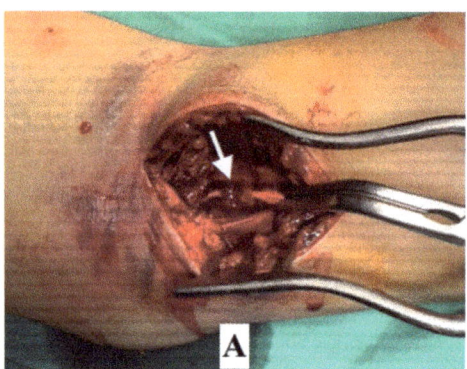
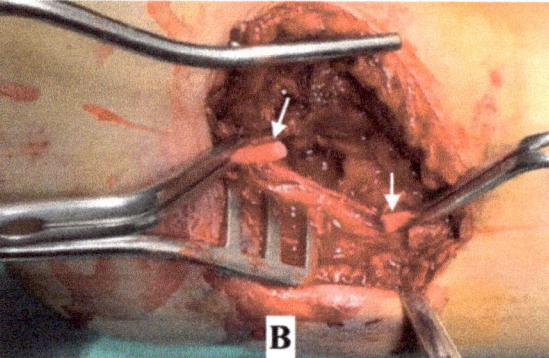

Figure 7. Physical injury to brachial artery and its surgical management. (**A**) Contusion, thrombosis and brachial artery nearly ruptured. (**B**) Damaged artery excised and directly anastomosed.

4.5. Limitations

Several limitations need to be noted in this article. First of all, in operating on these patients, it was most important to us to restore vascular circulation, the recovery of bone anatomy being secondary. Hence, although there is no anatomical perfection, the bones have been less displaced. Additionally, while there was a follow-up in this study, the period for evaluating patient outcomes was within one month following surgery. There are two main reasons for this which should be acknowledged. Firstly, the main purpose in our study was to focus on treating early-stage vascular damage. Secondly, because COVID-19 lockdowns have been continuously imposed in Vietnam and out-of-province patients are those who have been most affected by this, the re-examination of patients after surgery has been very difficult in our institution. Therefore, longer-term outcomes have not been evaluated in this study.

5. Conclusions

The majority of supracondylar humerus fractures with brachial artery injuries did not present with signs and symptoms of critical limb ischemia similar to peripheral vascular injuries in lower extremity; therefore, emergency management was not required in all cases. Diagnosis and treatment for pediatric supracondylar humerus fractures with vascular injury is a difficult and time-consuming procedure, especially in cases of transverse fractures. Two-thirds of patients who underwent surgery had no physical damage to the blood vessel wall and lumen. As a result of this study, we propose to apply a unique protocol in the management of pediatric supracondylar humerus fractures with brachial artery injuries with the aim of shortening treatment duration and minimizing the performance of unnecessary procedures and surgical treatments.

Author Contributions: Conceptualization, T.N.V.; methodology, T.N.V., S.H.D.P., L.H.V. and U.H.N.; validation, T.N.V., S.H.D.P. and U.H.N.; formal analysis, T.N.V. and L.H.V.; investigation, T.N.V., S.H.D.P., L.H.V. and U.H.N.; data curation, T.N.V. and L.H.V.; writing—original draft preparation, T.N.V., S.H.D.P. and L.H.V.; writing—review and editing, U.H.N.; visualization, T.N.V., S.H.D.P., L.H.V. and U.H.N.; supervision, U.H.N. All authors have read and agreed to the final version of the manuscript.

Funding: This research received no external funding.

Institutional Review Board Statement: The studies involving human participants were reviewed and approved by the Ethics Board of the Viet Duc University Hospital (2430/QĐ-VĐ), 12 December 2020.

Informed Consent Statement: Informed consent was obtained from all individual participants included in the study. If the participants are under the age of 18, or otherwise legally or medically unable to provide written informed consent, then consent was obtained from their parents or guardians.

Data Availability Statement: All the data that support the findings of this study are available from the corresponding author on reasonable request. Requests for access to these data should be made to Tu Ngoc Vu (Email: vungoctu@hmu.edu.vn).

Acknowledgments: We sincerely thank the patients, their families, the members working at Department of Cardiovascular and Thoracic Surgery and the Board of Directors of Viet Duc University Hospital for their support.

Conflicts of Interest: The authors declare no conflict of interest.

References

1. Saeed, W.; Waseem, M. *Elbow Fractures Overview*; StatPearls Publishing LLC.: Treasure Island, FL, USA, 2021.
2. Landin, L.A. Fracture patterns in children: Analysis of 8682 fractures with special reference to incidence, etiology and secular changes in a swedish urban population 1950–1979. *Acta Orthop. Scand. Suppl.* **1983**, *202*, 3–109. [CrossRef]
3. Louahem, D.; Cottalorda, J. Acute ischemia and pink pulseless hand in 68 of 404 gartland type III supracondylar humeral fractures in children: Urgent management and therapeutic consensus. *Injury* **2016**, *47*, 848–852. [CrossRef]
4. Franklin, C.C.; Skaggs, D.L. Approach to the pediatric supracondylar humeral fracture with neurovascular compromise. *Instr. Course Lect.* **2013**, *62*, 429–433.
5. Gosens, T.; Bongers, K.J. Neurovascular complications and functional outcome in displaced supracondylar fractures of the humerus in children. *Injury* **2003**, *34*, 267–273. [CrossRef]
6. Badkoobehi, H.; Choi, P.D.; Bae, D.S.; Skaggs, D.L. Management of the pulseless pediatric supracondylar humeral fracture. *J. Bone Jt. Surg. Am. Vol.* **2015**, *97*, 937–943. [CrossRef]
7. Sabharwal, S.; Tredwell, S.J.; Beauchamp, R.; MacKenzie, W.G.; Jakubec, D.M.; Cairns, R.; Leblanc, J.G. Management of pulseless pink hand in pediatric supracondylar fractures of humerus. *J. Pediatr. Orthop.* **1997**, *17*, 303–310. [CrossRef] [PubMed]
8. Lewis, H.G.; Morrison, C.M.; Kennedy, P.T.; Herbert, K.J. Arterial reconstruction using the basilic vein from the zone of injury in pediatric supracondylar humeral fractures: A clinical and radiological series. *Plast. Reconstr. Surg.* **2003**, *111*, 1159–1163. [CrossRef]
9. Clement, D. Assessment of a treatment plan for managing acute vascular complications associated with supracondylar fractures of the humerus in children. *J. Pediatr. Orthop.* **1990**, *10*, 97–100. [CrossRef] [PubMed]
10. Luria, S.; Sucar, A.; Eylon, S.; Pinchas-Mizrachi, R.; Berlatzky, Y.; Anner, H.; Liebergall, M.; Porat, S. Vascular complications of supracondylar humeral fractures in children. *J. Pediatr. Orthop. B* **2007**, *16*, 133–143. [CrossRef] [PubMed]
11. Abzug, J.M.; Kozin, S.H.; Zlotolow, D.A. *The Pediatric Upper Extremity*; Springer: Hoboken, NJ, USA, 2015.
12. Houshian, S.; Mehdi, B.; Larsen, M.S. The epidemiology of elbow fracture in children: Analysis of 355 fractures, with special reference to supracondylar humerus fractures. *J. Orthop. Sci.* **2001**, *6*, 312–315. [CrossRef] [PubMed]
13. Trí, P.Q. Nghiên cứu điều trị gãy trên lồi cầu xương cánh tay kiểu duỗi ở trẻ em bằng nắn kín và xuyên kim qua da dưới màn tăng sáng. Ph.D. Thesis, Đại Học Y Dược Thành Phố Hồ Chí Minh, Ho Chi Minh City, Vietnam, 2016.
14. Kwong, S.; Kothary, S.; Poncinelli, L.L. Skeletal development of the proximal humerus in the pediatric population: MRI features. *Am. J. Roentgenol.* **2014**, *202*, 418–425. [CrossRef] [PubMed]

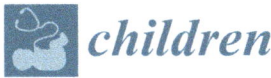

Review

Pediatric Supracondylar Humerus Fractures: Should We Avoid Surgery during After-Hours?

Sietse E. S. Terpstra [1,*], Paul T. P. W. Burgers [2], Huub J. L. van der Heide [3] and Pieter Bas de Witte [3]

1 Department of Rheumatology, Leiden University Medical Center, 2333 ZA Leiden, The Netherlands
2 Department of Orthopedics, University Medical Center Utrecht, Heidelberglaan 100, 3584 CX Utrecht, The Netherlands; paulepost@gmail.com
3 Department of Orthopedics, Leiden University Medical Center, 2333 ZA Leiden, The Netherlands; h.j.l.van_der_heide@lumc.nl (H.J.L.v.d.H.); p.b.de_witte@lumc.nl (P.B.d.W.)
* Correspondence: s.e.s.terpstra@lumc.nl; Tel.: +31-71-526-9111

Abstract: Pediatric supracondylar humerus fractures occur frequently. Often, the decision has to be made whether to operate immediately, e.g., during after-hours, or to postpone until office hours. However, the effect of timing of surgery on radiological and clinical outcomes is unclear. This literature review with the PICO methodology found six relevant articles that compared the results of office-hours and after-hours surgery for pediatric supracondylar humerus fractures. The surgical outcomes of both groups in these studies were assessed. One of the articles found a significantly higher "poor fixation rate" in the after-hours group, compared with office hours. Another article found more malunions in the "night" subgroup vs. the "all groups but night" group. A third article found a higher risk of postoperative paresthesia in the "late night" subgroup vs. the "day" group. Lastly, one article reported increased consultant attendance and decreased operative time when postponing to office hours more often. No differences were reported for functional outcomes in any of the articles. Consequently, no strong risks or benefits from surgical treatment during office hours vs. after-hours were found. It appears safe to postpone surgery to office hours if circumstances are not optimal for acute surgery, and if there is no medical contraindication. However, research with a higher level-of-evidence is needed make more definite recommendations.

Keywords: surgery; children; orthopedics; supracondylar humerus; night; fracture; reduction; after-hours

Citation: Terpstra, S.E.S.; Burgers, P.T.P.W.; van der Heide, H.J.L.; Witte, P.B.d. Pediatric Supracondylar Humerus Fractures: Should We Avoid Surgery during After-Hours?. *Children* **2022**, *9*, 189. https://doi.org/10.3390/children9020189

Academic Editor: Christiaan J. A. van Bergen

Received: 19 November 2021
Accepted: 28 January 2022
Published: 2 February 2022

Publisher's Note: MDPI stays neutral with regard to jurisdictional claims in published maps and institutional affiliations.

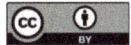

Copyright: © 2022 by the authors. Licensee MDPI, Basel, Switzerland. This article is an open access article distributed under the terms and conditions of the Creative Commons Attribution (CC BY) license (https://creativecommons.org/licenses/by/4.0/).

1. Introduction

Supracondylar humerus fractures account for 15% of all childhood fractures [1]. The incidence decreases sharply after the age of 10 due to skeletal maturation, and after the age of sixteen this fracture is very rare [1]. The classic trauma mechanism is a fall on the outstretched arm, resulting in an extension type fracture, which accounts for 97% of supracondylar humerus fractures [2]. A significant portion of these children need surgical treatment and fixation. However, there is debate in clinical practice whether or not to operate on these injuries during after-hours.

The main indications for acute treatment of supracondylar humerus fractures are traumatic neurovascular injury, open fractures and significant fracture dislocation [3,4]. Acute neurovascular injuries are reported in 17% of patients with a dislocated supracondylar humerus fracture [5]. Dislocation is reported in 54% and is often classified with the Gartland classification. Gartland type I indicates a fracture without dislocation, which generally can be treated conservatively. Gartland type II indicates partial dislocation, which more often requires reduction with or without fixation. Type III and IV indicate complete dislocation, where type IV also has periosteal disruption [6,7]. These type III and IV fractures are often associated with anterior interosseous nerve neuropraxia, brachial artery disruption, and other complications [1]. Both usually require closed or open reduction and fixation. Fixation is generally performed with multiple K-wire fixation [8].

Supracondylar humerus fractures are often managed at the day of admission, which can result in after-hours surgery [9]. After-hours surgery might provide additional risks for patients due to, for example, surgeon fatigue and the lack of a specialized team. In a recent publication on general orthopedic trauma, higher complication and mortality rates have been reported for surgery performed during after-hours [9]. But overall, the evidence for these alleged additional risks of after-hours surgery is limited. And in contrast, the hip fracture population has been investigated more extensively on after-hours surgery, showing no significant differences between results of office-hours and after-hours surgery [10]. However, these results cannot simply be extrapolated to the pediatric supracondylar humerus fracture patient group. Because of the lack of consensus on acute (after-hours) surgery on supracondylar humerus fractures, we investigated the following question: "Is it necessary and safe to perform surgery for pediatric supracondylar humerus fractures during after-hours?".

2. Materials and Methods

We performed a literature review using the PICO methodology [11]. The following research question was applied: in children under 18 years old with a supracondylar humerus fracture (P), does after-hours surgery (I), compared with surgery during office hours (C), result in different outcomes in follow-up in terms of successful surgical treatment, function and complications (O)?

A search strategy was built in collaboration with a librarian (J. W. Schoones, Leiden University Medical Center Walaeus library). This strategy was used for PubMed, Web of Science, Embase and Cochrane to find all relevant articles written in English and published in the past 10 years (Appendix A). All references of the identified studies were evaluated for relevant articles (cross-referencing).

Studies could be included based on the following criteria: comparative study (after-hours vs. office hours) including children with supracondylar humerus fractures, reporting on clinical outcomes in follow-up, as well as radiological outcomes (successful reduction) and complications. The first selection of articles after the literature search was performed with the screening of titles and abstracts. Of the remaining articles, the full texts were evaluated for inclusion based on our eligibility criteria. Quality of evidence of the included full texts was evaluated using the GRADE criteria [12]. Additionally, articles were assessed for risk of bias in their methods and outcomes using the ROBINS-I criteria. (Appendix B) [13].

3. Results

The search strategy resulted in fourteen articles on November 9th, 2021. After screening of the titles and abstracts by two authors (S.E.S.T. and P.B.d.W.), nine relevant articles were identified that compared office-hours and after-hours surgeries for pediatric supracondylar humerus fractures. After reading the full texts, six of these articles could be included; in the other three, there were no reported outcomes on follow-up, succesful surgical treatment, elbow function or complications. There was no disagreement between the authors. The quality of the six articles was regarded as sufficient according to the GRADE criteria [12].

All six articles articles retrospectively compared postoperative outcomes of pediatric patients who had surgery for supracondylar humerus fractures at different times of the day. Primary outcomes in the studies were reduction quality [14–19], malunion rate [15], loss of reduction [17] and complications [16]. Also, functional outcomes in follow-up were assessed in three articles [14–16]. Other reported secondary outcomes were length of hospital stay, duration of surgery, rate of open surgical reduction and complications. Outcomes of the six articles are summarized in Table 1.

Table 1. Outcomes and results of the included articles.

	Patients in Office-Hours Group	Patients in After-Hours Group	Primary Outcome *	Other Outcomes	Primary Result	Secondary Results	Risk of Bias According to the ROBINS-I Criteria [13]
Aydogmus et al. [14] 2017	47	44	poor fixation	surgical method, placement of any medial pins, operative time, any postoperative neurovascular complication, successful reduction rate, successful fixation rate, any induced deformity and rate of loss of function	significantly poorer fixation in the after-hours group vs. office hours. (4/47 (9%) vs. 17/44 (39%)) ($p = 0.005$))	no significant differences between groups	serious risk
Paci et al. [15] 2018	77	186	malunion	surgeon subspecialty, operative time, range of motion, carrying angle and other clinical outcomes.	more malunion in the "night" subgroup vs. the "all groups but night" group (2/26 (8%) vs. 2/236, (1%, $p = 0.05$)	more surgeries performed by a fellow during after-hours, compared with office hours: 72/77 (93%) vs. 95/186 (49%, $p < 0.001$), more Gartland type III/IV fractures in the after-hours group compared with office hours: 40/77 (73%) versus 129/186 (57%, $p = 0.01$).	moderate risk
Wendling-Keim et al. [16] 2019	52	47	Complications	-	significantly more paresthesia in the 22:00–2:00 group (3/9, 33.3%) vs. the 7:30 –16:40 group (6/52, 11.5%) ($p = 0.01$)	-	serious risk
Balakumar et al. [17] 2012	37	40	loss of reduction	number of pins used and technical quality of pinning	no significant difference in loss of reduction in the office hours vs. after-hours group (7/37, (19%) vs. 7/40, (18%) $p = 1.00$)	no significant differences between groups	serious risk

Table 1. *Cont.*

	Patients in Office-Hours Group	Patients in After-Hours Group	Primary Outcome *	Other Outcomes	Primary Result	Secondary Results	Risk of Bias According to the ROBINS-I Criteria [13]
Okkaoglu et al. [18] 2021	79	71	reduction quality	operative time, open reduction rate and time to surgery	no significant differences in any measures of reduction quality ($p > 0.05$)	More time to surgery during office hours; 14.0 h (SD 35.2) vs. 6.0 h (SD 3.5, $p < 0.001$)	moderate risk
Tuomilehto et al. [19] 2018	100	100	pin fixation quality	number of complications, number of open reductions and operative time	no significant difference in sufficient pin fixation quality for office hours versus after-hours (42% vs. 55% ($p = 0.08$))	operative time <60 min: 67% vs. 84% after implementation postponement protocol ($p = 0.01$)	serious risk

* not all articles explicitly mentioned their primary and secondary outcomes. In this case, the most relevant outcome to our topic was assessed as primary outcome. SD = Standard Deviation, h = hours, min = minutes.

Aydoğmus et al. [14] compared a group of 91 children (age 0–11) diagnosed with a Gartland type III fracture without neurovascular injury in the period of January 2012 to October 2014. Of the 91 patients, 47 were operated on during office hours (8:00–17:00), and 44 during after-hours (17:00–8:00). Surgical technique was chosen by the treating surgeon. Follow-up was weekly in the first month, followed by once every three months for at least one year.

Primary outcome was "poor fixation," defined as pins crossing the fracture line, pins not placed bicortically, and/or pins for which the entry points were very close to each other. A significant difference in poor fixation rate was found between the groups: 4/47 patients (9%) in the office-hours group had a poor fixation, compared with 17/44 (39%) in the after-hours group ($p = 0.005$). The authors stated that a lack of sleep is often present when performing surgical treatment at night, which might lead to this higher rate. For the secondary outcomes including surgical method, placement of any medial pins, operative time, neurovascular complications, successful reduction rate, successful fixation rate, range of motion, waiting time to surgical treatment and any induced deformity, no differences were found. No reoperations were performed for any of the patients during follow-up. Potential differences in surgeon training levels and severity of the fractures between both groups were not reported. The authors concluded that surgical treatment should be performed during office hours instead of after-hours by adequately rested surgical staff.

Paci et al. [15] included 263 patients with an uncomplicated Gartland type II, III or IV fracture diagnosed between 1 August 2002 to 31 July 2014. 263 patients with an average age of 5 years were included. Of these, 77 (29%) had surgical treatment and fixation during office hours, which was defined as 6:00–16:00 from Monday to Friday. This group was compared with 186 (71%) procedures performed during after-hours, subdivided into evening (16:00–23:00), night (23:00–6:00) and weekend (Saturdays and Sundays, 6:00–16:00).

Primary outcome was the rate of malunion, defined as a clinically significant deformity, resulting in a change in treatment or follow-up plan. Secondary outcomes included operative time, range of motion, carrying angle and functional flexion and extension. Functional flexion was defined as ≥ 130 degrees, and functional extension as ≤ 30 degrees. A normal carrying angle was defined as 0–19 degrees of elbow valgus. On final follow-up radiographs, the Baumann angles were measured and considered normal if between 64 and 81 degrees. No significant differences were found for any of the primary and secondary outcomes after an average follow-up of 135 days. The authors reported no malunions among 77 cases in the office-hours group vs. 4 malunions of 186 (2.3%) in the after-hours group ($p = 0.3$). However, when comparing all groups to the "night" subgroup, a borderline significant difference was found for malunion: 2/236 (0.9%) in the "all groups but night" group, compared with 2/26 (9%) in the "night" group ($p = 0.05$). This outcome might be at least partially associated with the fact that there were significantly more Gartland type III/IV fractures in the after-hours group: 40/77 (73%) vs. 129/186 (57%) in the office hours group ($p = 0.01$). Furthermore, the authors found that it was more likely to have surgical treatment performed by a fellow during after-hours, compared with office hours: 72/77 (93%) vs. 95/186 (49%, $p < 0.001$). Therefore, the authors concluded that late night surgical treatment performed between 23:00 and 05:59 may be associated with a higher rate of malunion, relating it to fatigue of the surgeon, variation in training and practice patterns of the operating surgeon and experience of supporting staff. Regarding secondary outcomes, the authors reported 55/55 (100%) functional extension in the office hours group vs. 126/128 (98%) in the after-hours group ($p = 1.00$), and 68% having functional flexion in the office hours group vs. (72%) in the after-hours group ($p = 0.6$). Based on these findings, the authors caution surgeons against operating during late night hours without urgent indication.

Wendling-Keim et al. [16]. compared 97 patients aged 0 to 18 years (mean age 5.8 years) with displaced supracondylar humerus fractures requiring osteosynthesis. Unstable Gartland type II as well as Gartland type III and IV fractures were included during a five-year period. The primary outcome was complication rate during hospital stay as well as during long-term follow-up. Complications were broadly defined, including, for example, impaired range of motion, paresthesia and wound infections. Timing of surgical treatment was recorded and stratified: daytime (7:30–16:30, 52 patients (53.6%)), early evening (16:31–22:00, 36 patients (37.1%)), late evening (22:00–2:00, 9 patients, (9.3%)) and night (2:00–7:30, no patients). The authors found that the incidence of paresthesia was significantly higher in the 22:00–2:00 group (3 out of 9 patients, 33.3%) compared with the 7:30–16:40 shift (6 out of 52 patients, 11.5%) ($p = 0.01$). No other differences in complication rates were found between office-hours and after-hours groups. Also, the authors found no association between the rate of complications and experience of the surgeon using an analysis of variance test ($p > 0.05$). It was not mentioned whether there were differences in Gartland classification between groups.

Balakumar et al. [17] analyzed 77 pediatric supracondylar humerus fracture procedures from July 2004 to October 2009. Mean age was 7.8 years. These fractures were divided into 37 cases with surgery during office hours (8:00–20:00) and 40 during after-hours (20:00–8:00). Ten Gartland type II fractures and 67 Gartland type III fractures were included.

The primary outcome was loss of reduction during follow-up. Secondary outcomes were number of pins used and technical quality of the pinning: i.e., adequate initial reduction, number of cortical purchases, lateral only pinning, technical errors and reduction quality (which was sufficient in case of anterior humeral line passing through the middle of the capitellum, restoration of Baumann angle and an intact medial and lateral column). Outcome evaluation was done by reviewing the intraoperative radiographs and comparing these to those acquired immediately after surgical treatment and at three weeks postoperatively. Four different pinning constructions were used, namely (a) two lateral pins; (b) three lateral pins; (c) crossed pins with one medial and one lateral entry pin; and (d) two lateral and one medial entry pin. A multivariate logistic regression analysis was performed to analyze individual factors causing loss of reduction.

No significant difference in terms of loss of reduction was found between the office hours and the after-hours group: seven cases were found with a loss of reduction after three weeks in both the office-hours and the after-hours group, i.e., 7/37 (19%) vs. 7/40 (18%, $p = 1.00$). The article did not report any differences in secondary outcomes between both groups. Assessing the patient group with loss of reduction, lateral pinning (odds ratio: 7.73, $p = 0.029$) and technical errors (odds ratio: 57.63, $p = 0.001$) were associated with loss of reduction. No associations were found with number of pins used, adequate initial surgical treatment, number of cortical purchases and technical quality of pinning. The Gartland classifications and surgeon level of experience were not reported separately for the office-hours and after-hours group.

The authors suggest that loss of reduction following fracture fixation is closely related to technical errors, which often results in inadequate reduction. However, as these technical errors were evenly distributed between office hours and after-hours, the authors concluded that timing of the procedure was not associated with loss of reduction.

Okkaoglu et al. [18] investigated 150 Gartland type III fracture surgeries (mean age 5.9 years (Standard Deviation (SD) 2.6). Open fractures, fractures associated with vascular injury and compartment syndrome and flexion type fractures were excluded. Of all patients, 79 underwent surgical reduction during office hours (8:00–17:00) and 71 during after-hours (of which 51 during the evening (17:00–24:00) and 20 during the night (24:00–8:00)). The office-hours surgery group partially consisted of fractures admitted during office hours, and partially of fractures postponed from after-hours. All surgeries were performed by an experienced orthopedic surgeon within 24 h of admission. The main outcome was reduction quality on postoperative radiographs, which was assessed with the lateral capitellohumeral angle (defined as acceptable: 22–70 degrees), Baumann angle (56–86 degrees) and anterior humeral line (crossing mid-third of capitellum). Other outcomes were operative time and open reduction rate.

No significant differences in patient characteristics were found between the office-hours and after-hours groups, and no significant differences were found for reduction quality, open reduction rate and mean operative time between office-hour and after-hours surgeries. Therefore, surgical outcomes were regarded as comparable between the office-hours and after-hours groups by the authors. Time from admission to surgery, however, was significantly longer for the office-hours group (14.0 (SD 5.1) vs. 6.0 (3.5) hours ($p < 0.01$)). No information on long term follow-up or functional outcomes was reported.

Based on this information, the authors concluded that it is generally safe to postpone surgery to office hours if there is no indication for acute surgery (open fractures, neurovascular impairment, compartment syndrome). However, the authors caution against very long time from admission to surgery (>24 h) as their data does not provide information on this topic.

Tuomilehto et al. [19] assessed 200 fractures (mean age 7.1 years, range 1.8 to 14.1, 15.5% Gartland type II, 83.5% Gartland type III). Of these fractures, timing of surgery for the first 100 patients depended on circumstances, and could therefore be during the night (24:00–7:00) (12% of surgeries). For the next 100 patients, a protocol was implemented postponing night-time surgery to office hours. During this period, only fractures with compromised circulation were treated during after-hours (2%). Main outcomes were pin fixation quality, number of open reductions, radiographic alignment, and postoperative complications. Pin fixation quality was regarded sufficient if both K-wires punctured both bone fragments and if pins were not crossing at the fracture line. Radiographic alignment was regarded sufficient if the Baumann angle was within $\pm 10°$ of reported normal range, and the anterior humeral line crossed the capitellum with no signs of malrotation.

The authors found no significant differences between the two treatment groups before vs. after implementation, respectively: adequate pin fixation quality (42% vs. 55% ($p = 0.08$), Gartland classification (79% Gartland III vs. 88%, $p = 0.13$), Bauman angle (55% normal vs. 70% normal, $p = 0.07$)), nerve injury (14 vs. 21, $p = 0.26$), other complications (5 vs. 3 infections ($p = 0.72$), and other outcomes. No information on long term follow-up or functional outcomes was reported. It is important to note that in the postponed group, the consultant was more often the primary surgeon (43% vs. 27% ($p = 0.02$)). Additionally, in the postponed group, mean operative time decreased by 11 min (no statistics reported) and the percentage of operations shorter than 60 min decreased from 67% to 84% ($p = 0.01$).

The authors concluded that postponing supracondylar humerus surgeries to office hours may not make a difference for the patients if surgery is performed within the first 24 h, while being beneficial in terms of consultant attendance and operative time.

4. Discussion

Obtaining immediate reduction and supposedly optimal clinical outcome are often arguments to perform acute surgical treatment, even during after-hours, for pediatric supracondylar humerus fractures. However, most surgeons prefer to postpone surgery to office hours, as it is generally assumed that after-hours surgery provides additional risks for patients [20]. We found six relevant retrospective articles reporting on outcomes of office-hours and after-hours surgery in pediatric patients with supracondylar fractures.

4.1. Primary Outcomes

Aydogmus et al. [14] found a significantly higher "poor fixation" rate in the after-hours group, compared with the office-hours group. However, this higher rate of "poor fixation" was not associated with loss of range of motion in the after-hours group during follow-up. Paci et al. [15] demonstrated a borderline significant difference in malunion rates when comparing their "all groups but night" subgroups with the "night" (23:00–6:00) subgroup, with the latter demonstrating a higher malunion rate. However, there was a significantly higher Gartland classification in the concerning night group, compared with the other groups. Therefore, more severe fractures appear to have been treated with minimal delay, i.e., during after-hours, if deemed necessary by the surgeon (confounding by indication).

In addition, more surgeries were performed by a fellow at night (performance bias). Both are potential confounders for the identified inferior outcomes of the "night" group. In the article of Wendling-Keim [16], surgical treatment from 22:00–2:00, compared with 7:30–16:40 was associated with a higher rate of paresthesia. The studies of Balakumar et al. [17], Okkaoglu et al. [18] and Tuomilehto et al. [19] found no significant differences between office hours and after-hours for reduction quality, loss of reduction and pin fixation quality.

4.2. Secondary Outcomes

No clinically or statistically significant differences were described between office and after-hours groups with regards to range of motion, carrying angle, surgical method, functional flexion and extension and any induced deformity. However, the study of Tuomilehto did show a decrease in operative time in the postponed/office-hours group (11 min), which coincided with the consultant orthopedic surgeon being more often the primary surgeon in this group (43% vs. 27% ($p = 0.02$)).

4.3. Early vs. Delayed Surgical Treatment

The aforementioned results suggest that the influence of timing of surgery on radiological and functional outcomes in pediatric supracondylar humerus fractures is limited. Still, in order to draw more definite conclusions about this topic, it is also important to assess differences in outcomes between direct surgical treatment and delayed surgical treatment, regardless of day and night. This is due to the fact that postponing surgical treatment to office hours implies a delay in surgical treatment. However, in our literature evaluation the articles of Aydogmus et al. [14], Wendling-Keim et al. [16] and Okkaoglu [18] assessed waiting time, but reported no association between waiting time and inferior radiological or clinical outcomes. Furthermore, an extensive review was published on delaying supracondylar humerus fracture surgery, regardless of day and night [21]. This review assessed the outcomes of 1735 patients from 12 articles, and evaluated the functional outcomes of early surgical treatment compared with delayed surgical treatment. The findings of this review are in accordance with our results, as the authors found no strong evidence that delaying surgical treatment influences the outcomes of surgery negatively or positively. This was confirmed by a more recent article of Shon et al. on Gartland type III fractures, in which no differences were reported for clinical outcomes of early and delayed surgery, as long as performed within 24 h [22].

4.4. Strengths and Limitations of This Study

To our knowledge, this is the first review that compares the outcomes of surgical treatment during office hours vs. after hours for pediatric supracondylar humerus fractures. There are some factors that should be taken into consideration when interpreting our results. As for all review studies, our study is as strong as its included literature. First of all, only six relevant articles were found. All of these are retrospective and with methodological limitations. Also, four out of six articles have a serious risk of bias according to the ROBINS-I criteria. Furthermore, the aforementioned confounding by indication is likely to be present. Paci et al. [15] reported this effect and was the only study making an effort to minimize this bias by using multivariable logistic regression in order to control for differences in baseline characteristics. The aforementioned performance bias is also likely to be present in the included articles. The studies of Aydogmus et al. [14] and Tuomilehto et al. [19] indeed found more surgeries performed by a fellow during after-hours compared with office hours. Wendling-Keim et al. [16] reported no significant difference, however, in the rate of complications between more and less experienced surgeons. The other studies did not report on this topic. Other limitations to the current study are that all six studies have relatively small patient groups, and quite heterogeneous outcome measures.

4.5. Conclusions and Recommendations

We found weak evidence for inferior reduction quality and more complications when performing after-hours surgery, which might be caused by confounding by indication. Clinical implications of this weak evidence seem limited: no significant differences were reported in any of the articles for other outcomes in follow-up, including complications and postoperative elbow function. Postponing surgery to office-hours generally coincides with the consultant surgeon more often as the primary surgeon, and with shorter operative time. Additionally, literature comparing acute vs. delayed surgery of pediatric supracondylar humerus fractures reveals no significant influence on surgical outcome.

In conclusion, it appears generally safe to postpone surgery for Gartland type II, III and IV fractures to office hours if circumstances are not optimal for surgery (e.g., no dedicated surgeon available), and if there is no medical contraindication. However, as literature on this topic is scarce and subject to various biases, more research with a higher level-of-evidence is needed to make more definite conclusions and recommendations for clinical practice. Long-term results, functional scores and the influence of surgeon experience would be key topics for further research on supracondylar humerus fractures.

Author Contributions: Conceptualization: S.E.S.T., P.T.P.W.B., P.B.d.W. and H.J.L.v.d.H.; methodology: S.E.S.T., P.T.P.W.B., P.B.d.W. and H.J.L.v.d.H.; validation: S.E.S.T., P.T.P.W.B., P.B.d.W. and H.J.L.v.d.H.; formal analysis: S.E.S.T.; investigation: S.E.S.T., P.T.P.W.B., P.B.d.W. and H.J.L.v.d.H.; data curation: S.E.S.T.; writing—original draft preparation: S.E.S.T.; writing—review and editing: P.T.P.W.B., P.B.d.W. and H.J.L.v.d.H.; visualization: S.E.S.T.; supervision: S.E.S.T., P.T.P.W.B., P.B.d.W. and H.J.L.v.d.H.; project administration: S.E.S.T. All authors have read and agreed to the published version of the manuscript.

Funding: This research received no external funding.

Institutional Review Board Statement: Not applicable.

Informed Consent Statement: Not applicable.

Data Availability Statement: Not applicable.

Acknowledgments: We thank J. W. Schoones, librarian of the Leiden University Medical Center, for help with our PICO search strategy.

Conflicts of Interest: The authors declare no conflict of interest.

Appendix A.

Pubmed Search strategy of the present study (conducted April 2021)

((("supracondylar humerus fracture"[tw] OR "supracondylar humerus fractures"[tw] OR "supracondylar humeral fracture"[tw] OR "supracondylar humeral fractures"[tw] OR (("Humeral Fractures"[Mesh] OR "humerus fracture"[tw] OR "humerus fractures"[tw] OR "humeral fracture"[tw] OR "humeral fractures"[tw]) AND ("supracondylar"[tw] OR supracondyl*[tw])) OR supracondyl*[tw]) AND ("Night Care"[mesh] OR "night"[tw] OR "nights"[tw] OR "nighttime"[tw] OR "night time"[tw] OR night*[tw] OR "overtime"[tw] OR "after-hours"[tw] OR "Sleep Deprivation"[mesh] OR "Shift Work Schedule"[mesh] OR "office hours"[tw] OR "daytime"[tw] OR nocturnal*[tw]) AND ("child"[tw] OR "Child"[Mesh] OR "child"[tw] OR "children"[tw] OR "Infant"[Mesh] OR "infant"[tw] OR "infants"[tw] OR "infancy"[tw] OR "newborn"[tw] OR "newborns"[tw] OR "new-born"[tw] OR "new-borns"[tw] OR "neonate"[tw] OR "neonates"[tw] OR "neonatal"[tw] OR "neonate"[tw] OR "neo-nates"[tw] OR "neo-natal"[tw] OR "neonatology"[tw] OR "NICU"[tw] OR "premature"[tw] OR "prematures"[tw] OR "pre-mature"[tw] OR "pre-matures"[tw] OR "preterm"[tw] OR "pre-term"[tw] OR "postnatal"[tw] OR "post-natal"[tw] OR "baby"[tw] OR "babies"[tw] OR "suckling"[tw] OR "sucklings"[tw] OR "toddler"[tw] OR "toddlers"[tw] OR "childhood"[tw] OR "schoolchild"[tw] OR "schoolchildren"[tw] OR "childcare"[tw] OR "child-care"[tw] OR "young"[tw] OR "youngster"[tw] OR "youngsters"[tw] OR "preschool"[tw] OR "pre-school"[tw] OR "kid"[tw] OR "kids"[tw] OR "boy"[tw] OR "boys"[tw]

OR "girl"[tw] OR "girls"[tw] OR "Adolescent"[Mesh] OR "adolescent"[tw] OR "adolescents"[tw] OR "adolescence"[tw] OR "pre-adolescent"[tw] OR "pre-adolescents"[tw] OR "pre-adolescence"[tw] OR "schoolage"[tw] OR "schoolboy"[tw] OR "schoolboys"[tw] OR "schoolgirl"[tw] OR "schoolgirls"[tw] OR "pre-puber"[tw] OR "pre-pubers"[tw] OR "pre-puberty"[tw] OR "prepuber"[tw] OR "prepubers"[tw] OR "prepuberty"[tw] OR "puber"[tw] OR "pubers"[tw] OR "puberty"[tw] OR "puberal"[tw] OR "teenager"[tw] OR "teenagers"[tw] OR "teens"[tw] OR "youth"[tw] OR "youths"[tw] OR "underaged"[tw] OR "under-aged"[tw] OR "Pediatrics"[Mesh] OR "Pediatric"[tw] OR "Pediatrics"[tw] OR "Paediatric"[tw] OR "Paediatrics"[tw] OR "PICU"[tw] OR ("child"[all fields] NOT child[au]) OR children*[all fields] OR schoolchild*[all fields] OR "infant"[all fields] OR "infants"[all fields] OR "infancy"[all fields] OR adolesc*[all fields] OR pediat*[all fields] OR paediat*[all fields] OR neonat*[all fields] OR toddler*[all fields] OR "teen"[all fields] OR "teens"[all fields] OR teenager*[all fields] OR preteen*[all fields] OR newborn*[all fields] OR postneonat*[all fields] OR postnatal*[all fields] OR "puberty"[all fields] OR preschool*[all fields] OR suckling*[all fields] OR "juvenile"[all fields] OR "new born"[all fields] OR "new borns"[all fields] OR new-born*[all fields] OR neo-nat*[all fields] OR neonat*[all fields] OR perinat*[all fields] OR underag*[all fields] OR "under age"[all fields] OR "under aged"[all fields] OR youth*[all fields] OR pubescen*[all fields] OR prepubescen*[all fields] OR "prepuberty"[all fields] OR "school age"[all fields] OR "schoolage"[all fields] OR "school ages"[all fields] OR schoolage*[all fields] OR "one year old"[tw] OR "two year old"[tw] OR "three year old"[tw] OR "four year old"[tw] OR "five year old"[tw] OR "six year old"[tw] OR "seven year old"[tw] OR "eight year old"[tw] OR "nine year old"[tw] OR "ten year old"[tw] OR "eleven year old"[tw] OR "twelve year old"[tw] OR "thirteen year old"[tw] OR "fourteen year old"[tw] OR "fifteen year old"[tw] OR "sixteen year old"[tw] OR "seventeen year old"[tw] OR "eighteen year old"[tw] OR "1 year old"[tw] OR "2 year old"[tw] OR "3 year old"[tw] OR "4 year old"[tw] OR "5 year old"[tw] OR "6 year old"[tw] OR "7 year old"[tw] OR "8 year old"[tw] OR "9 year old"[tw] OR "10 year old"[tw] OR "11 year old"[tw] OR "12 year old"[tw] OR "13 year old"[tw] OR "14 year old"[tw] OR "15 year old"[tw] OR "16 year old"[tw] OR "17 year old"[tw] OR "18 year old"[tw] OR "two years old"[tw] OR "three years old"[tw] OR "four years old"[tw] OR "five years old"[tw] OR "six years old"[tw] OR "seven years old"[tw] OR "eight years old"[tw] OR "nine years old"[tw] OR "ten years old"[tw] OR "eleven years old"[tw] OR "twelve years old"[tw] OR "thirteen years old"[tw] OR "fourteen years old"[tw] OR "fifteen years old"[tw] OR "sixteen years old"[tw] OR "seventeen years old"[tw] OR "eighteen years old"[tw] OR "2 years old"[tw] OR "3 years old"[tw] OR "4 years old"[tw] OR "5 years old"[tw] OR "6 years old"[tw] OR "7 years old"[tw] OR "8 years old"[tw] OR "9 years old"[tw] OR "10 years old"[tw] OR "11 years old"[tw] OR "12 years old"[tw] OR "13 years old"[tw] OR "14 years old"[tw] OR "15 years old"[tw] OR "16 years old"[tw] OR "17 years old"[tw] OR "18 years old"[tw]))

Appendix B. Risk of Bias of the Articles Included According to the ROBINS-I Criteria

Article	Aydogmus et al.	Paci et al.	Wendling-Keim et al.	Balakumar et al.
Pre-intervention				
Bias due to confounding	Moderate risk	Moderate risk	Moderate risk	Serious risk
Bias in selection of participants into the study	Low risk	Low risk	Low risk	Low risk
At intervention				
Bias in classification of interventions	Serious risk	Moderate risk	Serious risk	Serious risk
Post-intervention				
Bias due to deviations from intended interventions	Low risk	Low risk	Low risk	Low risk
Bias due to missing data	Low risk	Low risk	Low risk	Low risk
Bias in measurement of outcomes	Moderate risk	Moderate risk	Low risk	Moderate risk
Bias in selection of the reported result	Low risk	Low risk	Low risk	Low risk
Total risk of bias score	Serious risk	Moderate risk	Serious risk	Serious risk

References

1. Saeed, W.; Waseem, M. *Elbow Fractures Overview*; StatPearls: Treasure Island, FL, USA, 2019.
2. Barr, L.V. Paediatric supracondylar humeral fractures: Epidemiology, mechanisms and incidence during school holidays. *J. Child. Orthop.* **2014**, *8*, 167–170. [CrossRef] [PubMed]
3. Marson, B.; Craxford, S.; Price, K.R.; Ollivere, B.J. Interventions for treating supracondylar elbow fractures in children. *Cochrane Database Syst. Rev.* **2020**. [CrossRef]
4. Scherl, S.A.; Schmidt, A. Pediatric trauma: Getting through the night. *Instr. Course Lect.* **2010**, *59*, 455–463. [PubMed]
5. Tomaszewski, R.; Wozowicz, A.; Wysocka-Wojakiewicz, P. Analysis of Early Neurovascular Complications of Pediatric Supracondylar Humerus Fractures: A Long-Term Observation. *BioMed Res. Int.* **2017**, *2017*, 1–5. [CrossRef] [PubMed]
6. Gartland, J.J. Management of supracondylar fractures of the humerus in children. *Surg. Gynecol. Obstet.* **1959**, *109*, 145–154. [PubMed]
7. Leitch, K.; Kay, R.; Femino, J.; Tolo, V.; Storer, S.; Skaggs, D. Treatment of Multidirectionally Unstable Supracondylar Humeral Fractures in Children. *J. Bone Jt. Surg.* **2006**, *88*, 980–985. [CrossRef] [PubMed]
8. Sahu, R.L. Percutaneous K-wire fixation in paediatric Supracondylar fractures of humerus: A retrospective study. *Niger. Med. J.* **2013**, *54*, 329–334. [CrossRef] [PubMed]
9. Halvachizadeh, S.; Teuber, H.; Cinelli, P.; Allemann, F.; Pape, H.-C.; Neuhaus, V. Does the time of day in orthopedic trauma surgery affect mortality and complication rates? *Patient Saf. Surg.* **2019**, *13*, 1–8. [CrossRef] [PubMed]
10. Chacko, A.T.; Ramirez, M.; Ramappa, A.J.; Richardson, L.C.; Appleton, P.T.; Rodriguez, E.K. Does Late Night Hip Surgery Affect Outcome? *J. Trauma: Inj. Infect. Crit. Care* **2011**, *71*, 447–453. [CrossRef] [PubMed]
11. Santos, C.M.D.C.; Pimenta, C.A.D.M.; Nobre, M.R.C. The PICO strategy for the research question construction and evidence search. *Rev. Latino-Am. Enferm.* **2007**, *15*, 508–511. [CrossRef] [PubMed]
12. What is GRADE? Available online: https://bestpractice.bmj.com/info/toolkit/learn-ebm/what-is-grade/ (accessed on 20 June 2021).
13. Sterne, J.A.C.; Hernán, M.A.; Reeves, B.C.; Savović, J.; Berkman, N.D.; Viswanathan, M.; Henry, D.; Altman, D.G.; Ansari, M.T.; Boutron, I.; et al. ROBINS-I: A tool for assessing risk of bias in non-randomised studies of interventions. *BMJ* **2016**, *355*, i4919. [CrossRef] [PubMed]
14. Aydoğmuş, S.; Duymuş, T.M.; Keçeci, T.; Adiyeke, L.; Kafadar, A.B. Comparison of daytime and after-hours surgical treatment of supracondylar humeral fractures in children. *J. Pediatr. Orthop. B* **2017**, *26*, 400–404. [CrossRef] [PubMed]
15. Paci, G.M.; Tileston, K.R.; Vorhies, J.S.; Bishop, J.A. Pediatric Supracondylar Humerus Fractures: Does After-Hours Treatment Influence Outcomes? *J. Orthop. Trauma* **2018**, *32*, e215–e220. [CrossRef] [PubMed]
16. Wendling-Keim, D.S.; Binder, M.; Dietz, H.; Lehner, M. Prognostic Factors for the Outcome of Supracondylar Humeral Fractures in Children. *Orthop. Surg.* **2019**, *11*, 690–697. [CrossRef] [PubMed]
17. Madhuri, V.; Balakumar, B. A retrospective analysis of loss of reduction in operated supracondylar humerus fractures. *Indian J. Orthop.* **2012**, *46*, 690–697. [CrossRef] [PubMed]

18. Okkaoglu, M.C.; Ozdemir, F.E.; Ozdemir, E.; Karaduman, M.; Ates, A.; Altay, M. Is there an optimal timing for surgical treatment of pediatric supracondylar humerus fractures in the first 24 h? *J. Orthop. Surg. Res.* **2021**, *16*, 1–6. [CrossRef] [PubMed]
19. Tuomilehto, N.; Sommarhem, A.; Salminen, P.; Nietosvaara, A.Y. Postponing surgery of paediatric supracondylar humerus fractures to office hours increases consultant attendance in operations and saves operative room time. *J. Child. Orthop.* **2018**, *12*, 288–293. [CrossRef] [PubMed]
20. Carter, C.T.; Bertrand, S.L.; Cearley, D.M. Management of pediatric type III supracondylar humerus fractures in the United States: Results of a national survey of pediatric orthopaedic surgeons. *J. Pediatr. Orthop.* **2013**, *33*, 750–754. [CrossRef] [PubMed]
21. Farrow, L.; Ablett, A.D.; Mills, L.; Barker, S. Early versus delayed surgery for paediatric supracondylar humeral fractures in the absence of vascular compromise: A systematic review and meta-analysis. *Bone Joint J.* **2018**, *100-B*, 1535–1541. [CrossRef] [PubMed]
22. Shon, H.-C.; Kim, J.W.; Shin, H.-K.; Kim, E.; Park, S.-J.; Park, J.K.; Song, S.; Park, J.H. Does the timing of surgery affect outcomes of gartland type III supracondylar fractures in children? *Pediatr. Traumatol. Orthop. Reconstr. Surg.* **2019**, *7*, 25–32. [CrossRef]

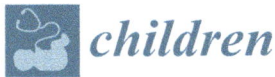

Article

Diagnosis and Treatment of Children with a Radiological Fat Pad Sign without Visible Elbow Fracture Vary Widely: An International Online Survey and Development of an Objective Definition

Maximiliaan A. Poppelaars [1,*], Denise Eygendaal [2], Bertram The [1], Iris van Oost [3] and Christiaan J. A. van Bergen [1]

1. Department of Orthopaedic Surgery, Amphia Hospital, 4818 CK Breda, The Netherlands; bthe@amphia.nl (B.T.); cvanbergen@amphia.nl (C.J.A.v.B.)
2. Department of Orthopaedic and Sports Medicine, Erasmus Medical Centre, 3015 GD Rotterdam, The Netherlands; d.eygendaal@erasmusmc.nl
3. Foundation for Orthopaedic Research, Care & Education, Amphia Hospital, 4818 CK Breda, The Netherlands; ivanoost@amphia.nl
* Correspondence: mpoppelaars3@amphia.nl

Abstract: Children often present at the emergency department with a suspected elbow fracture. Sometimes, the only radiological finding is a 'fat pad sign' (FPS) as a result of hydrops or haemarthros. This sign could either be the result of a fracture, or be due to an intra-articular haematoma without a concomitant fracture. There are no uniform treatment guidelines for this common population. The aims of this study were (1) to obtain insight into FPS definition, diagnosis, and treatment amongst international colleagues, and (2) to identify a uniform definition based on radiographic measurements with optimal cut-off points via a receiver operating characteristic (ROC) curve. An online international survey was set up to assess the diagnostic and treatment strategies, criteria, and definitions of the FPS, the probability of an occult fracture, and the presence of an anterior and/or posterior FPS on 20 radiographs. Additionally, the research team performed radiographic measurements to identify cut-off values for a positive FPS, as well as test–retest reliability and inter-rater reliability via intraclass correlation coefficients (ICC). A total of 133 (paediatric) orthopaedic surgeons completed the survey. Definitions, further diagnostics, and treatments varied considerably amongst respondents. Angle measurements of the fat pad as related to the humeral axis line showed the highest reliability (test–retest ICC, 0.95 (95% CI 0.88–0.98); inter-rater ICC, 0.95 (95% CI 0.91–0.98)). A cut-off angle of 16° was defined a positive anterior FPS (sensitivity, 1.00; specificity, 0.87; accuracy, 99%), based on the respondents' assessment of the radiographs in combination with the research team's measurements. Any visible posterior fat pad was defined as a positive posterior FPS. This study provides insight into the current diagnosis and treatment of children with a radiological fat pad sign of the elbow. A clear, objective definition of a positive anterior FPS was identified as a $\geq 16°$ angle with respect to the anterior humeral line.

Keywords: fat pad sign (FPS); children; elbow; survey; receiver operating characteristic (ROC); intraclass correlation coefficients (ICC); anterior fat pad sign (AFPS); posterior fat pad sign (PFPS)

Citation: Poppelaars, M.A.; Eygendaal, D.; The, B.; van Oost, I.; van Bergen, C.J.A. Diagnosis and Treatment of Children with a Radiological Fat Pad Sign without Visible Elbow Fracture Vary Widely: An International Online Survey and Development of an Objective Definition. *Children* 2022, 9, 950. https://doi.org/10.3390/children9070950

Academic Editor: Vito Pavone

Received: 30 May 2022
Accepted: 22 June 2022
Published: 25 June 2022

Publisher's Note: MDPI stays neutral with regard to jurisdictional claims in published maps and institutional affiliations.

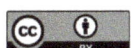

Copyright: © 2022 by the authors. Licensee MDPI, Basel, Switzerland. This article is an open access article distributed under the terms and conditions of the Creative Commons Attribution (CC BY) license (https://creativecommons.org/licenses/by/4.0/).

1. Introduction

Children often present at the emergency department with suspicion of a fracture in the elbow. The cumulative incidence of bone fracture during childhood is 40% for boys and 28% for girls between 6–16 years [1]. Approximately 28% of all paediatric fractures are elbow fractures [2]. Paediatric elbow fractures occur in approximately 25% at the distal humerus, but overall, the numbers of various types of elbow fractures vary [3,4] A prolonged time interval between injury and treatment could result in negative treatment outcomes. Unrecognised or misdiagnosed fractures presenting more than 3 weeks after the injury could result in malunion, delayed union, or non-union. [5]

The standard method of imaging are radiographs in anteroposterior and lateral directions to detect a potential fracture. Sometimes, the only finding is a fat pad sign (FPS) as a result of hydrops or haemarthros without a visible fracture. The FPS is an intra-articular, but extrasynovial, joint effusion in which the fat pad becomes elevated. Physiologically, a small anterior fat pad is usually visible. In contrast, the posterior fat pad is located in the olecranon fossa and only becomes visible in case of joint effusion. The trauma to the elbow causes intra-articular bleeding, resulting in the fat pad moving away from the joint and thus becoming visible as a triangular shape on the lateral radiographic view [6]. In such a case, the anterior and/or posterior FPS (AFPS, PFPS) could be a sign of an occult fracture [7,8].

Currently, there is no clear definition for the FPS, which may result in variations in diagnosis and treatment [9]. Usually, these children are treated with plaster and are scheduled for an orthopaedic and possibly radiographic follow-up [10]. In a number of cases, this may lead to overtreatment. Unnecessary immobilisation has disadvantages, including disability, healthcare costs, muscle atrophy, and demineralisation of the bone [10]. On the other hand, there are also fractures that require low-threshold surgical treatment, e.g., displaced lateral condyle fractures [11]. Other recent findings in the literature are the frequently missed injuries around the elbow, called the TRASH (the radiographic appearance seemed harmless) lesions [12]. Those lesions should warrant additional imaging methods, such as ultrasound, MRI, or CT, for correct diagnosis. Misdiagnosis is accountable for a large part of the complications [10]. The incidence and types of occult fractures in children with a positive FPS is difficult to assess, as the variety of definitions of FPS currently in use is high [9]. A clearer definition is mandatory to formulate a proper treatment rationale.

The aim of this study was first to assess—through an international online survey—the definition, work-up, and treatment of children with a positive FPS without visible fracture that are currently in use. Second, this study aimed to develop a clear, objective definition of an FPS that is based on radiographic measurements and international agreement on the presence of an FPS.

2. Materials and Methods

An online international survey was set up to assess the criteria and definitions of the AFPS and PFPS, the probability of occult fractures, diagnostic and treatment strategies, and the presence or absence of the FPS on 20 radiographs. The survey was distributed amongst members of the European Paediatric Orthopaedic Society (EPOS) and the European Society for Surgery of the Shoulder and the Elbow (SECEC), as well as national orthopaedic trauma, paediatric orthopaedic, and upper limb societies. Open questions, multiple-choice questions, and radiographs were built into the online platform of Survey Monkey (Supplementary Materials). The study was approved by the medical research ethic committee of Utrecht (MEC-U) on 2 April 2021 under registration number W21.087.

In addition, the respondents indicated whether the AFPS and/or PFPS was present (yes/no) on 20 radiographs. The radiographs were selected from a local database of elbow radiographs of children (10 females, 7 right side, age 7–16) between 2018 and 2021, and ranged from no visible FPS to an extreme FPS without other visible pathology. Only answers of the responders who fully completed the online survey were analysed.

Furthermore, radiographic measurements were performed on the same radiographs by the research team to identify cut-off values for a positive FPS. Three paediatric orthopaedic trauma and elbow surgeons and two trained researchers (blinded to the respondents' answers) independently measured two possible objective measures of an FPS on each of the 20 radiographs, namely, (1) the angle between the fat pad and humerus, and (2) the size of the fat pad relative to the humerus diameter (Figure 1). The averages of the five researchers' measurements were used as the final measurement of each radiograph. The radiographs were measured again eight weeks later by the first author in a different order; the author was blinded to the first series of measurements to assess test–retest reliability.

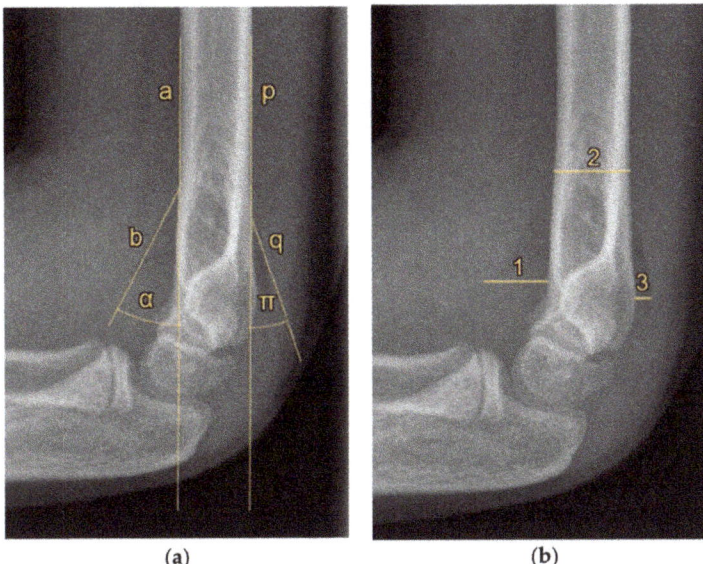

(a) (b)

Figure 1. Radiographic measurements of the anterior and posterior fat pad signs. (**a**) Angle measurements. a: line along the anterior side of the humerus shaft; b: line indicating the anterior fat pad; α: angle measurement of the anterior fat pad; p: line along the posterior side of the humerus shaft; q: line indicating the posterior fat pad; π: angle measurement of the posterior fat pad. (**b**) Distance measurements—1: maximum perpendicular distance of the anterior fat pad to the humerus; 2: humerus diameter measured at the proximal level of the anterior fat pad; 3: maximum perpendicular distance of the posterior fat pad to the humerus. The anterior fat pad distance was indicated by 1 divided by 2; the posterior fat pad distance was indicated by 3 divided by 2.

Descriptive statistics were described for the outcomes of the survey. The test–retest and interobserver reliability of the radiographic measurements were analysed with use of intraclass correlation coefficients (ICC) [13]. The measurements with the highest ICCs (i.e., angle or distance measurements) were plotted against the percentages of positive answers to the presence or absence of an FPS by the respondents for each radiograph. This was performed in order to determine the measurement values at which the majority of professionals agreed about the presence of the AFPS and PFPS.

Further analysis was carried out with use of receiver operating characteristic (ROC) curves to determine the optimal cut-off value of a positive AFPS with corresponding sensitivity and specificity. For the purpose of the definition development, three agreement levels on the presence of an FPS were analysed with ROC curves (i.e., 50%, 60%, and 70% of the respondents). The agreement level with the highest area under the curve (AUC) was chosen to determine the optimal cut-off value. All analyses were performed using the software package SPSS (IBM SPSS, version 28, Armonk, NY, USA).

3. Results

There were a total of 198 respondents who started the survey, of whom 133 completed the survey entirely. The distribution of experience of the responding physicians was fairly widespread (Table 1). The most common subspecialty was paediatric orthopaedic surgery ($n = 49$).

Table 1. Respondent characteristics (n = 133).

Survey Questions	Responses, n (%)
How many paediatric elbow injuries do you treat annually?	
<10	36 (27.1)
10–20	41 (30.8)
20–50	35 (26.3)
>50	21 (15.8)
How many years have you been in practice as an (orthopaedic or trauma) surgeon?	
0	14 (10.5)
1–5	31 (23.3)
6–10	18 (13.6)
>10	70 (52.6)
What is your expertise?	
Paediatric orthopaedic surgeon	49 (36.7)
Orthopaedic upper limb surgeon	28 (21.1)
Orthopaedic trauma surgeon	19 (14.3)
Orthopaedic resident	18 (13.5)
General orthopaedic surgeon	13 (9.8)
General trauma surgeon	1 (0.8)
Other	5 (3.8)

3.1. Definition

The definitions of the FPS that the respondents listed varied considerably. The most commonly used terms included (sail) sign, dark shape, black shadow, elevated capsule, and darkened shade.

3.2. Probability of Occult Fracture

The survey showed that in the case of a positive FPS, it was expected that there is an occult fracture in an average of 73.3% (SD 18.2%) of cases. The estimated fracture rate was not significantly dependent on the respondents' clinical experience.

3.3. Diagnosis and Treatment

A supracondylar humerus fracture was considered the most common fracture in case of a positive fat pad sign without visible fracture, followed by radial head and neck fractures (Table 2). Most participants used repeated radiography after 1 week in the further diagnostic work-up. Some participants replied 'other' (n = 15), mostly described by 'depending on clinical examination'. Regarding standard treatment, the majority (n = 70) used plaster or a cast, but again, a wide variety was observed.

Table 2. Diagnosis and treatment (n = 133).

Survey Questions	Responses, n (%)
What is the most probable fracture in case of a positive fat pad sign without visible fracture?	
Supracondylar	87 (65.4)
Radial head	18 (13.5)
Radial neck	11 (8.3)
Lateral condyle fracture	6 (4.5)
Medial epicondyle	5 (3.8)
Other	4 (3.0)
Olecranon	2 (1.5)
What is your usual further diagnostic work-up?	
Repeat radiographs after 1 week	42 (31.6)
No further imaging	35 (26.3)
Repeat radiographs on indication	30 (22.6)
Other	15 (11.3)
CT	7 (5.2)
MRI	4 (3.0)

Table 2. Cont.

Survey Questions	Responses, n (%)
What is your standard treatment?	
Plaster/casting	70 (52.6)
Other	25 (18.8)
No standard treatment	11 (8.3)
Pressure bandage	11 (8.3)
Functional treatment (i.e., no immobilisation)	8 (6.0)
Sling	8 (6.0)

3.4. Radiographic Evaluation

The reliability of the angular and distance measurements of the AFPS and PFPS are shown in Table 3.

Table 3. Intraclass correlation coefficients (ICCs) for radiographic measurements of the anterior (AFPS) and posterior fat pad sign (PFPS).

	Intraclass Correlation Coefficient	95% Confidence Interval
Anterior angle measurement (α) *		
Test–retest	0.95	0.88–0.98
Interobserver	0.95	0.91–0.98
Posterior angle measurement (π) *		
Test–retest	0.91	0.41–0.99
Interobserver	0.95	0.91–0.98
Perpendicular ratios AFPS (1/2) *		
Test–retest	0.76	0.42–0.91
Interobserver	0.74	0.38–0.89
Perpendicular ratios PFPS (3/2) *		
Test–retest	0.91	0.47–0.99
Interobserver	0.89	0.71–0.93

* See Figure 1 for corresponding measurements.

As the AFPS angle measurements (α) and the PFPS angle measurement (π) were most reliable, these were used to determine cut-off values of the proposed definitions.

An overview of radiographic angle measurements and corresponding percentages of positive answers for the presence of an AFPS is shown in Figure 2.

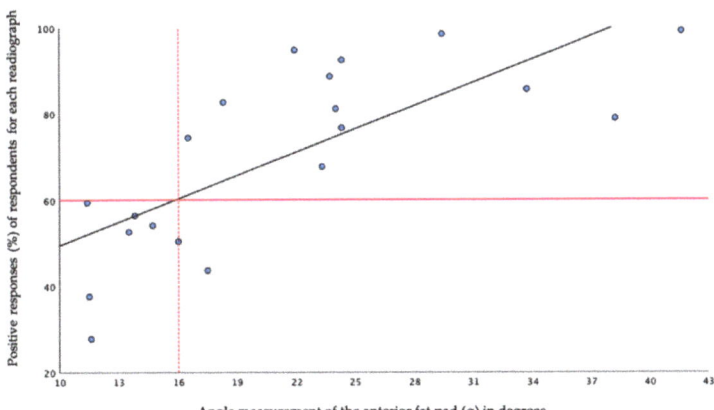

Figure 2. Scatter plot showing the mean angle measurements plotted against the percentages of positive respondents for the presence of an AFPS, assessed on the 20 radiographs. The horizontal red line indicates the 60% level of agreement of the respondents. The vertical dotted red line shows the mean angle at which at least 60% of the respondents indicated the presence of the AFPS.

The analysed agreement levels of 50%, 60%, and 70% corresponded with an AUC of 0.84 (95% CI 0.64–1.00), 0.99 (95% CI 0.96–1.00), and 0.96 (95% CI 0.96–1.00), respectively. The 60% level of agreement was thus chosen to define the cut-off values of objective FPS definitions, because of the highest AUC. For the AFPS, this resulted in a cut-off value of 16° for a positive AFPS (see Figure 2).

Out of the 20 radiographs, there were 5 measurable posterior fat pads (angle π, 15.6–23.9°). The percentages of positive respondents for the visible posterior fat pads was high (72.9–100%), while those of the invisible posterior fat pads were low (0.8–34.6%). Therefore, if a posterior fat pad was visible, it was defined as positive.

The accompanying ROC curve for the objective AFPS definition of 16° had an AUC of 0.99 (95% CI 0.96–1.00) (Figure 3). Thus, the model will be able to classify 99% correctly in a given randomly selected positive AFPS and a randomly selected negative AFPS. The overall accuracy of determining the presence of a AFPS with a cut-off value of 16° was 99% (sensitivity 1.00, specificity 0.87). The ROC curve for the PFPS had an AUC of 1.00 (95% CI 1.00–1.00) (sensitivity 1.00, specificity 1.00).

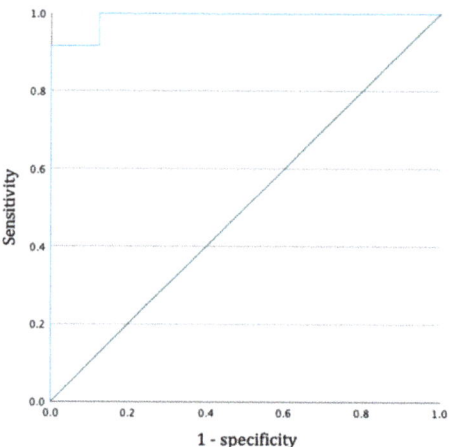

Figure 3. Receiver operating characteristic (ROC) curve for the 16-degree cut-off value of the anterior fat pad sign (α).

4. Discussion

Norell first described the radiological fat pad sign of the elbow [14] in 1954. As stated in previous research, neglected paediatric elbow fractures could result in serious long-term consequences [5,11]. Today, the FPS after a traumatic event in children is still a subject within orthopaedics that lacks clarity in terms of definition, additional imaging, and guidelines for treatment. The first objective of this study was to provide more insight into the variety of definitions, work-ups, and treatments of children with a positive FPS in a large group of orthopaedic surgeons. The responses to the survey amongst the orthopaedic community varied widely. The results of the present study form an important basis in the process of developing more uniform diagnostic and treatment guidelines for children with a positive FPS without visible fracture.

Another notable result of the survey was the high expected probability of an occult fracture in the case of a positive FPS. The orthopaedic surgeons indicated, on average, that in 73.3% (SD 18.2%) of the cases with a positive FPS, they assumed the presence of an occult fracture. However, these figures are somewhat lower in the published literature. Kappelhof et al., in a meta-analysis, showed that a fracture is actually present in only 45% of children with a positive FPS and no visible fracture, based on further imaging [9].

An objective definition of a positive fat pad sign is not available in the literature [9]. Likewise, the variety in answers on definitions in the survey also highlight the need for a uniform and objective definition of an FPS. Therefore, the second aim of the study was to develop an objective definition of a positive FPS. It was found that a cut-off angle of 16° relative to the anterior humerus line indicates a positive anterior fat pad, with high reliability (ICC, 95%) and accuracy (AUC, 99%). A posterior fat pad sign was defined as any visible posterior fat pad on the lateral elbow radiograph. These findings are a first but important step towards more uniform diagnostic and treatment protocols.

A potential limitation of this study is that the development of the objective FPS definition is based on the judgements of experts with 60% agreement. At the start of the study, a range of agreements was set up in order to determine the optimal cut-off value. As described previously, determining consensus via expert panels is still a challenging element of diagnostic research [15]. By determining a cut-off value in this way, an attempt was made to do so as accurately as possible. Because of the high number of participants (n = 133), we believe these judgements reflect the general assessment of the FPS on paediatric elbow radiographs and, therefore, are the best alternative to a reference standard diagnostic method. Furthermore, the 20 radiographs, with a full range from no FPS to an extreme FPS, are considered a representative sample of the actual population. The sample could, therefore, be used reliably to assess the degree of maximum uncertainty in order to establish the optimal cut-off value for the definition of a positive FPS.

The current study provides opportunities for future research to improve the care for the investigated population. One question is whether the projection of the radiological images will affect the appearance of the FPS. Furthermore, the severity of the FPS can be studied in relation to occult fractures in children. Finally, enhanced imaging may assist physicians in optimizing patient-specific diagnoses and treatments.

5. Conclusions

Definitions, diagnoses, and treatments of children with a positive FPS vary considerably in the orthopaedic community. This study provides a clear and objective AFPS definition of a 16-degree angle relative to the humerus line.

Supplementary Materials: The following are available online at https://www.mdpi.com/article/10.3390/children9070950/s1, Online Survey.

Author Contributions: Conceptualization, D.E. and C.J.A.v.B.; methodology, M.A.P.; formal analysis, M.A.P.; writing—original draft preparation, all authors; writing—review and editing, D.E., B.T., I.v.O. and C.J.A.v.B.; supervision, C.J.A.v.B.; project administration, C.J.A.v.B. All authors have read and agreed to the published version of the manuscript.

Funding: This research received no external funding.

Institutional Review Board Statement: Not applicable.

Informed Consent Statement: Not applicable.

Acknowledgments: We would like to thank the following colleagues, who kindly completed the online survey: J. Aguilar-Gonzalez; T. Alves-da-Silva; J. Amaya; A. Andreacchio; A. Angelliaume; J. Arcângelo; H. Arro; A. Balslev-Clausen; S. Bekmez; A.T. Besselaar; J.H.J.M. Bessems; N. Boeijink; J.B. Bolder; A. Borgo; G. Casellas-Garcia; N. Catena; M. Chomicki; I. Coifman; A. Cosentino; P. Cundy; J.M. de Beus; P.B. de Witte; I. De Rus; I. Delniotis; A.M. Demirtas; L.W. Diederix; P. Domos; F.U. Verstraelen; E. Gonen; M. Grigoras; V.A. Groen; N. Guindani; V. Halvorsen; R. Houben; A.P.J. Joosten; G. Jozsa; L. Kaas; A.E.B. Kleipool; T. Kraal; M.J. Kraus; P. Lascombes; W.B. Lehman; J.K.G. Louwerens; N. Lutz; K.C. Mahabier; S. Marangoz; M. Mario; B. Marson; F. Martinez; A.K. Mosterd; E.M. Nelissen; W.H. Nijhuis; S. Nota; D.E. O'Briain; J. Ovesen; P. Paolo; A. Pitsounis; A. Popchenko; A.R. Poublon; N. Pouliart; F.T.H.G. Rahusen; R. Rolink; Y. Saglam; M. Salom; E. Samara; M.M. Scarlat; O.S. Schmidt; M. Schultz; R. Schwartz; R.M. Schwend; G. Sforza; J. Snel; D.W. Sommerfeldt; A.J. Spaans; W. Spierenburg; V. Spiteri; M. Synder; C. Thevenin-Lemoine; M. Thüsing; F. Toft; J.J. Tolk; A. van Noort; A.L. van der Zwan; C.M. van den Broek; J. van de Breevaart; J.C. van Egmond.; J.H. van Linge; J.P.J. van Dijsseldonk; L. van der Heijden; M. van der Pluijm; M.J.A. van Steijn; M.P.J. van den Bekeroml; O.A.J. van der Meijden; R.P. van Hove; S.C. van Veen; T.M. van Raaij; D.R. Rad; W.M. van Wijhe;

M. van Lotten; A.M.J.S. Vervest; C.P.J. Visser; A.J.H. Vochteloo; H. Weel; S.J. Westerbos; and R.L. Wimberly.

Conflicts of Interest: The authors declare no conflict of interest.

References

1. NVVH. Fracturen Bij Kinderen—Richtlijn—Richtlijnendatabase. Available online: https://richtlijnendatabase.nl/richtlijn/fracturen_bij_kinderen/startpagina.html (accessed on 6 March 2019).
2. Hussain, S.; Dar, T.; Beigh, A.Q.; Dhar, S.; Ahad, H.; Hussain, I.; Ahmad, S. Pattern and epidemiology of pediatric musculoskeletal injuries in Kashmir valley, a retrospective single-center study of 1467 patients. *J. Pediatric Orthop. B* **2015**, *24*, 230–237. [CrossRef] [PubMed]
3. Gogola, G.R. Pediatric Humeral Condyle Fractures. *Hand Clin.* **2006**, *22*, 77–85. [CrossRef] [PubMed]
4. Yousefzadeh, D.K.; Jackson, J.H. Lipohemarthrosis of the Elbow Joint. *Radiology* **1978**, *128*, 643–645. [CrossRef] [PubMed]
5. Trisolino, G.; Antonioli, D.; Gallone, G.; Stallone, S.; Zarantonello, P.; Tanzi, P.; Olivotto, E.; Stilli, L.; Di Gennaro, G.L.; Stilli, S. Neglected Fractures of the Lateral Humeral Condyle in Children; Which Treatment for Which Condition? *Children* **2021**, *8*, 56. [CrossRef] [PubMed]
6. Blumberg, S.M.; Kunkov, S.; Crain, E.F.; Goldman, H.S. The predictive value of a normal radiographic anterior fat pad sign following elbow trauma in children. *Pediatric Emerg. Care* **2011**, *27*, 596–600. [CrossRef] [PubMed]
7. Skaggs, D.L.; Mirzayan, R. The Posterior Fat Pad Sign in Association with Occult Fracture of the Elbow in Children. *J. Bone Jt. Surg.* **1999**, *81*, 1429–1433. [CrossRef] [PubMed]
8. Al-Aubaidi, Z.; Torfing, T. The role of fat pad sign in diagnosing occult elbow fractures in the pediatric patient. *J. Pediatric Orthop. B* **2012**, *21*, 514–519. [CrossRef] [PubMed]
9. Kappelhof, B.; Roorda, B.; Poppelaars, M.A.; The, B.; Eygendaal, D.; Mulder, T.; van Bergen, C.J.A. *Occult Fractures in Children with a Radiological Fat Pad Sign the Elbow: A Meta-Analysis*; Amphia Hospital: Breda, The Netherlands, 2007.
10. Major, N.M.; Crawford, S.T. Elbow Effusions in Trauma in Adults and Children. *Am. J. Roentgenol.* **2002**, *178*, 413–418. [CrossRef] [PubMed]
11. Tan, S.; Dartnell, J.; Lim, A.; Hui, J.H. Paediatric lateral condyle fractures: A systematic review. *Arch. Orthop. Trauma Surg.* **2018**, *138*, 809–817. [CrossRef] [PubMed]
12. Patwardhan, S.; Omkaram, S. Trash lesions around the elbow: A review of approach to diagnosis and management. *Indian J. Orthop.* **2021**, *55*, 539–548. [CrossRef] [PubMed]
13. Koo, T.K.; Li, M.Y. A guideline of selecting and reporting intraclass correlation coefficients for reliability research. *J. Chiropr. Med.* **2016**, *15*, 155–163. [CrossRef] [PubMed]
14. Norell, H.-G. Roentgenologic visualization of the extracapsular fat. *Acta Radiol.* **1954**, *42*, 205–210. [CrossRef] [PubMed]
15. Bertens, L.C.; Broekhuizen, B.D.; Naaktgeboren, C.A.; Rutten, F.H.; Hoes, A.W.; van Mourik, Y.; Reitsma, J.B. Use of expert panels to define the reference standard in diagnostic research: A systematic review of published methods and reporting. *PLoS Med.* **2013**, *10*, e1001531. [CrossRef] [PubMed]

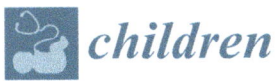

Systematic Review

Pediatric Radial Neck Fractures: A Systematic Review Regarding the Influence of Fracture Treatment on Elbow Function

Lisette C. Langenberg [1,2,3], Kimberly I. M. van den Ende [3], Max Reijman [3], G. J. (Juliën) Boersen [3] and Joost W. Colaris [3,*]

1. Centre for Orthopedic Research Alkmaar (CORAL), 1815 JD Alkmaar, The Netherlands; lc.langenberg@nwz.nl
2. Department of Orthopedic Surgery, Noordwest Ziekenhuisgroep, 1815 JD Alkmaar, The Netherlands
3. Department of Orthopedic Surgery and Sports Medicine, Erasmus MC University Medical Center Rotterdam, P.O. Box 2040, 3000 CA Rotterdam, The Netherlands; kimvandenende@gmail.com (K.I.M.v.d.E.); m.reijman@erasmusmc.nl (M.R.); j.boersen@erasmusmc.nl (G.J.B.)
* Correspondence: j.colaris@erasmusmc.nl

Abstract: Background: This review aims to identify what angulation may be accepted for the conservative treatment of pediatric radial neck fractures and how the range of motion (ROM) at follow-up is influenced by the type of fracture treatment. Patients and Methods: A PRISMA-guided systematic search was performed for studies that reported on fracture angulation, treatment details, and ROM on a minimum of five children with radial neck fractures that were followed for at least one year. Data on fracture classification, treatment, and ROM were analyzed. Results: In total, 52 studies (2420 children) were included. Sufficient patient data could be extracted from 26 publications (551 children), of which 352 children had at least one year of follow-up. ROM following the closed reduction (CR) of fractures with <30 degrees angulation was impaired in only one case. In fractures angulated over 60 degrees, K-wire fixation (Kw) resulted in a significantly better ROM than intramedullary fixation (CIMP; Kw 9.7% impaired vs. CIMP 32.6% impaired, $p = 0.01$). In more than 50% of cases that required open reduction (OR), a loss of motion occurred. Conclusions: CR is effective in fractures angulated up to 30 degrees. There may be an advantage of Kw compared to CIMP fixation in fractures angulated over 60 degrees. OR should only be attempted if CR and CRIF have failed.

Keywords: pediatric radial neck fracture; radial neck angulation; elbow motion

1. Introduction

Although radial neck fractures in children occur frequently, there is no consensus on the optimal treatment. The indication to perform a (surgical) reduction varies widely; some authors advise striving for anatomical reduction of the radial neck, and others accept up to 60° of fracture angulation [1–7].

Several treatment options are available. Closed reduction (CR) without fixation, closed reduction with intramedullary pinning (CIMP) with or without pin rotation, K-wire leverage and K-wire pinning (Kw), and open reduction or combinations of the aforementioned options may be used. There is no consensus yet on the fracture angulation threshold for surgical intervention and which surgical technique should be used.

Loss of motion is reported to be the most important cause of a poor outcome [8]. Therefore, the purpose of this systematic review was to compare the elbow function following different types of treatment in relation to the angulation of the pediatric radial neck fracture. With this research, we aimed to find out which treatment modality for different types of pediatric radial neck fractures results in the best elbow function.

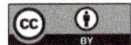

2. Materials and Methods

This study followed the guidelines of the Preferred Reporting Items for Systematic Reviews and Meta-Analyses (PRISMA). The protocol for this systematic review is registered in the PROSPERO database http://www.crd.york.ac.uk/PROSPERO/ (accessed on 7 May 2022), (registration number CRD42018088696).

2.1. Search Strategy

A health science librarian of our institution, with extensive experience in the conduct of literature searching for systematic reviews, assisted in designing and performing the search [9]. The following databases were searched: Embase, Cochrane Central Register, Medline, Web of Science, PubMed Publisher, and Google Scholar. The following main keywords were used: radial neck fracture, angulation, elbow, outcome, pronation, and supination. The search strategy for each database is outlined in Appendix A of this paper. The databases were searched from inception to 17 November 2021 (Figure 1).

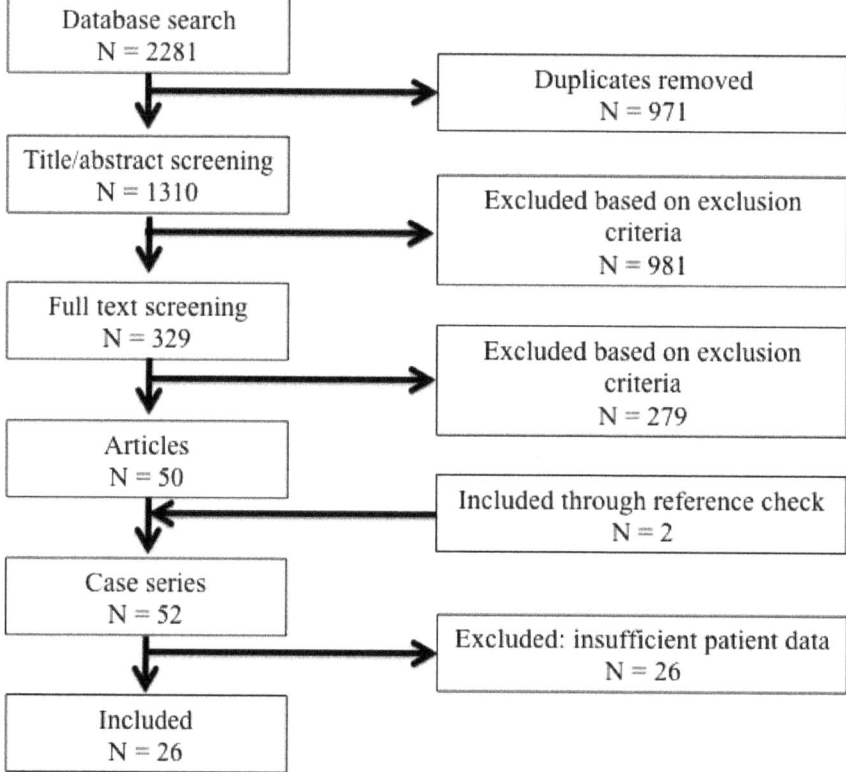

Figure 1. PRISMA-guided systematic search.

2.2. Study Selection

The results from all databases were combined, and duplicate titles were removed. Two authors (K.I.M.v.d.E. and G.J.B.) screened all titles, abstracts, and full articles independently. The inclusion and exclusion criteria are listed in Table 1. Disagreements were solved by discussion, and a final decision was made by a third reviewer (J.W.C.) if there was disagreement. Patients with less than one year of follow-up were excluded.

Table 1. Inclusion and exclusion criteria.

Inclusion Criteria	Exclusion Criteria
Prospective or retrospective follow-up study	Review/meta-analysis
≥5 children with radial neck fractures	Age > 16 years
Fracture angulation should be reported	Elbow prosthesis
Radiological imaging at presentation	Animals
Outcome: range of motion at follow-up	Less than one year follow-up
Outcome linked to fracture angulation and treatment	
Language: English, Dutch	

2.3. Risk of Bias Assessment

The risk of bias was assessed by using the prognostic checklist adapted from the Cochrane handbook for systematic reviews, chapter 7 [10] (see Table 2). Each study was scored for selection bias, information bias, and confounding. Two authors (K.I.M.v.d.E. and G.J.B.) assessed the quality of the included studies independently. If consensus was not reached after discussion, a third reviewer (M.R.) was consulted. Finally, article quality was screened using the MINORS criteria; an overview is listed in Table 3.

Table 2. Risk of bias assessment based on adapted Cochrane checklist.

Author	Selectionbias	Informationbias	Confounding
Al-Aubaidi (2012) [11]	green	orange	red
Bilal (2021) [12]	green	green	orange
Brandão (2010) [13]	green	green	green
evik (2018) [14]	green	green	green
Cha (2012) [15]	green	green	green
Cossio (2014) [16]	green	green	green
Endele (2010) [17]	green	orange	green
Falciglia (2014) [8]	orange	green	orange
Fowles (1986) [18]	green	green	green
Futami (1995) [19]	red	red	green
Gutierrez-de la Iglesia (2015) [20]	orange	green	orange
Jones (1971) [21]	green	green	green
Klitscher (2009) [22]	green	green	green
Koca (2017) [23]	green	green	green
Massetti (2020) [24]	green	green	green
Metaizeau (1993) [25]	green	green	green
Monson (2009) [26]	orange	green	orange
Shah (2020) [27]	green	green	green
Stiefel (2001) [28]	green	green	orange
Tanagho (2015) [29]	orange	red	orange
Tarallo (2013) [30]	green	green	green
Tibone (1981) [31]	green	green	green
Ugutmen (2010) [32]	green	green	green
Walcher (2000) [33]	green	green	green
Yallapragada (2020) [34]	green	orange	orange
Zhang (2016) [35]	green	orange	red

Scores: green = low risk, orange = moderate risk, red = high risk.

Table 3. Part a: Overview of included articles, part b: MINORS criteria.

(a)

Author	Year	Fracture Classification	Injury Type	N	1y FU	Mean Age in Years (Range)	Mean Follow-Up in Years (Range)	Outcome
Al-Aubaidi [11]	2012	Steele	all pt w/open physis treated with metaizeau	16	16	12 (9–15)	3.3 (1.3–6.3)	DASH
Bilal [12]	2021	>30°	>30°,intramedullary nailing (TEN)	15	15	10.1 (6.4–15.8)	2.1 (1.3–3)	Tan&Mahadev
Brandão [13]	2010	O'Brien	O'Brien type 3	28	26	8.6 (6–13)	4.3 (1.7–10)	radiologic union, ROM
evik [14]	2018	Judet	Judet 3/4	20	20	9.75 (4–13)	2.9 (1.1–7)	ROM
Cha [15]	2012	Judet	Judet 3/4	13	13	10.4 (6–13)	3.5 (2.4–4.4)	flynn score
Cossio [16]	2014	Judet	Judet 3/4	9	9	9.1 (6–12)	2.2 (1–3)	Tibone
Endele [17]	2010	Judet	all RN# in a retrospective period	54	42	8 (1–13)	4 (0.5–11)	ROM
Falciglia [8]	2014	O'Brien	all RN# in a retrospective period without success of CR or KW	24	24	7.1 (4.3–10.2)	7.1 (3.2–12.1)	MEPS
Fowles [18]	1986	<20°, >20°	all RN# in a retrospective period	23	17	9.1 (5–13)	1.5 (0.7–2.8)	ROM
Futami [19]	1995	none	angulated RN# (not specified)	10	10	9 (6–13)	u	Tibone and Stolz
Gutierrez-de la Iglesia [20]	2015	Judet	Judet 3/4	51	0	8 (3–15)	1.2 (0.7–3.3)	Tibone and Stolz, Ursei
Jones [21]	1971	15–29°, 30–59°, 60–90°	all RN# in a retrospective period	34	18	10 (5–13)	5 (1–14)	Steele
Klitscher [22]	2009	Judet	Judet 3/4	28	0	8 (5–11)	2.7 (0.5–5.6)	MEPS, Metaizeau
Koca [23]	2017	Judet	Judet 3	11	11	7.7 (6–10)	2.0 (1.7–2.7)	Leung/Peterson
Massetti [24]	2020	judet	Judet 3/4	20	0	7.8 (2–11)	0.7–3.8	MEPS
Metaizeau [25]	1993	Judet	Judet 3/4	47	47	10.7 (5–13)	4 (ns)	MEPS
Monson [26]	2009	Degrees	all RN# in a retrospecitve period	6	6	9.5 (6–11)	0.36	Morrey, Metaizeau, Steinberg, Rodriguez-Merchan
Shah [27]	2020	Judet	Judet 4	10	10	8.6 (6–12)	1 (0.8–1.3)	ROM
Stiefel [28]	2001	Judet	Judet 4	6	6	8.4 (7–10.8)	u (0.75–2.5)	Own rating system
Tanagho [29]	2015	Steele	isolated metaphyseal RN# >30°	9	9	9.6 (u)	1.6 (u)	Own rating system
Tarallo [30]	2013	Judet	Judet 3/4	20	20	11 (6–16)	3.5 (1.3–5.3)	MEPS, Metaizeau
Tibone [31]	1981	Degrees	all RN# in a retrospective period	23	23	9.2 (4–14)	3.15 (2.0–8.0)	ROM
Ugutmen [32]	2010	Judet	RN# with open growth plates	16	16	8 (6–13)	2 (1.5–3.3)	Metaizeau
Walcher [33]	2000	Judet	Judet 2/3, failed CR	5	0	7 (u)	3 (u)	ROM, own rating system

Table 3. Cont.

(a)

Author	Year	Fracture Classification	Injury Type	N	1y FU	Mean Age in Years (Range)	Mean Follow-Up in Years (Range)	Outcome
Yallapragada [34]	2020	Judet	Judet 3/4	21	0	8 (u)	0.4 (0.3–0.5)	OES, Metaizeau MEPS
Zhang [35]	2016	Judet	Judet 3/4	50	0	8.4 (5.6–13)	2 (u)	
				569	352	8.96	2.69	

(b)

Author	Year	MINORS Total	Aim	Consecutive Cases	End Points	Bias	Follow-Up	Lost to FU	Study Size
Al-Aubaidi [11]	2012	7	1	2	1	0	2	1	0
Bilal [12]	2021	6	1	1	2	1	2	0	0
Brandão [13]	2010	10	2	2	2	1	2	1	0
evik [14]	2018	10	2	2	2	2	2	0	0
Cha [15]	2012	10	2	2	2	2	2	0	0
Cossio [16]	2014	8	1	1	2	2	2	0	0
Endele [17]	2010	9	1	1	2	1	2	2	0
Falciglia [8]	2014	8	2	1	2	1	1	1	0
Fowles [18]	1986	8	1	2	1	0	2	2	0
Futami [19]	1995	2	0	0	0	0	2	0	0
Gutierrez-de la Iglesia [20]	2015	8	2	1	2	1	2	0	0
Jones [21]	1971	8	1	1	1	1	2	2	0
Klitscher [22]	2009	9	1	2	2	1	2	1	0
Koca [23]	2017	8	2	1	2	1	2	0	0
Massetti [24]	2020	5	2	1	1	2	1	0	0
Metaizeau [25]	1993	7	2	1	2	1	1	0	0
Monson [26]	2009	3	1	1	1	0	0	0	0
Shah [27]	2020	4	0	2	1	1	1	0	0
Stiefel [28]	2001	4	2	1	1	0	0	0	0
Tanagho [29]	2015	4	1	1	0	0	1	1	0
Tarallo [30]	2013	8	2	1	2	1	2	0	0

Table 3. Cont.

(a)

Author	Year	Fracture Classification	Injury Type	N	1y FU	Mean Age in Years (Range)	Mean Follow-Up in Years (Range)	Outcome
Tibone [31]	1981	9	1	2	2	1 2	1 1	0
Ugutmen [32]	2010	5	1	1	1	1 1	0	0
Walcher [33]	2000	4	1	1	0	1 1	0	0
Yallapragada [34]	2020	4	1	1	1	1 1	0	0
Zhang [35]	2016	6	2	1	1	0 2	0	0

u = unknown; RN# = radial neck fractures; ROM = range of motion; MEPS = Mayo Elbow Performance Score; OES = Oxford Elbow Score.

Data regarding study design, number of children, age, fracture classification, type of surgical intervention or conservative therapy, range of motion (ROM) at presentation, ROM at follow-up, and complications were extracted by one reviewer (K.I.M.v.d.E.). Characteristics are listed in Table 3. The primary outcome was ROM of the elbow at follow-up.

2.4. Data Analysis

Each study was analyzed for individual patient data on preoperative angulation, method of treatment, and postoperative range of motion. Data regarding radial neck angulation ($\leq 30°$, 31–60°, and >60°) and treatment were extracted from articles or obtained from authors. If published articles provided insufficient patient data to be included for the data analysis, the authors were contacted with a request for individual data if contact details were available.

For each received treatment, the ROM at follow-up was evaluated (Table 4). Four different treatment groups were identified: no reduction or closed reduction only (CR); closed reduction followed by internal fixation (CRIF), either with K-wire fixation (Kw) or closed intramedullary pin fixation (CIMP); or open reduction (OR). If there was no full range of motion at follow-up (defined as at least 5 degrees of impairment in any direction described by the authors), the outcome was scored "impaired". Differences in outcomes for several groups were statistically analyzed using the Chi-Square Fisher Exact test ($p < 0.05$) using the software SPSS Statistics for Windows, Version 27.0 (IBM Corp. Released 2020. IBM, Armonk, NY, USA).

3. Results

Of the 2281 publications found by our search, 52 series of pediatric radial neck fractures were of potential interest. Other than evik et al. [14], Cha et al. [15], and Cossio et al. [16], all studies showed some risk of bias. Selection bias was seen in 10 papers, information bias in 15 papers, and confounding in 18 papers (see Tables 2 and 3).

Twenty-six case series provided sufficient data regarding angulation at trauma, treatment details, and elbow ROM at follow-up [36–60]. The main characteristics of the included studies are listed in Table 3. All studies had a retrospective design. In total, 551 pediatric cases could be included, ranging from 5 to 54 children per study [8,11,13–18,20–23,25,26,28–33,35]. All fractures were divided into three groups based on the degrees of fracture angulation following the classifications of O'Brien and Judet [5,7]: $\leq 30°$ (35 cases), 31–60° (247 cases), and >60° (269 cases). In total, 352 of these patients had a follow-up of at least one year. Results are depicted in Table 4, which includes data from nineteen articles [8,11,13–16,21,23,25,30–32].

Table 4. Data analysis of 352 pediatric patients who sustained a radial neck fracture and had at least 1 year follow-up.

Fracture Angle	N (%)	Treatment Groups	N with Loss of Motion (% of Treatment)	N (% of Angulation Group)
$\leq 30°$	25 (7.1)	CR	1 (7.7)	13 (52.0)
		CRIF	0	11 (44.0)
		CIMP	0	11 (44.0)
		Kw	0	0
		OR	1 (100)	1 (4.0)
		Group sum	*2 (8.0)*	
31–60°	152 (43.2)	CR	7 (63.6)	11 (7.2)
		CRIF	12 (9.4)	127 (83.6)
		CIMP	10 (9.5) NS$	105 (69.1)
		Kw	2 (9.1) NS$	22 (14.5)
		OR	7 (50)	14 (9.2)
		Group sum	*26 (17.1)*	

Table 4. Cont.

Fracture Angle	N (%)	Treatment Groups	N with Loss of Motion (% of Treatment)	N (% of Angulation Group)
>60°	175 (49.7)	CR	0	0
		CRIF	33 (26.4)	123 (70.3)
		CIMP	30 (32.6) *@	92 (52.6)
		Kw	3 (9.7) *@	31 (17.7)
		OR	31 (59.6)	52 (29.7)
		Group sum	64 (36.6)	
>30° (31–60° and >60° combined)	327 (92.9)	CR	7 (63.6) *^	11 (3.4)
		CRIF	45 (18.0) *^	250 (76.5)
		CIMP	40 (20.3) ^{NS}#	197 (60.2)
		Kw	5 (9.4) ^{NS}#	53 (16.2)
		OR	38 (55.1)	66 (20.2)
		Group sum	90 (27.5)	

CR = closed reduction without fixation or immobilization only; CRIF = closed reduction internal fixation; OR = open reduction; CIMP = retrograde intramedullar fixation; Kw = percutaneous fixation with K-wire. N = number of patients; *: significant difference; ^{NS}: non-significant difference. $^{\$}$: In the group angulated 31–60, there is no significant difference between Kw and CIMP, $p = 0.950$. ^: In the >30 angulated patients, there is a significant difference between CR (without fixation) and CRIF (CIMP and Kw) fixation; $p < 0.001$. #: In the >30 angulated patients, there is no significant difference between IM fixation or Kw fixation, $p = 0.007$. @: In the >60 angulated patients, there is a significant difference between Kw and CIMP; $p = 0.001$.

Treatment options consisted of cast immobilization without reduction; closed reduction [26,27], which may be aided by leverage of a percutaneous pin [61]; K-wire fixation (either transcapitellar [18,62], across the fracture [41], by percutaneous K-wire leverage and pinning [15,16,19,29,33,46,49,52]); intramedullary K-wire [24,32]; Nancy nail or Titanium elastic nail (TEN) [11,13,22,23,25,28,34,36,54,55] combined techniques such as CIMP assisted by Kw leverage [14,17,30,43,50,53,57]; open reduction only [8]; or the description of several treatments [20,21,31,35,37–39,42,45,47,56,59,60]. Some included (slight) adjustments to established techniques [12,58].

Children with a fracture angulation of ≤30° who were treated with CR showed loss of motion in 7.7% at follow-up. In fractures angulated over 30 degrees, 63.6% of conservatively treated children had impaired ROM (7/11 cases). The outcome following CR was significantly worse compared to patients treated with CRIF (either Kw fixation or CIMP), in angulation >30 degrees (CR 7/11 (63.6%) impaired vs. CRIF 45/250 (18.0%) p-value < 0.001).

A closed reduction with intramedullary pinning was most frequently performed (250 patients in total) in both the 31–60° and >60° group. If only the groups over 30 degrees angulation are compared, there was a significantly better outcome following K-wire fixation than following CIMP (Kw vs. CIMP 5/53 (9%) vs. 40/197 (20%); p-value < 0.001). This is also true for a separate analysis of the >60° group (K-wire vs. CIMP 3/31 (9.7%) vs. 30/92 (32.6%) impaired, p-value of 0.001), but a separate analysis of Kw vs. CIMP in the 31–60 group yields a non-significant difference (Table 4). Overall, there was no significant difference between Kw and CIMP.

Open reduction resulted in an impaired range of motion in about 60% of cases. All but one OR had been performed in fractures angulated over 30°. Nine separate articles published data on open reductions (OR), but the numbers were too small for a statistical analysis. Following OR, there had been 7 fractures without fixation, 11 with IM fixation, and 18 with K-wire fixation; 3 were not described in detail.

4. Discussion

To our knowledge, this is the first systematic review that performed a pooled analysis that focused on range of motion as an outcome following pediatric radial neck fracture treatment. Overall pediatric radial neck fractures resulted in impaired elbow function in 26% of cases. Radial neck fractures with an angulation of ≤30° demonstrated good results with CR. Fractures angulated >60° showed the least ROM impairment if K-wires were used. Open reduction had been mostly used in severely angulated fractures and often ended in an impaired elbow function.

In the literature, there is a wide variety of different scales and ratings to report radial neck fracture outcomes [63]. Only a few authors used a validated outcome scale, such as the Mayo Elbow Performance Scale (MEPS) or the (quick)DASH (Table 3). Many used their own rating system to judge the clinical or radiological outcome, which led to low comparability. Thereby, most authors only published the mean outcomes of certain groups of patients or mixed outcomes of several fracture classifications. Data pooling of individual patient cases and a meta-analysis for various treatments and their outcomes were hence impossible; the only analysis that could be performed on the extracted data was an evaluation of the outcome of range of motion based on fracture classification.

4.1. CR and Indication for Fracture Reduction

All children who were treated with immobilization or closed reduction only received a long arm cast (or collar and cuff sling under the clothes [21]). In the studies of Fowles and Kassab [18] and Jones and Esah [21], the elbows were immobilized for 3 weeks. For all other conservative treatments, the duration of immobilization was unclear [20,26,31].

Overall, no manipulation was performed when the initial angle was ≤30°, and closed reduction was indicated when the initial angle was >30°. An exception is an article by Jones [21] that advised fracture reduction when angulation exceeded 15 degrees. Closed reduction was always unsuccessful in radial neck fractures angulated over 60°, following a study that evaluated the success rate of closed radial neck fracture reduction in the emergency ward [64]. The same article stated that delayed reduction that was attempted over 24 h following trauma, may be prone to failure.

Closed reduction of a radial neck fracture may be challenging and might result in residual angulation or re-displacement. In a series of 48 fractures that were reduced by closed manipulation without fixation, as many as 36 fractures remained slightly or severely unreduced [45]. The quality of the cast may play a role, which may be calculated using the casting index (CI) [65,66].

Closed reduction without osteosynthesis in fractures angulated >30 degrees showed loss of motion at follow-up in over 60% of cases (N = 11). A recent review therefore advised to consider the percutaneous fixation of a successful closed reduction [63]. Malunion was the main reason for loss of motion in this group [42,43,51]. Some stated that closed manipulation may be attempted in fractures angulated as much as 45 degrees, but if residual angulation exceeds 20 degrees, intramedullary pin fixation should be considered [25]. Others concluded that closed reduction should be considered unsuccessful if residual angulation is over 15 degrees [21].

Closed reduction may be aided by percutaneous K-wire manipulation [28,29,52,67]. Some authors, however, stated that the manipulation by the K-wire in proximity to the physis may cause abnormalities to the physis or risk of neurological damage, and advised against it [32]. Small series were published which demonstrated other options to facilitate reduction: a forceps may be introduced ulnar to the radial neck [58], or a small elevator may be introduced at the fracture site [19]. Nevertheless, in the series that described an elevator-assisted reduction technique, a premature physis fusion occurred in 4/10 patients.

4.2. Choice of Treatment and Relation to Postoperative ROM

Although one of the case series showed favorable results of CIMP [30], our combined analysis shows that there is a better ROM following K-wire fixation compared to CIMP fixation, which is significant in fractures angulated >60 degrees. Potentially, this difference may be explained by the low number of patients reported in single case series, which renders a high risk of bias.

4.3. Open Reduction (OR)

OR should only be performed when closed reduction fails. For example, the introduction of an intramedullary device may be challenging if angulation exceeds 80° [68]. A small incision (<3 cm) is recommended [20], the annular ligament should be preserved, and instruments that could damage the radial head during reduction should be avoided. The use of a "Joy stick" K-wire in the proximal fragment to aid fracture reduction is favored over the use of clamps to prevent potential damage to the posterior interosseous nerve (PIN) [69].

Poor results following OR may be caused by damage of the blood supply [70], proximal radioulnar joint adhesion [8], or periarticular ossification [57,71]. Potentially, the focal damage to tissues due to trauma plays a role [8]. Nevertheless, interposing soft tissue makes open reduction necessary in some cases [32]. In all fracture angulation groups, loss of motion was seen in about half of the children treated with open reduction. We therefore agree with Klitscher et al. [22], who stated: "Every manipulative technique should be tried before open reduction is chosen". However, there may be bias because OR was sometimes described as the last available option when closed reduction failed.

Although some authors stated that if the radial head was stable following OR, fixation was not always necessary [8], this is disputed by our high percentage of loss of ROM in non-fixated fractures after OR. Given the fact that this percentage is significantly lower in the CRIF groups, fixation by an intramedullary nail or K-wire fixation should be considered, even after OR.

The results of this systematic review are subject to some limitations. First of all, the overall level of evidence is low. Almost all articles were level 4, and some were level 3. The overall quality of included articles is mediocre, with a risk of selection bias in 10 articles, information bias in 15 articles, and confounding bias in 18 articles. Several articles described a new or modified surgical technique without a power analysis for group size [32,33], and without a statistical analysis to compare to traditional techniques or a clear comparative design. The low incidence of displaced radial neck fractures and subsequently small cohort sizes played a role. The scores for the MINORS criteria were low for all studies, mainly due to the retrospective character of all case series that were included.

Secondly, this article only focuses on fracture angulation without considering the effect of fracture translation or rotation. In addition, associated injuries, such as ipsilateral olecranon fracture, ipsilateral fracture of the medial epicondyle, or elbow instability, were not registered; however, they can be present in 50% of children suffering a radial neck fracture [31,39]. The influence of the presence of a more extensive injury on the choice of treatment for the radial neck fracture [17] or the postoperative outcome [25,40] is still subject to discussion [18]. Some authors stated ROM would not be impaired [42]; others disagreed and showed a less favorable prognosis when associated injuries were present [17,39,42,48].

Thirdly, growth can behave like a friend or an enemy in children and might affect the outcomes. Nevertheless, a radial neck fracture is near the minimal active proximal physis, which results in less correction than in distal radius fractures. To minimize the influence of correction by growth, we only included children with a minimal follow-up of one year.

The influence of immobilization in the non-conservative groups could not be calculated. There was no evidence that postoperative immobilization had any advantages [57,72], and the worse outcome in ROM was seen when the elbow was immobilized for more than three weeks [37]. It is noteworthy that almost none of the included studies mentioned physiotherapy. Only Wang et al. [57] described "exercises under supervision (...) 1 day after operation", and Walcher et al. [33] mentioned physiotherapy only in one complex case.

5. Conclusions

This systematic review shows that conservative treatment with or without the closed reduction of pediatric radial neck fractures with primary angulation up to 30° results in good elbow function. In radial neck fractures with an angulation of >60°, closed reduction followed by K-wire fixation may have an advantage over intramedullary fracture fixation, but this difference is not significant in fractures angulated 31–60°. Open reduction should only be performed if closed reduction fails, and caution should be taken not to (further) damage the physis and radial head vascularization.

Author Contributions: K.I.M.v.d.E., G.J.B., J.W.C. and L.C.L. performed study selection and quality assessment. K.I.M.v.d.E. and L.C.L. performed data extraction and data analysis. L.C.L. and M.R. performed the statistical analysis. M.R. and J.W.C. supervised methodological accuracy and the writing of the manuscript. All authors have read and agreed to the published version of the manuscript.

Funding: The fee for publication of this article was partially paid by the CORAL (Centre for Orthopaedic Research Alkmaar) research fund, and partially by the orthopaedic surgery research fund of the Erasmus Medical Center, Rotterdam, the Netherlands.

Institutional Review Board Statement: Not applicable.

Informed Consent Statement: Not applicable.

Data Availability Statement: Access to the database may be requested by email via the corresponding author.

Acknowledgments: We thank W.M. Bramer, medical librarian, for his support in the systematic search. We thank the Centre for Orthopedic Research Alkmaar (CORAL), The Netherlands, and D. Eygendaal for their support in publishing this article.

Conflicts of Interest: The authors have no conflicts of interest to declare.

Appendix A

Literature search on 17 November 2021:

Embase.com

(('radius fracture'/de AND ('elbow'/de OR 'radioulnar joint'/de)) OR (((Radial OR radius OR forearm*) NEAR/6 (neck OR elbow OR proximal*) NEAR/6 (fracture* OR trauma* OR injur*))):ab,ti) AND ('body posture'/de OR 'movement (physiology)'/de OR 'motor dysfunction'/de OR (pronation* OR supination* OR motion* OR rotat* OR movement* OR (elbow* NEAR/6 (perform* OR kinematic* OR kinetic* OR function* OR dysfunction*)) OR Broberg OR Morrey):ab,ti)

Medline Ovid

(("Radius Fractures"/ AND ("elbow"/ OR "Elbow Joint"/)) OR (((Radial OR radius OR forearm*) ADJ6 (neck OR elbow OR proximal*) ADJ6 (fracture* OR trauma* OR injur*)).ab,ti.) AND ("Pronation"/ OR "Supination"/ OR "movement"/ OR "Movement Disorders"/ OR (pronation* OR supination* OR motion* OR rotat* OR movement* OR (elbow* ADJ6 (perform* OR kinematic* OR kinetic* OR function* OR dysfunction*)) OR Broberg OR Morrey).ab,ti.)

Cochrane

(((((Radial OR radius OR forearm*) NEAR/6 (neck OR elbow OR proximal*) NEAR/6 (fracture* OR trauma* OR injur*))):ab,ti) AND ((pronation* OR supination* OR motion* OR rotat* OR movement* OR (elbow* NEAR/6 (perform* OR kinematic* OR kinetic* OR function* OR dysfunction*)) OR Broberg OR Morrey):ab,ti)

Web of science

TS=(((((Radial OR radius OR forearm*) NEAR/5 (neck OR elbow OR proximal*) NEAR/5 (fracture* OR trauma* OR injur*)))) AND ((pronation* OR supination* OR motion* OR rotat* OR movement* OR (elbow* NEAR/5 (perform* OR kinematic* OR kinetic* OR function* OR dysfunction*)) OR Broberg OR Morrey)))

PubMed publisher

(("Radius Fractures"[mh] AND ("elbow"[mh] OR "Elbow Joint"[mh])) OR (((Radial OR radius OR forearm*[tiab]) AND (neck OR elbow OR proximal*[tiab]) AND (fracture*[tiab] OR trauma*[tiab] OR injur*[tiab])))) AND ("Pronation"[mh] OR "Supination"[mh] OR "movement"[mh] OR "Movement Disorders"[mh] OR (pronation*[tiab] OR supination*[tiab] OR motion*[tiab] OR rotat*[tiab] OR movement*[tiab] OR (elbow*[tiab] AND

(perform*[tiab] OR kinematic*[tiab] OR kinetic*[tiab] OR function*[tiab] OR dysfunction*[tiab])) OR Broberg OR Morrey)) AND publisher[sb]
Google scholar
"Radial I radius neck fracture I fractures" I "proximal Radial I radius fracture I fractures" pronation I supination

References

1. Steinberg, E.; Salama, R.; Wientroub, S. Radial Head and Neck Fractures in Children. *J. Paediatr. Orthop.* **1988**, *8*, 35–40. [CrossRef] [PubMed]
2. Newman, J. Displaced Radial Neck Fractures in Children. *Injury* **1977**, *2*, 114–121. [CrossRef]
3. Kojima, K.; Baumgaertner, M.; Trafton, P.; Ring, D.; Kloen, P. Proximal Forearm 21-A2.2: AO Foundation. Available online: https://www2.aofoundation.org/wps/portal/surgery?bone=Radius&segment=Proximal&classification=21-A2.2&showPage=indication (accessed on 21 June 2021).
4. Tibrewal, S.; Saha, S.; Haddo, O. Percutaneous K-Wire Butress Technique for Displaced Radial Neck Fracture. *Orthop. Traumatol. Rehabil.* **2013**, *15*, 169–174.
5. O'Brien, P. Injuries Involving the Proximal Radial Epiphysis. *Clin. Orthop. Relat. Res.* **1965**, *41*, 51–58.
6. Randomisli, T.; Rosen, A. Controversies Regarding Radial Neck Fractures in Children. *Clin. Orthop. Relat. Res.* **1998**, *353*, 30–39. [CrossRef]
7. Judet, J.; Judet, R.; Lefranc, J. Fracture of the Radial Head in the Child. *Ann. Chir.* **1962**, *16*, 1377–1385.
8. Falciglia, F.; Giordano, M.; Aulisa, A.; Di Lazzaro, A.; Guzzanti, V. Radial Neck Fractures in Children: Results When Open Reduction Is Indicated. *Pediatr. Orthop.* **2014**, *34*, 756–762. [CrossRef]
9. Bramer, W.M.; Rethlefsen, M.L.; Kleijnen, J.; Franco, O.H. Optimal Database Combinations for Literature Searches in Systematic Reviews: A Prospective Exploratory Study. *Syst. Rev.* **2017**, *6*, 245. [CrossRef]
10. Higgins, J.P.T.; Thomas, J.; Chandler, J.; Cumpston, M.; Li, T.; Page, M.J. (Eds.) Cochrane Handbook for Systematic Reviews of Interventions Version 6.3 (Updated February 2022). Available online: www.training.cochrane.org/handbook (accessed on 10 March 2021).
11. Al-Aubaidi, Z.; Pedersen, N.W.; Nielsen, K.D. Radial Neck Fractures in Children Treated with the Centromedullary Métaizeau Technique. *Injury* **2012**, *43*, 301–305. [CrossRef]
12. Bilal, Ö.; Murat Kalender, A.; Karsli, B.; Kilinçoğlu, V.; Kinaş, M.; Dündar, N. Radiological and Functional Outcomes of Modified Metaizeau Technique in Displaced Radial Neck Fractures. *Acta. Orthop. Belg.* **2021**, *87*, 235–241. [CrossRef]
13. Brandão, G.F.; Soares, C.B.; Teixeira, L.E.M.; Boechat, L.D.C. Displaced Radial Neck Fractures in Children: Association of the Métaizeau and Böhler Surgical Techniques. *J. Pediatr. Orthop.* **2010**, *30*, 110–114. [CrossRef] [PubMed]
14. Çevik, N.; Cansabuncu, G.; Akalın, Y.; Otuzbir, A.; Öztürk, A.; Özkan, Y. Functional and Radiological Results of Percutaneous K-Wire Aided Métaizeau Technique in the Treatment of Displaced Radial Neck Fractures in Children. *Acta. Orthop. Traumatol. Turc.* **2018**, *52*, 428–434. [CrossRef] [PubMed]
15. Cha, S.M.; Shin, H.D.; Kim, K.C.; Han, S.C. Percutaneous Reduction and Leverage Fixation Using K-Wires in Paediatric Angulated Radial Neck Fractures. *Int. Orthop.* **2012**, *36*, 803–809. [CrossRef] [PubMed]
16. Cossio, A.; Cazzaniga, C.; Gridavilla, G.; Gallone, D.; Zatti, G. Paediatric Radial Neck Fractures: One-Step Percutaneous Reduction and Fixation. *Injury* **2014**, *45*, S80–S84. [CrossRef] [PubMed]
17. Endele, S.M.; Wirth, T.; Eberhardt, O.; Fernandez, F.F. The Treatment of Radial Neck Fractures in Children According to Métaizeau. *J. Pediatr. Orthop. Part B* **2010**, *19*, 246–255. [CrossRef]
18. Fowles, J.V.; Kassab, M.T. Observations Concerning Radial Neck Fractures in Children. *J. Pediatr. Orthop.* **1986**, *6*, 51–57. [CrossRef] [PubMed]
19. Futami, I.; Tsukamoto, Y.; Itoman, M. Percutaneous Reduction of Displaced Radial Neck Fractures. *J. Shoulder Elb. Surg.* **1995**, *4*, 162–167. [CrossRef]
20. Gutiérrez-De La Iglesia, D.; Pérez-López, L.M.; Cabrera-González, M.; Knörr-Giménez, J. Surgical Techniques for Displaced Radial Neck Fractures: Predictive Factors of Functional Results. *J. Pediatr. Orthop.* **2017**, *37*, 159–165. [CrossRef]
21. Jones, E.R.; Esah, M. Displaced Fractures of the Ncek of the Radius in Children. *J. Bone Jt. Surg. Br.* **1971**, *53*, 429–439. [CrossRef]
22. Klitscher, D.; Richter, S.; Bodenschatz, K.; Hückstädt, T.; Weltzien, A.; Müller, L.P.; Schier, F.; Rommens, P.M. Evaluation of Severely Displaced Radial Neck Fractures in Children Treated with Elastic Stable Intramedullary Nailing. *J. Pediatr. Orthop.* **2009**, *29*, 698–703. [CrossRef]
23. Koca, K.; Erdem, Y.; Neyişci, Ç.; Erşen, Ö. Intramedullary Elastic Nailing of the Displaced Radial Neck Fractures in Children. *Acta. Orthop. Traumatol. Turc.* **2017**, *51*, 451–454. [CrossRef] [PubMed]
24. Massetti, D.; Marinelli, M.; Facco, G.; Falcioni, D.; Giampaolini, N.; Specchia, N.; Gigante, A.P. Percutaneous K-Wire Leverage Reduction and Retrograde Transphyseal k-Wire Fixation of Angulated Radial Neck Fractures in Children. *Eur. J. Orthop. Surg. Traumatol.* **2020**, *30*, 931–937. [CrossRef] [PubMed]
25. Metaizeau, J.; Lascombes, P.; Lemelle, J.; Finlayson, D.; Prevot, J. Reduction and Fixation of Displaced Radial Neck Fractures by Closed Intramedullary Pinning. *J. Paediatr. Orthop.* **1993**, *13*, 355–360. [CrossRef] [PubMed]

26. Monson, R.; Black, B.; Reed, M. A New Closed Reduction Technique for the Treatment of Radial Neck Fractures in Children. *J. Pediatr. Orthop.* **2009**, *29*, 243–247. [CrossRef] [PubMed]
27. Shah, M.M.; Gupta, G.; Rabbi, Q.; Bohra, V.; Wang, K.K. Close Reduction Technique for Severely Displaced Radial Neck Fractures in Children. *Indian J. Orthop.* **2021**, *55*, 109–115. [CrossRef] [PubMed]
28. Stiefel, D.; Meuli, M.; Altermatt, S. Fractures of the Neck of the Radius in Children. Early Experience with Intramedullary Pinning. *J. Bone Jt. Surg. Br.* **2001**, *83*, 536–541. [CrossRef]
29. Tanagho, A.; Ansara, S. Percutaneous Reduction and Fixation Using Two K-Wires in Paediatric Angulated Radial Neck Fractures. *J. Hand Microsurg.* **2016**, *7*, 314–316. [CrossRef]
30. Tarallo, L.; Mugnai, R.; Fiacchi, F.; Capra, F.; Catani, F. Management of Displaced Radial Neck Fractures in Children: Percutaneous Pinning vs. Elastic Stable Intramedullary Nailing. *J. Orthop. Traumatol.* **2013**, *14*, 291–297. [CrossRef]
31. Tibone, J.; Stoltz, M. Fractures of the Radial Head and Neck in Children. *J. Bone Jt. Surg.* **1981**, *63*, 100–106. [CrossRef]
32. Ugutmen, E.; Ozkan, K.; Ozkan, F.U.; Eceviz, E.; Altintas, F.; Unay, K. Reduction and Fixation of Radius Neck Fractures in Children with Intramedullary Pin. *J. Pediatr. Orthop. Part B* **2010**, *19*, 289–293. [CrossRef]
33. Walcher, F.; Rose, S.; Mutschler, W.; Marzi, I. Minimally Invasive Technique for Reduction and Stabilization of Radial Head and Radial Neck Fractures in Children. A Description of a Modified Technique and an Overview of the Literature. *Eur. J. Trauma* **2000**, *26*, 85–89. [CrossRef]
34. Yallapragada, R.K.; Maripuri, S.N. Radial Neck Fractures in Children: A Surgical Tip Using the Metaizeau Technique to Improve Stability of the Reduction. *J. Orthop.* **2020**, *17*, 127–133. [CrossRef] [PubMed]
35. Zhang, F.Y.; Wang, X.D.; Zhen, Y.F.; Guo, Z.X.; Dai, J.; Zhu, L.Q. Treatment of Severely Displaced Radial Neck Fractures in Children with Percutaneous K-Wire Leverage and Closed Intramedullary Pinning. *Medicine* **2016**, *95*, e2346. [CrossRef] [PubMed]
36. Baddula, A.R.; Thirupathi, G. A Retrospective Analysis of Management of Pediatric Radial Neck Fractures by Metaizeau Technique. *J. Dent. Med. Sci.* **2018**, *17*, 19–21. [CrossRef]
37. Badoi, A.; Frech-Dörfler, M.; Häcker, F.M.; Mayr, J. Influence of Immobilization Time on Functional Outcome in Radial Neck Fractures in Children. *Eur. J. Pediatr. Surg.* **2016**, *26*, 514–518. [CrossRef]
38. Baghdadi, S.; Shah, A.S.; Lawrence, J.T.R. Open Reduction of Radial Neck Fractures in Children: Injury Severity Predicts the Radiographic and Clinical Outcomes. *J. Shoulder Elb. Surg.* **2021**, *30*, 2418–2427. [CrossRef]
39. Basmajian, H.G.; Choi, P.D.; Huh, K.; Sankar, W.N.; Wells, L.; Arkader, A. Radial Neck Fractures in Children: Experience from Two Level-1 Trauma Centers. *J. Pediatr. Orthop. Part B* **2014**, *23*, 369–374. [CrossRef]
40. Bastard, C.; Le Hanneur, M.; Pannier, S.; Fitoussi, F. Radial Neck Fractures in Children Secondary to Horse-Riding Accidents: A Comparative Study. *Orthop. Traumatol. Surg. Res.* **2020**, *106*, 1293–1297. [CrossRef]
41. Biyani, A.; Mehara, A.; Bhan, S. Percutaneous Pinning for Radial Neck Fractures. *Injury* **1994**, *25*, 169–171. [CrossRef]
42. De Mattos, C.B.; Ramski, D.E.; Kushare, I.V.; Angsanuntsukh, C.; Flynn, J.M. Radial Neck Fractures in Children and Adolescents: An Examination of Operative and Nonoperative Treatment and Outcomes. *J. Pediatr. Orthop.* **2016**, *36*, 6–12. [CrossRef]
43. Du, X.; Yu, L.; Xiong, Z.; Chen, G.; Zou, J.; Wu, X.; Xiong, B.; Wang, B. Percutaneous Leverage Reduction with Two Kirschner Wires Combined with the Métaizeau Technique versus Open Reduction plus Internal Fixation with a Single Kirschner-Wire for Treating Judet IV Radial Neck Fractures in Children. *J. Int. Med. Res.* **2019**, *47*, 5497–5507. [CrossRef] [PubMed]
44. Dietzel, M.; Scherer, S.; Esser, M.; Kirschner, H.J.; Fuchs, J.; Lieber, J. Fractures of the Proximal Radius in Children: Management and Results of 100 Consecutive Cases. *Arch. Orthop. Trauma Surg.* **2021**. [CrossRef] [PubMed]
45. Henrikson, B. Isolated Fractures of the Proximal End of the Radius in Children. Epidemiology, Treatment and Prognosis. *Acta Orthop. Scand.* **1969**, *40*, 246–260. [CrossRef] [PubMed]
46. Jiang, H.; Wu, Y.; Dang, Y.; Qiu, Y. Closed Reduction Using the Percutaneous Leverage Technique and Internal Fixation with K-Wires to Treat Angulated Radial Neck Fractures in Children-Case Report. *Medicine* **2017**, *96*, e5806. [CrossRef]
47. Kiran, M.; Bruce, C.; George, H.; Garg, N.; Walton, R. Intramedullary Devices in the Management of Judet III and IV Paediatric Radial Neck Fractures. *Chin. J. Traumatol. Engl. Ed.* **2018**, *21*, 34–37. [CrossRef]
48. Lindham, S.; Hugosson, C. The Significance of Associated Lesions Including Dislocation in Fractures of the Neck of the Radius in Children. *Acta Orthop.* **1979**, *50*, 79–83. [CrossRef]
49. Okçu, G.; Aktuglu, K. Surgical Treatment of Displaced Radial Neck Fractures in Children with Metaizeau Technique Çocuklarda Ayrılmış Radius Boyun Kırıklarının Metaizeau Tekniği Ile Cerrahi Tedavisi. *Turk. J. Trauma Emerg. Surg.* **2007**, *13*, 122–127.
50. Qiao, F.; Jiang, F. Closed Reduction of Severely Displaced Radial Neck Fractures in Children. *BMC Musculoskelet. Disord.* **2019**, *20*, 567. [CrossRef]
51. Rodriguez Merchan, E. Percutaneous Reduction of Displaced Radial Neck Fractures in Children Nov. *J. Trauma* **1994**, *37*, 812–814. [CrossRef]
52. Steele, J.A.; Kerr, H. Angulated Radial Neck Fractures in Children, a Prospective Study of Percutaneous Reduction. *J. Bone Jt. Surg.* **1992**, *74*, 760–764. [CrossRef]
53. Su, Y.; Jin, C.; Duan, X.; Wang, J.; Li, K. Treatment of Displaced Radial Neck Fractures under Ultrasonographic Guidance in Children. *Int. Orthop.* **2020**, *44*, 2337–2342. [CrossRef]
54. Trabelsi, A.; Khalifa, M.A.; Brahem, R.; Jedidi, M.; Bouattour, K.; Osman, W.; Ayeche, M.L. Ben Radial Neck Fracture in Children: Anatomic and Functional Results of Metaizeau Technique. *Pan. Afr. Med. J.* **2020**, *36*, 1–10. [CrossRef] [PubMed]

55. Ursei, M.; Sales De Gauzy, J.; Knorr, J.; Abid, A.; Darodes, P.; Cahuzac, J.P. Surgical Treatment of Radial Neck Fractures in Children by Intramedullary Pinning. *Acta. Orthop. Belg.* **2006**, *72*, 131–137. [PubMed]
56. Vocke, A.; Von Laer, L. Treatment and Prognosis of Displaced Proximal Radius Fractures. *Tech. Orthop.* **2000**, *15*, 58–66. [CrossRef]
57. Wang, J.; Chen, W.; Guo, M.; Su, Y.; Zhang, Y. Percutaneous Reduction and Intramedullary Fixation Technique for Displaced Pediatric Radial Neck Fractures. *J. Pediatr. Orthop. Part B* **2013**, *22*, 127–132. [CrossRef]
58. Watkins, C.J.; Yeung, C.M.; Rademacher, E.; Kramer, D.E. Percutaneous Leverage Technique for Reduction of Radial Neck Fractures in Children: Technical Tips. *J. Child. Orthop.* **2020**, *14*, 118–124. [CrossRef]
59. Xia, A.; You, C.; Han, J.; Wu, D.; Xia, Y.; Wang, J. Comparison of Different Treatments for Children with Radial Neck Fracture and Analysis of Prognostic Factors. *Arch. Orthop. Trauma Surg.* **2021**. [CrossRef]
60. Zimmerman, R.M.; Kalish, L.A.; Hresko, M.T.; Waters, P.M.; Bae, D.S. Surgical Management of Pediatric Radial Neck Fractures. *J. Bone Jt. Surg. Ser. A* **2013**, *95*, 1825–1832. [CrossRef]
61. Rodriguez Merchan, E. Displaced Fractures of the Head and Neck of the Radius in Children: Open Reduction and Temporary Transarticular Internal Fixation. *Orthopedics* **1991**, *14*, 697–700. [CrossRef]
62. Ali, A.A. Outcome of Transcapitellar K-Wire Fixation for Radial Neck Fractures. *Mustansiriya Med. J.* **2014**, *13*, 26–32.
63. Kumar, S.; Mishra, A.; Odak, S.; Dwyer, J. Treatment Principles, Prognostic Factors and Controversies in Radial Neck Fractures in Children: A Systematic Review. *J. Clin. Orthop. Trauma* **2020**, *11*, S456–S463. [CrossRef] [PubMed]
64. Kong, J.; Lewallen, L.; Elliott, M.; Jo, C.H.; Mcintosh, A.L.; Ho, C.A. Pediatric Radial Neck Fractures: Which Ones Can Be Successfully Closed Reduced in the Emergency Department? *J. Pediatr. Orthop.* **2021**, *41*, 17–22. [CrossRef] [PubMed]
65. Sengab, A.; Krijnen, P.; Schipper, I.B. Risk Factors for Fracture Redisplacement after Reduction and Cast Immobilization of Displaced Distal Radius Fractures in Children: A Meta-Analysis. *Eur. J. Trauma Emerg. Surg.* **2020**, *46*, 789–800. [CrossRef] [PubMed]
66. Maccagnano, G.; Notarnicola, A.; Pesce, V.; Tafuri, S.; Mudoni, S.; Nappi, V.; Moretti, B. Failure Predictor Factors of Conservative Treatment in Pediatric Forearm Fractures. *BioMed Res. Int.* **2018**, *2018*, 5930106. [CrossRef]
67. Pesudo, J.; Aracil, J.; Barcelo, M. Leverage Method in Displaced Fractures of the Radial Neck in Children. *Clin. Orthop. Relat. Res.* **1982**, *169*, 215–218. [CrossRef]
68. Devgan, A.; Singh, R.; Kumar, S.; Verma, V.; Magu, N.; Siwach, R. Indirect Reduction and Intramedullary Pinning in Severely Displaced Radial Neck Fractures in Children. *Int. J. Clin. Med.* **2011**, *2*, 75–78. [CrossRef]
69. Demetri, L.; Young, C.; Patterson, J.T.; Kandemir, U.; Morshed, S.; Immerman, I.; Lee, N.H. Management of Metadiaphyseal Proximal Radius Fractures. *Tech. Hand Up. Extrem. Surg.* **2021**, *25*, 156–164. [CrossRef] [PubMed]
70. Hemmer, J.; Happiette, A.; Muller, F.; Barbier, D.; Journeau, P. Prognostic Factors for Intramedullary Nailing in Radial Neck Fracture in Children. *Orthop. Traumatol. Surg. Res.* **2020**, *106*, 1287–1291. [CrossRef]
71. Eberl, R.; Singer, G.; Fruhmann, J.; Saxena, A.; Hoellwarth, M. Intramedullary Nailing for the Treatment of Dislocated Pediatric Radial Neck Fractures. *Eur. J. Pediatr. Surg.* **2010**, *20*, 250–252. [CrossRef] [PubMed]
72. Hilgert, R.; Dallek, M.; Rueger, J. Die Minimal-Invasive Behandlung Massiv Dislozierter Kindlicher Radiushalsfrakturen Durch Perkutane Joystick-Reposition Und Prevot-Nagelung Minimal Invasive Treatment of Massively Dislocated Radial Neck Fractures in Children by Percutaneous Joystick Repos. *Unfallchirurg* **2002**, *105*, 116–119. [CrossRef]

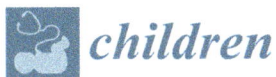

Article

Is a Parry Fracture—An Isolated Fracture of the Ulnar Shaft—Associated with the Probability of Abuse in Children between 2 and 16 Years Old?

Kyra Hermans [1], Duncan Fransz [2,3,*], Lisette Walbeehm-Hol [4], Paul Hustinx [1] and Heleen Staal [2]

1 Department of Trauma Surgery, Zuyderland Medical Center, 6419 PC Heerlen, The Netherlands
2 Department of Orthopaedic Surgery, Maastricht University Medical Center, 6229 HX Maastricht, The Netherlands
3 Department of Orthopaedic Surgery, Zuyderland Medical Center, 6419 PC Heerlen, The Netherlands
4 Department of Pediatrics, Zuyderland Medical Center, 6419 PC Heerlen, The Netherlands
* Correspondence: dpfransz@gmail.com

Abstract: A parry fracture is an isolated fracture of the ulnar shaft. It occurs when the ulna receives the full force of an impact when the forearm is raised to protect the face. The aim of this study is to assess a possible association between a parry fracture and the probability of abuse in children. In this retrospective, observational, multicenter study, we identified patients between 2 and 16 years old who had been treated for an isolated ulnar shaft fracture. Patient characteristics were registered, anonymized radiographs were rated, and charts were screened for referral to a child protective team. A total of 36 patients were analyzed. As no referrals were registered during follow-up, the primary outcome was changed to a perpendicular force as trauma mechanism. Univariable regression analysis and independent t-test both showed no significant association between patient factors or radiographic classification, and the reported trauma mechanism. We were unable to determine an association between a parry fracture and the probability of abuse. Since trauma mechanism does have a biomechanical effect on the fracture type, we would advise that a very clear reconstruction (and documentation) of the trauma mechanism should be established when a parry fracture is identified on radiographs.

Keywords: non-accidental trauma; self-defense; violence; adolescent; dexterity; biomechanics

1. Introduction

A very specific type of forearm fracture, a so-called 'parry' (or 'nightstick') fracture, has been associated with interpersonal and extramural violence in the field of paleopathology [1]. A parry fracture is an isolated fracture of the ulnar shaft (see Figure 1) and can occur when the ulna (which is more exposed than the radius when arms are raised as a means of defense) receives the full force of a blunt force attack [2]. Due to the mechanism of trauma that is required to cause such a fracture, it might therefore be associated with (child) abuse.

The proportion of fractures attributed to abuse is highest in infants younger than 1 year (24.9%). This proportion decreases to 7.2% in children 12 to 23 months and 2.9% in children 24 to 35 months of age [3]. Recognizing abusive injuries is critical to preventing further injury and even death of the child [4]. Failure to identify child abuse at the time of initial presentation leaves the victim with a 30–50% chance of recurrent abuse [5].

Unfortunately, distinguishing between non-inflicted fractures and those caused by abuse can be challenging, particularly in children and even more so when they are older than two years. The dependency relationship with the perpetrator ensures that it is difficult to determine whether there is abuse or not. When children are able to relate the situation, there is a fair chance that they will keep silent out of loyalty to the parents or out of fear of the perpetrator [6].

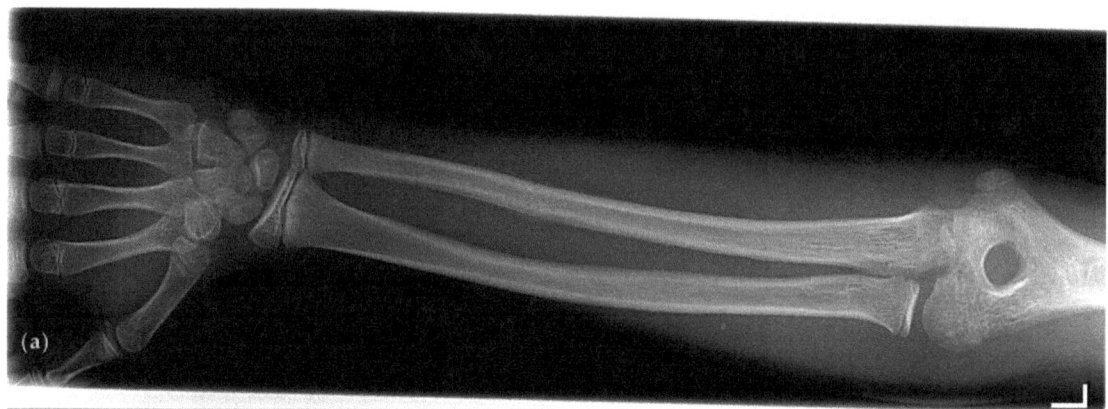
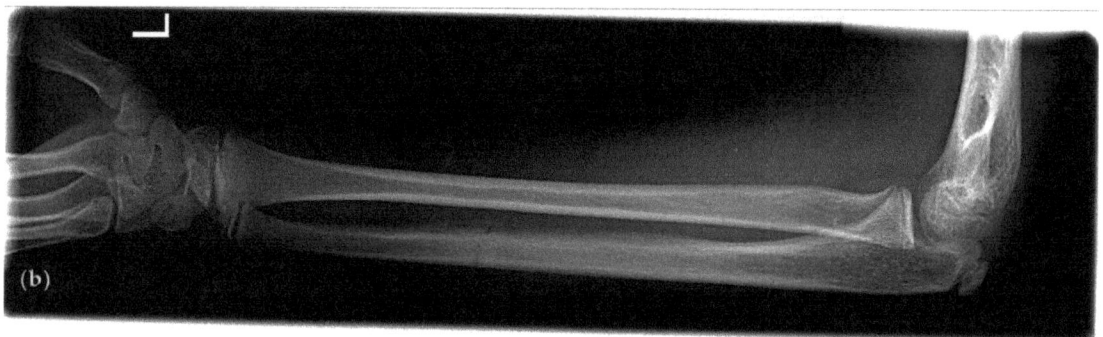

Figure 1. A typical example of an isolated fracture of the left ulna that meets all four parry fracture criteria according to Judd [1]: absence of radial involvement, transverse fracture line, distal from midshaft, and minimal displacement. Radiographs are shown in (**a**) anteroposterior projection; (**b**) lateral projection.

No specific type of fracture, on its own, can distinguish an abusive from a non-abusive cause [6,7]. However, various red flags regarding fracture characteristics have been proposed. These include presentation to the emergency department with multiple fractures, fractures in various states of healing, metaphyseal corner fractures, long bones fractures in children who are not of walking age, spine fractures, scapular fractures, rib fractures, epiphyseal separations, swelling not proportional to injury type (i.e., less swelling than would be expected for an acute fracture), and fractures reported as "falls from a bed or couch" in those less than one year of age [7,8].

When specifically looking into forearm fractures, fractures of the radius and/or ulna are uncommon in infants because they cannot meet the conditions necessary to cause this fracture [3]. In an older child, forearm fractures most often occur from falling onto an arm that is outstretched to break the fall [3]. In a retrospective study on 47 children (2–17 years old) with a forearm fracture that had been screened by a child protective team, no particular type of forearm fracture was inherently indicative of child abuse [9].

However, thus far, no study has investigated a possible association between a parry fracture and abuse in children. Therefore, we set out to analyze a possible relation between isolated ulnar shaft fractures and the probability of abuse in patients between 2 and 16 years old.

2. Materials and Methods

2.1. Data Collection

For this retrospective study, we identified patients between 2 and 16 years old who were treated for a forearm fracture at the emergency department (ED) or outpatient clinic (OC) at Zuyderland Medical Center or at Maastricht University Medical Center between 1 January 2008 and 1 January 2018.

2.1.1. Radiographs

We retrieved radiology reports for the identified patients, and for those reports that described an isolated fracture of the ulna, the corresponding radiographs were collected. Patients with fractures of the Monteggia type, or with ulnar shaft fractures that were accompanied by any type of radial fracture, were excluded.

2.1.2. Patients

For the remaining patients, we retrieved patient characteristics from their charts. Age at presentation, sex, fractured side, previous fractures, presentation location (ED or OC), trauma mechanism (as described by patient or parent), and delay (days since trauma) were registered. Patients were excluded if osteogenesis imperfecta (brittle bone disease) or any other bone metabolism disorder had been previously diagnosed.

As primary outcome, we recorded if patients had been referred to a child protective team for further evaluation up to 1 January 2021.

2.2. Data Analysis

Three assessors (trauma surgeon, pediatric orthopedic surgeon, and pediatrician) reviewed and scored all data individually.

2.2.1. Radiographic Classification

The classification of anonymized radiographs was done according to the AO Pediatric classification [10] and to the paleopathology parry (P3) fracture criteria [1]. If a fracture met all four of the below criteria, it was regarded as a P3 fracture:

1. the absence of radial involvement;
2. a transverse fracture line ($\leq 45°$);
3. a location below the midshaft (<0.5 adjusted distance to the lesion's center); and
4. either minor unalignment ($\leq 10°$) in any plane or horizontal apposition from the diaphysis (<50%).

Classification was done twice, the second time after a repeated randomization.

2.2.2. Chart Assessment

None of the included patients had been referred to a child protective team for further evaluation. Therefore, we had to formulate an alternative primary outcome. As any retrospective interpretation of the available information on an ED or OC chart would introduce several forms of bias, we decided to select the reported trauma mechanism as the primary outcome. If the chart stated that the child fell (from an object or during an activity), we regarded the trauma mechanism as a parallel force. If the chart stated that someone exerted a force upon the arm, we regarded the trauma mechanism as a perpendicular, direct force.

2.3. Statistical Analysis

All statistical analyses were performed using IBM SPSS Statistics for Mac (IBM Corp., version 21.0, Armonk, NY, USA).

For each radiograph, a resultant classification was compiled from the 3 (assessors) × 2 (repetitions) assessments. If the resultant remained inconclusive (i.e., majority rule), the assessment of a fourth assessor served as the decider. To assess the agreement within and between the assessors regarding the different radiographic classifications, we calculated Cohen's kappa [11]. This method corrects for agreement based on chance and is well suited for categorical variables. A value above 0.6 is regarded as substantial agreement.

We used univariable binary logistic regression analysis to quantify the association between potential determinants (patient characteristics and fracture classifications) and the dependent variable (an evident perpendicular force as trauma mechanism). The patient characteristics 'age' and 'delay' were entered as continuous variables, all others were entered as dichotomous. Though strictly not a continuous variable, we did consider the AO Pediatric classification as continuous (in contrast to categorical), since a 'higher' classification essentially implies a more serious injury. Whether or not a parry fracture was apparent was entered as a dichotomous variable.

We also compared mean values between the two groups (i.e., fall versus direct trauma) with an independent samples t-test. For both statistical tests, we considered a p-value < 0.05 as an indication of statistical significance.

3. Results

3.1. Data Collection

Between 1 January 2008 and 1 January 2018, a total of 42 patients were treated at the ED or OC for an isolated ulna shaft fracture. Six patients had to be excluded from further analysis: five patients did not have any information at all in their charts, however the radiographs and radiology reports were available; one patient had missing radiographs. The patient characteristics for the 36 included patients are shown in Table 1, an overview of the various reported trauma mechanisms is shown in Table 2.

Table 1. Characteristics of the included patients (n = 36).

Determinant	n (%)	mean ± SD (Range)
Age (years)		8.9 ± 3.8 (2.3–15.4)
Sex (male)	23 (64%)	
Side (right)	15 (42%)	
Previous fracture (yes)	3 (8%)	
Delay (yes)	8 (22%)	9.3 ± 3.9 (1–14) *

* The mean ± SD when there was a delay in presentation of the fracture, in days.

Table 2. Overview of reported trauma mechanisms (n = 36).

Fall from	n	Fall during	n
bicycle	1	cartwheeling	1
bouncy castle	2	dancing	1
chair	1	field hockey	1
climbing frame	3	gymnastics	2
couch	1	handball	1
gymnastic vault	2	playing with old rubber tire	1
hoverboard	1	playing in the mud	1
pony	1	soccer	1
sandbox	1		
sidewalk	1	**Direct Trauma**	**n**
slide	2	kicked by other kid	2
small pole	1	kicked by pony	1
standing	1	other kid fell on arm	1
swing	1	other kid stepped on arm	2

In two cases, there was notion of a fall, but without a cause.

3.2. Data Analysis

In Table 3, the results for the fracture classifications as evaluated by the assessors are shown. For both classifications, assessment by a fourth assessor was necessary in three cases to break the tie.

Table 3. Fracture classifications and the contributing assessments.

Classification		Contributing Assessments (%)	
AO Pediatric	n	yes	no
Bowing (1.1)			
Greenstick (2.1)	9	69	31
Complete transverse 1 (4.1)	10	75	25
Complete transverse 2 (4.2)			
Complete oblique or spiral 1 (5.1)	15	68	32
Complete oblique or spiral 2 (5.2)	2	75	25
Paleopathology			
Parry fracture	14	77	23
No parry fracture	22	89	11

Percentages were calculated based on 3 (assessors) × 2 (repetitions) × n assessments. For instance, of all the fractures that were classified as a 'Complete transverse 1' according to the AO Pediatric (i.e., n = 10), 25% of the assessments did not classify the fracture as such. Assessment by a fourth assessor was necessary in three cases for each the AO Pediatric classification (this resulted in 2 × 5.1 and 1 × 4.1) and the paleopathology criteria (2 × yes, 1 × no).

As none of the patients had been referred to a child protective team for further evaluation by the 1 January 2021, we decided to select the reported trauma mechanism as the primary outcome. In Table 2, the distinction between a parallel (fall, n = 30) and an evident perpendicular force (direct, n = 6) is apparent.

3.3. Statistical Analysis

The agreement within and between assessors is available as Supplemental Data. The intra-observer agreement was higher than the inter-observer agreement. In general, the agreement between assessors was fair to moderate [12], with the P3 criteria scoring higher than the AO Pediatric classification.

Regression analysis showed no significant association between patient characteristics and fracture classifications, and an evident perpendicular force as trauma mechanism (Table 4). Similarly, the t-test did not show a significant difference between group means (Table 5).

Table 4. Univariable binary logistic regression analysis.

	Exp(B) [95% C.I.]	p-Value
Age	1.289 [0.980–1.695]	0.069
Sex	1.158 [0.182–7.384]	0.877
Side	0.229 [0.240–2.198]	0.201
Previous fracture	2.800 [0.212–37.03]	0.434
Delay	1.029 [0.846–1.251]	0.778
AO Pediatric	1.055 [0.554–2.011]	0.870
Paleopathology	4.667 [0.720–30.23]	0.106

Age (years), delay (days), and AO Pediatric classification were entered as continuous variables. The other variables were entered as dichotomous; sex (0 = female), side (0 = left), previous fracture (0 = none), and paleopathology criteria (0 = no).

Table 5. Means, standard deviation, and *p*-value when comparing groups of the patients that suffered from a fall with patients that suffered from a direct impact.

	Fall (*n* = 30)	Direct (*n* = 6)	*p*-Value
Age	8.41 ± 3.78	11.71 ± 3.10	0.053
Sex	0.63 ± 0.49	0.67 ± 0.52	0.881
Side	0.47 ± 0.51	0.17 ± 0.41	0.183
Previous fracture	0.07 ± 0.25	0.17 ± 0.41	0.433
Delay	1.97 ± 4.06	2.50 ± 5.65	0.784
AO Pediatric	3.73 ± 1.34	3.83 ± 1.72	0.874
Paleopathology	0.30 ± 0.47	0.67 ± 0.52	0.093

Age (years), delay (days), and AO Pediatric classification were entered as continuous variables. The other variables were entered as dichotomous; sex (0 = female), side (0 = left), previous fracture (0 = none), and paleopathology criteria (0 = no).

4. Discussion

In this study, we were unable to determine an association between a parry fracture and the probability of abuse. We selected our patient group based on fracture type, and as it turned out, this group did not include children who had been referred to a child protective team for further evaluation during the follow-up period.

This finding is in accordance with a previous study that showed that no particular type of forearm fracture was specific for abuse in children younger than 18 months [9]. However, while not addressing the parry fracture specifically, transverse fractures were seen in 45% (5/11) of the abusive fractures, compared to 28% (9/32) of non-inflicted fractures [9].

As our group sizes were small, no statistical difference was expected to be found. However, it seems that age, side, and the P3 criteria are somewhat related to the trauma mechanism, albeit non-significantly (Tables 4 and 5).

In general, specific fracture types are caused by a particular application of force. Transverse fractures are caused by a bending load perpendicular to the bone, spiral fractures by torsion along its long axis, and oblique fractures by a combination of both [13]. The reported direct mechanisms (Table 2) are comparable to a direct blow when the forearm is raised to protect the face, as is the case with a parry fracture [1]. Therefore, we would advise that a very clear reconstruction of the trauma mechanism should be established, especially if a parry fracture is identified on a radiograph. Even more importantly, these details should be written down in the charts. We found that the limited information for both medical history and physical examination highlighted another known problem: the ED documentation of pediatric injury is quite insufficient, making child abuse very difficult to suspect [14].

The possible effect of age is most likely due to the different activities older kids undertake, predisposing them to this trauma mechanism.

The current study showed 58% of ulnar fractures on the left side, which was to be expected in the case of a fall. Children tend to favor their left hand to protect themselves when they fall; sometimes the dominant hand is engaged in some activity. The left arm also seems to fracture more easily because of greater fragility, immaturity, and suboptimal neuromuscular coordination, rendering the left arm less suited to managing the situation [15]. However, in the case of abuse, the left side also fractures more often. In a study on a total 124 unclaimed cadavers prone to abuse, the left ulna was the most affected long bone of the upper limb. This may be explained by a right-sided attack [2].

This study had several limitations. In contrast to a previous study [9], the basis of our study was a specific type of forearm fracture. As it turned out, our sample did not include any cases where actual abuse was identified; none of the patients had been referred to a child protective team for further evaluations. Therefore, we were unable to answer our original research question, though we had a minimum follow-up of three years. However, the follow-up was limited to the hospital of initial presentation and subsequent presentation to another hospital therefore was not considered.

Even though the isolated ulnar shaft fracture is an uncommon fracture type (4% of the forearm fractures in children) [9], the current sample of 36 patients is perhaps still too small to identify associations between type of fracture and possible child abuse. A larger patient population would be desirable.

Since absence of proof is not proof of absence, future research should focus on identifying as many red flags regarding child abuse as possible. Perhaps the advent of machine learning and big data can further assist in this multifactorial domain of relatively low incidence but grave consequences. Failing to recognize abuse at the initial presentation leaves the victim with a 30–50% chance of recurrent abuse, as well as an increased risk of morbidity and mortality [5].

5. Conclusions

We were unable to determine an association between a parry fracture and the probability of abuse. If, however, the described trauma mechanism consisted of a perpendicular bending load, the resulting fracture often met the criteria for a parry fracture. Therefore, we would advise that a very clear reconstruction (and documentation) of the trauma mechanism should be established when a parry fracture is identified on radiographs.

Supplementary Materials: The following are available online at https://www.mdpi.com/article/10.3390/children8080650/s1: Table S1: Assessor agreement for the radiographic classifications.

Author Contributions: Conceptualization: K.H. and D.F.; methodology: D.F.; software: D.F.; validation: H.S., L.W.-H. and P.H.; formal analysis: D.F.; investigation: K.H.; resources: K.H. and D.F.; data curation: K.H.; writing—original draft preparation: K.H. and D.F.; writing—review and editing: H.S., L.W.-H. and P.H.; visualization: K.H.; supervision: D.F., P.H. and H.S.; project administration: K.H. All authors have read and agreed to the published version of the manuscript.

Funding: This research received no external funding.

Institutional Review Board Statement: The study was conducted according to the guidelines of the Declaration of Helsinki, and was approved by both participating hospitals (2018-0596 and 2018-0086, Zuyderland Medical Center granted on 21 August 2018 and Maastricht University Medical Center granted on 25 July 2018, respectively).

Informed Consent Statement: Not applicable.

Data Availability Statement: Not applicable.

Conflicts of Interest: The authors declare no conflict of interest.

References

1. Judd, M.A. The parry problem. *J. Arch. Sci.* **2008**, *35*, 1658–1666. [CrossRef]
2. Geldenhuys, E.M.; Burger, E.H.; Alblas, A.; Greyling, L.M.; Kotzé, S.H. The association between healed skeletal fractures indicative of interpersonal violence and alcoholic liver disease in a cadaver cohort from the Western Cape, South Africa. *Alcohol* **2016**, *52*, 41–48. [CrossRef] [PubMed]
3. Pierce, M.C.; Kaczor, K.; Lohr, D.; Richter, K.; Starling, S.P. A practical guide to differentiating abusive from accidental fractures: An injury plausibility approach. *Clin. Pediatric Emerg. Med.* **2012**, *13*, 166–177. [CrossRef]
4. Jenny, C.; Hymel, K.P.; Ritzen, A.; Reinert, S.E.; Hay, T.C. Analysis of missed cases of abusive head trauma. *J. Am. Med. Assoc.* **1999**, *281*, 621–626. [CrossRef] [PubMed]
5. Rosenfeld, E.H.; Johnson, B.; Wesson, D.E.; Shah, S.R.; Vogel, A.M.; Naik-Mathuria, B. Understanding non-accidental trauma in the United States: A national trauma databank study. *J. Pediatr. Surg.* **2020**, *55*, 693–697. [CrossRef]
6. Bilo, R.A.C.; Robben, S.G.F.; van Rijn, R.R. *Forensic Aspects of Pediatric Fractures: Differentiating Accidental Trauma from Child Abuse*, 1st ed.; Springer: Berlin/Heidelberg, Germany, 2009.
7. Kemp, A.M.; Dunstan, F.; Harrison, S.; Morris, S.; Mann, M.; Rolfe, K.; Datta, S.; Thomas, D.P.; Sibert, J.R.; Maguire, S. Patterns of skeletal fractures in child abuse: Systematic review. *BMJ* **2008**, *337*, a1518. [CrossRef] [PubMed]
8. Pandya, N.K.; Baldwin, K.; Wolfgruber, H.; Christian, C.W.; Drummond, D.S.; Hosalkar, H.S. Child abuse and orthopaedic injury patterns: Analysis at a level I pediatric trauma center. *J. Pediatr. Orthop.* **2009**, *29*, 618–625. [CrossRef] [PubMed]
9. Ryznar, E.; Rosado, N.; Flaherty, E.G. Understanding forearm fractures in young children: Abuse or not abuse? *Child Abus. Negl.* **2015**, *47*, 132–139. [CrossRef] [PubMed]

10. Slongo, T.; Audigé, L. *AO Pediatric Comprehensive Classification of Long-Bone Fractures (PCCF)*; AO Foundation: Davos, Switzerland, 2010.
11. Cohen, J. Weighted Kappa: Nominal scale agreement with provision for scaled disagreement or partial credit. *Psychol. Bull.* **1968**, *70*, 213–220. [CrossRef] [PubMed]
12. Viera, A.J.; Garrett, J.M. Understanding interobserver agreement: The kappa statistic. *Fam. Med.* **2005**, *37*, 360–363.
13. Flaherty, E.G.; Perez-Rossello, J.M.; Levine, M.A.; Hennrikus, W.L. Evaluating children with fractures for child physical abuse. *Pediatrics* **2014**, *133*, e477–e489. [CrossRef]
14. Castagnino, M.; Paglino, A.; Berardi, C.; Riccioni, S.; Esposito, S. Recording risk factors of physical abuse in children younger than 36 months with bone fractures: A 12-years retrospective study in an Italian general hospital emergency room. *Front. Pediatr.* **2020**, *8*, 183. [CrossRef]
15. Mortensson, W.; Thönel, S. Left-side dominance of upper extremity fracture in children. *Acta Orthop. Scand.* **1991**, *62*, 154–155. [CrossRef]

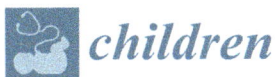

Case Report

Patient-Specific Guided Osteotomy to Correct a Symptomatic Malunion of the Left Forearm

Femke F. Schröder [1,2], Feike de Graaff [1,*] and Anne J. H. Vochteloo [1]

1. Orthopedisch Centrum Oost Nederland, Centre for Orthopaedic Surgery, 7555 DL Hengelo, The Netherlands; f.schroder@ocon.nl (F.F.S.); a.vochteloo@ocon.nl (A.J.H.V.)
2. Techmed Centre, Faculty of Science and Technology, University of Twente, 7522 NB Enschede, The Netherlands
* Correspondence: f.dgraaff@ocon.nl

Abstract: We present a case report of a 12-year old female with a midshaft forearm fracture. Initial conservative treatment with a cast failed, resulting in a malunion. The malunion resulted in functional impairment for which surgery was indicated. A corrective osteotomy was planned using 3D analyses of the preoperative CT-scan. Subsequently, patient-specific guides were printed and used during the procedure to precisely correct the malunion. Three months after surgery, the radiographs showed full consolidation and the patient was pain-free with full range of motion and comparable strength in both forearms. The current case report shows that a corrective osteotomy with patient-specific guides based on preoperative 3D analyses can help surgeons to plan and precisely correct complex malunions resulting in improved functional outcomes.

Keywords: forearm malunion; osteotomy; patient-specific guides; 3D

1. Introduction

Forearm fractures are common among children and are often treated with closed methods (i.e., closed reduction and cast immobilization). Although bones in young children are generally forgiving, they can heal in an abnormal position. i.e., a malunion. Malunions occur in about 15% of fractures, and can lead to, among other complaints, pain, carpal and distal radioulnar joint instability, reduced range of motion, and in the long term, osteoarthritis [1–3]. Corrective osteotomy, a surgical method to restore normal bone anatomy, should be considered if the malunion results in functional impairment [4].

Historically, corrective osteotomies were planned based on radiographs. These images can be sufficient in the case of simple fractures, as angular and translational deformities can generally be assessed in 2D. However, malunited forearm fractures are often complex, involving deformities in multiple anatomical planes. As found in a study of Miyake et al. [5], complex malunited forearm fractures seem to have rotational deformities in a range from 115 degrees of pronation to 15 degrees of supination. Plain 2D radiographs generally do not provide adequate information about rotational deformities and are therefore not suitable for the preoperative assessment of the malunion and planning of correction osteotomies [6,7].

In recent years, there has been an increased interest in the use of 3D analysis and printing in (paediatric) orthopaedics [8–10]. Nowadays, a corrective osteotomy is often preceded by preoperative planning based on 3D analyses of the malunion. The introduction of 3D preoperative planning and printing of patient-specific guides has significantly improved the interpretation of complex fractures. Several studies have shown that the correction of malunited forearm fractures can be precisely planned and performed using 3D analyses and printing of guides, which subsequently resulted in improved functional outcomes [11–15].

We present a case report of a 12-year old female with a malunited midshaft forearm fracture treated with patient-specific guided corrective osteotomies of radius and ulna. The

---

Citation: Schröder, F.F.; de Graaff, F.; Vochteloo, A.J.H. Patient-Specific Guided Osteotomy to Correct a Symptomatic Malunion of the Left Forearm. *Children* **2021**, *8*, 707. https://doi.org/10.3390/children8080707

Academic Editor: Christiaan J. A. van Bergen

Received: 9 July 2021
Accepted: 13 August 2021
Published: 17 August 2021

Publisher's Note: MDPI stays neutral with regard to jurisdictional claims in published maps and institutional affiliations.

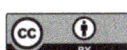

Copyright: © 2021 by the authors. Licensee MDPI, Basel, Switzerland. This article is an open access article distributed under the terms and conditions of the Creative Commons Attribution (CC BY) license (https://creativecommons.org/licenses/by/4.0/).

case is a perfect example of how preoperative planning and printing of patient-specific guides create the possibility to restore the preoperative anatomical position and function of complex malunited fractures.

2. Case Description

2.1. Patient Case and History

In June 2020, a 12-year old girl presented at the emergency department after falling on her left forearm while jumping on a trampoline. After physical examination, radiographs of the left forearm were obtained (Figure 1A). The patient was diagnosed with a mid-shaft antebrachial fracture without dislocation which was treated conservatively with a cast. During follow-up, the fracture consolidated, however, with a secondary displacement of the fracture. Conservative treatment was prolonged.

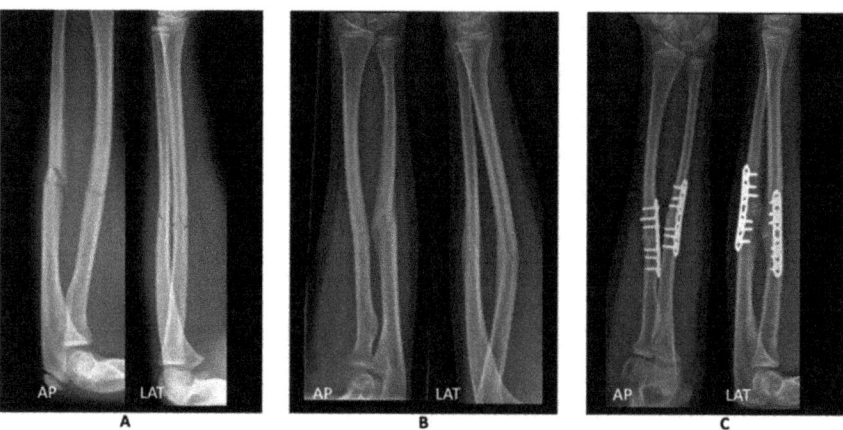

Figure 1. Radiographs of the forearm in anterior posterior (AP) and lateral (LAT) directions (**A**) at initial trauma, (**B**) 3 months after initial trauma where the fracture is consolidated and the arm shows bowing and dorsal angulation, and (**C**) after patient-specific guided correction.

Three months after the initial fracture, the arm was still painful and function of the forearm was limited (elbow flexion/extension 145-0-0, pronation/supination 10-0-10, palmar flexion/dorsal flexion 60-0-60). A video of the preoperative range of motion is added in the Supplementary Materials (Video S1). This complicated daily activities and sports. Radiographs (Figure 1B) showed bowing and dorsal angulation of both radius and ulna. The patient was diagnosed with a symptomatic malunion of the left forearm. Therefore, 3D preoperative analyses were performed and a corrective osteotomy using patient-specific sawing and drilling guides was scheduled: this process takes about a month. At the request of her parents, the operation was scheduled three months after the analyses. Pain and function of the forearm had not improved compared to three months post-fracture.

2.2. Preoperative Planning & Guide Design

First, a CT scan (slice thickness of 0.6 mm) of both forearms was made. Based on the CT data, 3D models (Figure 2A,B) of the left and right forearm were created using Mimics (Materialise, Leuven, Belgium) software. To obtain a 3D model, automatic threshold-based bone segmentation was performed. Afterwards, the segmentation of the bones was checked, made solid, and labelled.

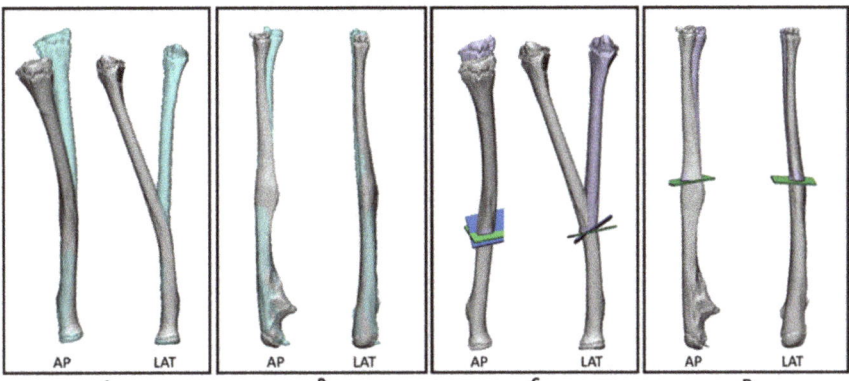

Figure 2. 3D models based on the preoperative CT scan in anterior posterior (AP) and lateral (LAT) position of (**A**) the injured left radius (grey) and the mirrored contralateral radius (blue), (**B**) the injured left ulna (grey) and the mirrored contralateral ulna (blue), (**C**) planned double osteotomy of the radius where the green and blue planes represent the first and second sawing planes, respectively. After correction, the injured radius (grey) can be repositioned towards the desired (purple) position, and (**D**) planned single osteotomy of the ulna with the green plane representing the sawing plane.

The uninjured contralateral forearm (right side) was mirrored over the injured forearm (left side) to use as a model of the anatomical desired position of the left forearm (Figure 2A,B). As a result, the rotational deviation of the injured side with respect to the uninjured side could be measured. Based on the centre of gravity of the radius, there was an increase of 15° of dorsal inclination, 11° of pronation, and 2° of radial deviation. For the ulna, the differences were smaller, with 2° of dorsal inclination, 8° of pronation, and 6° of ulnar deviation Then, a double osteotomy for the radial part and a single osteotomy of the ulnar part was performed (Figure 2C,D) and the distal parts of the radius and ulna were rotated and translated into the desired anatomic position (Figure 2C,D). The 3D preoperative analyses were discussed and authorised by a multidisciplinary team (orthopaedic surgeons and a technical physician).

Patient-specific guides were designed based on the preoperative 3D plan in 3-Matic 13.0 (Materialise, Leuven, Belgium) software. First, drilling guides were designed (Figure 3A). These guides direct the drilling of holes to eventually fixate the plate in the right position after the osteotomy. Second, the sawing guides were created. These guides are used to perform the osteotomies (Figure 3B). Additionally, both guides contained 3 holes for 1.4 mm K-wires for fixation of the guides during the procedure. Once the guides were created, the 3D models of the preoperative radius and ulna, and the postoperative desired radius and ulna, were made print ready. The 3D printed models of the pre- and postoperative radius and ulna were used during the procedure to assure the right position of the guides and fixation and to provide insight into the procedure.

Finally, the designed patient-specific guides were exported as a stereolithographic (STL) file and sent to a 3D printing company which 3D laser-printed the designed patient-specific guides from medically certified polyamide powder. The patient-specific guides were post-processed and packaged for hospital sterilisation and sterilized in house according to our standard clinical guidelines.

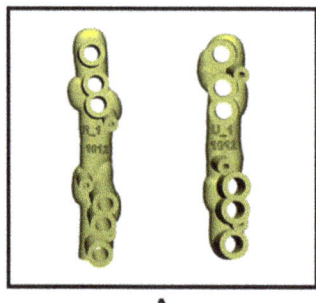 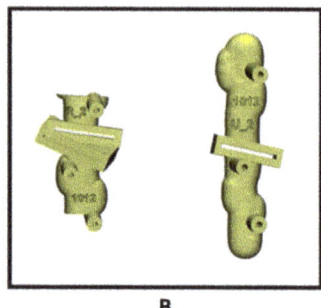

Figure 3. (**A**) Patient-specific drilling guides for the radius (left) and ulna (right), and (**B**) patient-specific saw guides for the radius (left) and ulna (right).

2.3. Surgical Procedure

The patient was operated under general anaesthesia. The left arm was positioned on an arm table and a tourniquet was applied. First, the radius was corrected through a volar Henry [16]. The patient-specific drilling guide was positioned on the radius. The position of the guide was confirmed using the surface anatomy of the bone and a 3D printed model of the radius. Once the position of the guide was verified, 1.4 mm K-wires were used to fixate the drilling guide. Subsequently, the screwholes were made in the radius through the guide. Subsequently, the drilling guide was replaced by the sawing guide using the same K-wires, and again the correct position of the guide was verified. The osteotomy was performed with an oscillating saw. The sawing guide and K-wires were removed and the radius was corrected to the planned position using a plate and screws.

The standard direct approach to the ulna was used, and similar to the correction of the radius, the patient-specific drill guide was used first, followed by the osteotomy guide. Subsequently, both guides were removed.

For both the radius and ulna, plates (2.4 mm straight LCP plates, Synthes) were placed on the pre-drilled holes and fixated with cortical and locking screws. The correction of the radius and ulna were verified under fluoroscopy. The range of motion was passively tested (elbow flexion/extension 145-0-0, pronation/supination 85-0-75, palmar flexion/dorsal flexion 80-0-80). The patient received an above elbow cast for 2 weeks.

2.4. Postoperative Results

The radial and ulnar corrections were evaluated using the CT-scan based 3D preoperative planning and postoperative radiographs of the forearm. After surgery, a CT scan was not obtained to avoid unnecessary radiation. To allow for image-based comparison, the preoperative 3D models were evaluated in the same view as the postoperative radiographs (Figure 4).

Clinically, the patient started visiting an experienced hand therapist (S.v.B.) every two weeks, starting at two weeks after surgery. Six weeks after surgery, the range of motion of the left forearm was comparable with the contralateral side (elbow flexion/extension 150-0-5, pronation/supination 90-0-90, palmar flexion/dorsal flexion 80-0-90). A video of the postoperative range of motion is added to the Supplementary Materials (Video S2). Three months after surgery, the patient was pain-free with full range of motion, and comparable grip strength of both hands. The radiographs showed full consolidation (Figure 1C).

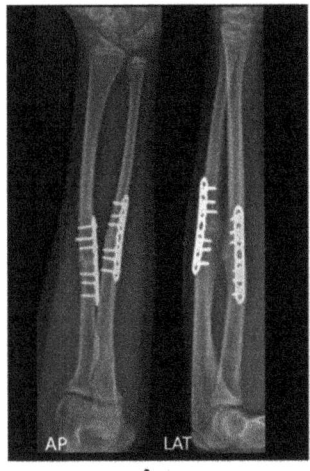 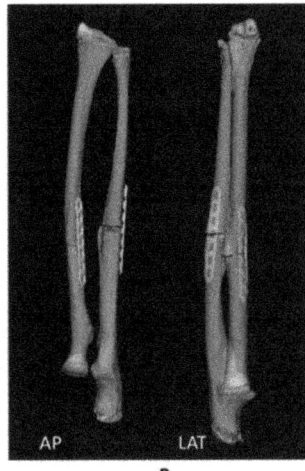

Figure 4. Comparison between (**A**) the postoperative radiographs and (**B**) the 3D planned postoperative position. Based on visual comparison, the correction was performed as planned.

3. Discussion and Conclusions

This case report presents the results of a corrective osteotomy of the forearm using 3D preoperative analysis and patient-specific guides in a patient with a malunited midshaft forearm fracture. The 3D preoperative analysis gives insight into the rotational and translational malalignment: without the planning and the drilling and sawing guides, it is almost impossible to perform a sufficient correction. The patient-specific guides ensure that the surgery will be performed according to plan, resulting in a correction in three planes of the malunion.

A corrective osteotomy may be considered when functional impairment persists as a result of a malunited fracture. In this specific case, the arm was painful, and the function of the forearm was limited three months after trauma. Although there has been debate about (the timing of) corrective osteotomies of malunions of forearm fractures in children, previous studies have shown favorable results. A review by Roth et al. (Roth et al. [17]), based on individual patient data of 11 cohort studies including 71 participants, revealed that corrective osteotomies provided a mean gain in forearm rotation of 77° (68° to 86°). In our case, we found an even better result, with full recovery of forearm rotation from 10° to 90°. Moreover, the study of Roth et al. revealed that both a younger age at osteotomy (median age 11 years at trauma) and a shorter time until osteotomy (median of 12 months between trauma and osteotomy) were associated with a better functional outcome. In our case, the patient was 12 years of age, with only 7 months between trauma and surgery. The relatively young age and short time between trauma and surgery may have contributed to the good functional outcome in our case study.

As mentioned earlier, malunited forearm fractures are often complex, involving deformities in multiple anatomical planes. The malunion presented here also included deviations in all anatomical planes for both the radius and ulna. These complex fractures are generally difficult to assess and plan based on plain 2D radiographs. Several studies have used 3D techniques to precisely plan and perform correction osteotomies of malunited forearm fractures. Byrne et al. [12] investigated the use of 3D planning and patient-specific guides in five consecutive patients with a diaphyseal forearm fracture and found an increase in both supination and pronation and a significant improvement in pain and grip strength. Miyake et al. [7] included 20 patients with a forearm malunion and found an improvement in angular deformity and an improvement in the mean arc of forearm motion. Kataoka et al. [14] investigated the use of computer-planning for the correction of malunited diaphyseal forearm fractures in four patients and found an improvement in angular deformity on X-ray, range of forearm rotation, and grip strength. These studies demonstrate that the use of 3D planning and printing of patient-specific guides helps surgeons to precisely perform corrective osteotomies of complex malunited fractures. This is supported by the findings of a review by Roth et al. [17], who showed that the use of 3D computer-assisted techniques is a predictor of superior functional outcome after corrective osteotomies of forearm malunions.

We are aware of the possible limitations of the current study in that it only describes the results of one patient. The results presented here, however, provide a complete picture of this specific case. Furthermore, one might consider the disadvantages of the use of 3D preoperative planning and patient-specific guides, as these techniques are cost and time-consuming. Another limitation is the necessity of a preoperative CT scan for 3D planning and printing. The additional dosage of the required CT scan compared to plain radiographs might be considered a problem, especially in children. Because of this, we have not obtained a postoperative CT scan to evaluate the performed corrective osteotomy. On the other hand, however, it has been shown that the use of 3D planning and printing reduces operating time, intraoperative blood loss, and fluoroscopic exposure [9].

The current case report shows that performing a corrective osteotomy with patient-specific guides based on preoperative 3D analyses for specific malunited fractures in children is of added value and makes it possible to precisely correct complex malunions of the forearm and closely mimic the pre-injured situation. The use of these computer-assisted techniques can help surgeons to plan and accurately perform corrective osteotomies resulting in improved functional outcomes.

Supplementary Materials: The following are available online at https://www.mdpi.com/article/10.3390/children8080707/s1, Video S1: preoperative range of motion and Video S2: postoperative range of motion.

Author Contributions: Conceptualization, F.F.S., F.d.G. and A.J.H.V.; writing—original draft preparation, F.F.S. and F.d.G.; writing—review and editing, F.F.S., F.d.G. and A.J.H.V. All authors have read and agreed to the published version of the manuscript.

Funding: This research received no external funding.

Institutional Review Board Statement: Ethical review and approval were waived for this study.

Informed Consent Statement: Written informed consent has been obtained from the patient and her parents to publish this paper.

Data Availability Statement: Since this is a case report all relevant data is presented in the result section.

Acknowledgments: The authors thank Simon van Benthem (S.v.B.), hand therapist, for performing the pre- and postoperative range of motion measurements.

Conflicts of Interest: The authors declare no conflict of interest.

References

1. Nagy, L.; Jankauskas, L.; Dumont, C.E. Correction of forearm malunion guided by the preoperative complaint. *Clin. Orthop. Relat. Res.* **2008**, *466*, 1419–1428. [CrossRef] [PubMed]
2. Fuller, D.J.; McCullough, C.J. Malunited fractures of the forearm in children. *J. Bone Jt. Surg. Br. Vol.* **1982**, *64*, 364–367. [CrossRef] [PubMed]
3. Trousdale, R.T.; Linscheid, R.L. Operative treatment of malunited fractures of the forearm. *J. Bone Jt. Surg. Am.* **1995**, *77*, 894–902. [CrossRef] [PubMed]
4. van Geenen, R.C.; Besselaar, P.P. Outcome after corrective osteotomy for malunited fractures of the forearm sustained in childhood. *J. Bone Jt. Surg. Br. Vol.* **2007**, *89*, 236–239. [CrossRef] [PubMed]
5. Miyake, J.; Oka, K.; Kataoka, T.; Moritomo, H.; Sugamoto, K.; Murase, T. 3-Dimensional deformity analysis of malunited forearm diaphyseal fractures. *J. Hand Surg. Am.* **2013**, *38*, 1356–1365. [CrossRef]
6. Vroemen, J.C.; Dobbe, J.G.; Strackee, S.D.; Streekstra, G.J. Positioning evaluation of corrective osteotomy for the malunited radius: 3-D CT versus 2-D radiographs. *Orthopedics* **2013**, *36*, e193–e199. [CrossRef] [PubMed]

7. Miyake, J.; Murase, T.; Oka, K.; Moritomo, H.; Sugamoto, K.; Yoshikawa, H. Computer-assisted corrective osteotomy for malunited diaphyseal forearm fractures. *J Bone Jt. Surg. Am.* **2012**, *94*, e150. [CrossRef] [PubMed]
8. Walenkamp, M.M.; de Muinck Keizer, R.J.; Dobbe, J.G.; Streekstra, G.J.; Goslings, J.C.; Kloen, P.; Strackee, S.D.; Schep, N.W. Computer-assisted 3D planned corrective osteotomies in eight malunited radius fractures. *Strateg. Trauma Limb. Reconstr.* **2015**, *10*, 109–116. [CrossRef] [PubMed]
9. Raza, M.; Murphy, D.; Gelfer, Y. The effect of three-dimensional (3D) printing on quantitative and qualitative outcomes in paediatric orthopaedic osteotomies: A systematic review. *EFORT Open Rev.* **2021**, *6*, 130–138. [CrossRef] [PubMed]
10. Levesque, J.N.; Shah, A.; Ekhtiari, S.; Yan, J.R.; Thornley, P.; Williams, D.S. Three-dimensional printing in orthopaedic surgery: A scoping review. *EFORT Open Rev* **2020**, *5*, 430–441. [CrossRef] [PubMed]
11. Bauer, A.S.; Storelli, D.A.R.; Sibbel, S.E.; McCarroll, H.R.; Lattanza, L.L. Preoperative Computer Simulation and Patient-specific Guides are Safe and Effective to Correct Forearm Deformity in Children. *J. Pediatric. Orthop.* **2017**, *37*, 504–510. [CrossRef] [PubMed]
12. Byrne, A.M.; Impelmans, B.; Bertrand, V.; Van Haver, A.; Verstreken, F. Corrective Osteotomy for Malunited Diaphyseal Forearm Fractures Using Preoperative 3-Dimensional Planning and Patient-Specific Surgical Guides and Implants. *J. Hand. Surg. Am.* **2017**, *42*, 836 e831–836 e812. [CrossRef] [PubMed]
13. Jeuken, R.M.; Hendrickx, R.P.M.; Schotanus, M.G.M.; Jansen, E.J. Near-anatomical correction using a CT-guided technique of a forearm malunion in a 15-year-old girl: A case report including surgical technique. *Orthop. Traumatol. Surg. Res.* **2017**, *103*, 783–790. [CrossRef] [PubMed]
14. Kataoka, T.; Oka, K.; Murase, T. Rotational Corrective Osteotomy for Malunited Distal Diaphyseal Radius Fractures in Children and Adolescents. *J. Hand. Surg. Am.* **2018**, *43*, 286.e281–286.e288. [CrossRef] [PubMed]
15. Miyake, J.; Murase, T.; Yamanaka, Y.; Moritomo, H.; Sugamoto, K.; Yoshikawa, H. Comparison of three dimensional and radiographic measurements in the analysis of distal radius malunion. *J. Hand. Surg. Eur. Vol.* **2013**, *38*, 133–143. [CrossRef]
16. Catalano, L.W., 3rd; Zlotolow, D.A.; Hitchcock, P.B.; Shah, S.N.; Barron, O.A. Surgical exposures of the radius and ulna. *J. Am. Acad. Orthop. Surg.* **2011**, *19*, 430–438. [CrossRef]
17. Roth, K.C.; Walenkamp, M.M.J.; van Geenen, R.C.I.; Reijman, M.; Verhaar, J.A.N.; Colaris, J.W. Factors determining outcome of corrective osteotomy for malunited paediatric forearm fractures: A systematic review and meta-analysis. *J. Hand. Surg. Eur. Vol.* **2017**, *42*, 810–816. [CrossRef]

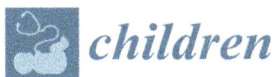

Article

Diagnostic Accuracy of 3D Ultrasound and Artificial Intelligence for Detection of Pediatric Wrist Injuries

Jack Zhang, Naveenjyote Boora, Sarah Melendez, Abhilash Rakkunedeth Hareendranathan and Jacob Jaremko *

Department of Radiology and Diagnostic Imaging, Walter C. Mackenzie Health Sciences Centre, University of Alberta, 8440-112 Street, Edmonton, AB T6G 2B7, Canada; jzzhang@ualberta.ca (J.Z.); naveenjy@ualberta.ca (N.B.); macdonel@ualberta.ca (S.M.); hareendr@ualberta.ca (A.R.H.)
* Correspondence: jjaremko@ualberta.ca; Tel.: +1-780-407-7923

Abstract: Wrist trauma is common in children, typically requiring radiography for diagnosis and treatment planning. However, many children do not have fractures and are unnecessarily exposed to radiation. Ultrasound performed at bedside could detect fractures prior to radiography. Modern tools including three-dimensional ultrasound (3DUS) and artificial intelligence (AI) have not yet been applied to this task. Our purpose was to assess (1) feasibility, reliability, and accuracy of 3DUS for detection of pediatric wrist fractures, and (2) accuracy of automated fracture detection via AI from 3DUS sweeps. Children presenting to an emergency department with unilateral upper extremity injury to the wrist region were scanned on both the affected and unaffected limb. Radiographs of the symptomatic limb were obtained for comparison. Ultrasound scans were read by three individuals to determine reliability. An AI network was trained and compared against the human readers. Thirty participants were enrolled, resulting in scans from fifty-five wrists. Readers had a combined sensitivity of 1.00 and specificity of 0.90 for fractures. AI interpretation was indistinguishable from human interpretation, with all fractures detected in the test set of 36 images (sensitivity = 1.0). The high sensitivity of 3D ultrasound and automated AI ultrasound interpretation suggests that ultrasound could potentially rule out fractures in the emergency department.

Keywords: 3D ultrasonography; wrist; fractures; pediatric; artificial intelligence

Citation: Zhang, J.; Boora, N.; Melendez, S.; Rakkunedeth Hareendranathan, A.; Jaremko, J. Diagnostic Accuracy of 3D Ultrasound and Artificial Intelligence for Detection of Pediatric Wrist Injuries. *Children* **2021**, *8*, 431. https://doi.org/10.3390/children8060431

Academic Editor: Vito Pavone

Received: 16 April 2021
Accepted: 18 May 2021
Published: 21 May 2021

Publisher's Note: MDPI stays neutral with regard to jurisdictional claims in published maps and institutional affiliations.

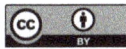

Copyright: © 2021 by the authors. Licensee MDPI, Basel, Switzerland. This article is an open access article distributed under the terms and conditions of the Creative Commons Attribution (CC BY) license (https://creativecommons.org/licenses/by/4.0/).

1. Introduction

Fractures are the third leading cause of pediatric hospitalizations in Canada [1]. Distal radius fractures account for up to 25% of fractures documented in children [2]. Distal radius fractures typically occur in children falling on an outstretched hand and involve the metaphysis or physis [2]. Depending on the area of injury, there can be a multitude of fracture patterns that affect treatment planning [3]. Therefore, when children present to primary care clinics or emergency department (ED) with suspected wrist fractures, radiographs are the standard of care as they allow for precise examination of the anatomy. In most hospitals, routine radiographs are performed on patients with wrist trauma, but only half of the imaging reveals fractures [4]. With the estimated cost of treating pediatric forearm fractures at $2 billion per year in the USA [5], streamlining care is desirable. Obtaining radiographs in ED typically involves sending the patient to a separate diagnostic imaging area, where they wait in an additional queue, and transferring them back, a process which can add hours to an ED visit. If clinicians could determine at bedside who has a fracture and requires an X-ray, systemwide radiation doses and costs could be reduced and ED visits shortened.

Ultrasound (US) is a ubiquitous but underutilized tool in the ED. It has the advantages of being inexpensive and portable while being able to reveal cortical disruption, periosteal fluid, and joint effusion to aid in detecting fractures. The use of US in pediatric distal radius fractures has been validated to have similar accuracy compared to radiography [6–11]. A recent meta-analysis identified 16 studies with 1204 patients, resulting in 97% sensitivity and 95% specificity [12]. More recent research has shown that a short 1–2 h training session is sufficient for physicians to perform the US scan [7,9]. 3D ultrasound (3DUS), essentially a high-quality sweep video obtained across the injured area, should more fully depict the fracture anatomy than a single 2D ultrasound image, but there are currently very few studies examining the role of 3DUS in pediatric fracture detection.

In general, 3DUS interpretation involves reviewing large amounts of image data, and its accuracy depends largely on the clinician's expertise. As a possible alternative to manual interpretation, we examined the feasibility of automatic interpretation of wrist ultrasound using AI. Our technique used an ensemble of convolutional neural networks (CNNs) that predicted the presence/absence of a fracture in a given image.

Accordingly, the aim of this study was to assess feasibility, reliability, and accuracy of 3DUS, interpreted by humans or automatically by AI, for detection of pediatric wrist fractures, in comparison to conventional radiographs. We hypothesized that these advanced tools allow use of ultrasound to detect fractures as accurately as radiographs.

2. Materials and Methods

2.1. Study Design

This was a prospective diagnostic study performed at a tertiary pediatric hospital. The study was approved by the institutional ethics committee (Pro00077093).

2.2. Study Protocol

A convenient sample of 30 children (age: 0–17 years) presenting to a tertiary pediatric hospital with unilateral upper extremity injuries to the wrist were identified at triage. Written informed consent was obtained from the parents (or the child if a mature minor > 16 years of age). Most US scans were performed in the waiting room prior to physician evaluation. Radiographs of the symptomatic limbs, as ordered by the EM physician at initial visit, and any follow-up imaging obtained over the next 30 days within our health region, were obtained from PACS, anonymized, and stored for blinded reading.

The inclusion criterion was tenderness in the distal radius region following trauma, such as falling on the arm. Exclusion criterion was inability to perform an ultrasound scan, such as due to an existing cast, laceration over scanning area, or open fractures. Children were not excluded based on severity of symptoms.

2.3. Imaging Technique and Training

Each child was seated, and their wrists were placed in a comfortable neutral position. Imaging was performed on a Philips IU22 machine using a 13 MHz 13VL5 probe for 3DUS. The child's injured limb was scanned on the dorsal and volar surfaces in both the sagittal and axial orientation. The operator centered the view on the distal 3 cm of the radius for all children in the different orientations and initiated the sweep. A 3.2 second automated sweep through a range of $\pm 15°$ to produce US slices of 0.2 mm thickness totaling 382 slices was performed. The non-injured wrists were similarly scanned. We thus had four sweeps of each wrist. The 3DUS probe was used to ensure consistent sweeps rather than imaging differences.

Training was deliberately kept minimal. The operators for scans were medical students (J.Z. and N.B.) with no prior experience with US. Each received 1 h of hands-on training by a pediatric MSK radiologist (J.J.) which consisted of primarily operating the IU22, a discussion on the basic anatomy of the distal forearm, and practice scanning the radiologist under supervision. Readers were given 5 examples of wrist fractures and 5 examples of non-fractured wrists for review prior to blinded reading.

2.4. Artificial Intelligence

CNNs have been gradually increasing in popularity for computer vision problems and are now the technique of choice due to success in image classification, as shown in competitions such as ImageNet [13]. CNN models consisting of convolutional layers and fully connected layers were trained to classify images frame-by-frame as either normal (category 0) or fractured (category 1). Convolutional layers are for detecting patterns, such as the edge of an uninjured bone, while fully connected layers interpret the detected patterns. For example, if the straight edge of a bone is suddenly disrupted, the fully connected layer might interpret that as a fracture. All frames were resized to match the network input size (128×128). Using a brute force approach, we trained several models with varying numbers of convolutional layers and fully connected layers and selected three networks that gave the highest accuracy to be part of the ensemble. The output of each ensemble represents the median prediction of the three CNNs included. The ranges of various network parameters used are summarized in Table 1. We trained separate ensembles for volar sagittal and dorsal sagittal scans.

Table 1. Networks were trained with all combinations of parameters and the top three networks in terms of validation set accuracy were included in the final ensemble model.

Network Parameter	Range of Values
Number of convolutional layers	2–5, step size = 1
Number of fully connected (FC) layers	1–2, step size = 1
Optimizers	Stochastic Gradient Descent (SGD), RMSprop, Adagrad, Adadelta, Adamax ADAM
Dropout	0–50%, step size = 10
Loss Function	Cross-entropy (CE)
Epochs	80

2.5. Statistical Analysis

3DUS readings of both injured and uninjured limbs were anonymized and read independently by a medical student (J.Z.), pediatric radiology fellow (S.M.), and pediatric MSK radiologist (J.J.). The radiographs were centrally re-reviewed by our pediatric MSK radiologist blinded to clinical data and compared to original reports. Sensitivity (SN), specificity (SP), positive and negative predictive value (PPV, NPV), and positive and negative likelihood radio (LR+, LR−) were calculated for human experts and AI using SPSS (SPSS Inc., v.22, Chicago, IL, USA). Interrater reliability was calculated as percentage agreement and Cohen's Kappa.

3. Results

We enrolled 30 children, resulting in 55 scans of individual limbs (five non-injured limbs could not be imaged due to logistical constraints in ED). The mean age was 9.9 years (range 3.8–14.8) and 70% of the participants were male. On radiographic review, unilateral arm radiographs of all 30 patients were assessed, revealing 19 distal forearm fractures. The blinded central re-review was in 100% agreement with original reports. Radiographic evidence of fracture was used as gold standard diagnosis.

3.1. Manual Interpretation

The diagnostic accuracy of 3DUS in identifying distal radius fractures in our dataset was 96.5% (95% CI 89–100%). Out of the 19 fractures, 19 were correctly identified by the radiologist and 18 were identified by the medical student and fellow. For limbs without fractures, we achieved an accuracy of 80% (95% CI 63–98%). Out of the 36 uninjured arms, the radiologist had 6 false positives while the medical student and fellow had 5 and 10 false positives, respectively. Overall, the three readers performed similarly with moderate to high interrater reliability (Cohen's kappa: J.J.–J.Z. 0.602, J.J.–S.M. 0.571, J.Z.–S.M. 0.536) [14]. By combining the three readers together, i.e., the diagnosis agreed upon by at least 2 readers, the combined reader had SN 1.00, SP 0.90 (Table 2).

Table 2. Statistical analysis of the individual readers and median combination of the individuals.

	J.J.	J.Z.	S.M.	Combined
Sensitivity	1.00 ± 0.00	0.95 ± 0.05	0.95 ± 0.05	1.00 ± 0.00
Specificity	0.83 ± 0.06	0.86 ± 0.06	0.74 ± 0.07	0.90 ± 0.05
Positive predictive value	0.76 ± 0.09	0.78 ± 0.09	0.64 ± 0.09	0.83 ± 0.08
Negative predictive value	1.00 ± 0.00	0.97 ± 0.03	0.97 ± 0.03	1.00 ± 0.00
Positive likelihood ratio	6.00	6.80	3.70	9.75
Negative likelihood ratio	0.00	0.06	0.07	0.00

The "combined reader" produced 4 false positives which were individually reviewed by the radiologist. Two scans were misclassified due to 3DUS artifacts and the other two scans represented possible subtle fractures that were not identified on radiographs (Figure 1). The combined reader did not have any false negatives (Figure 2).

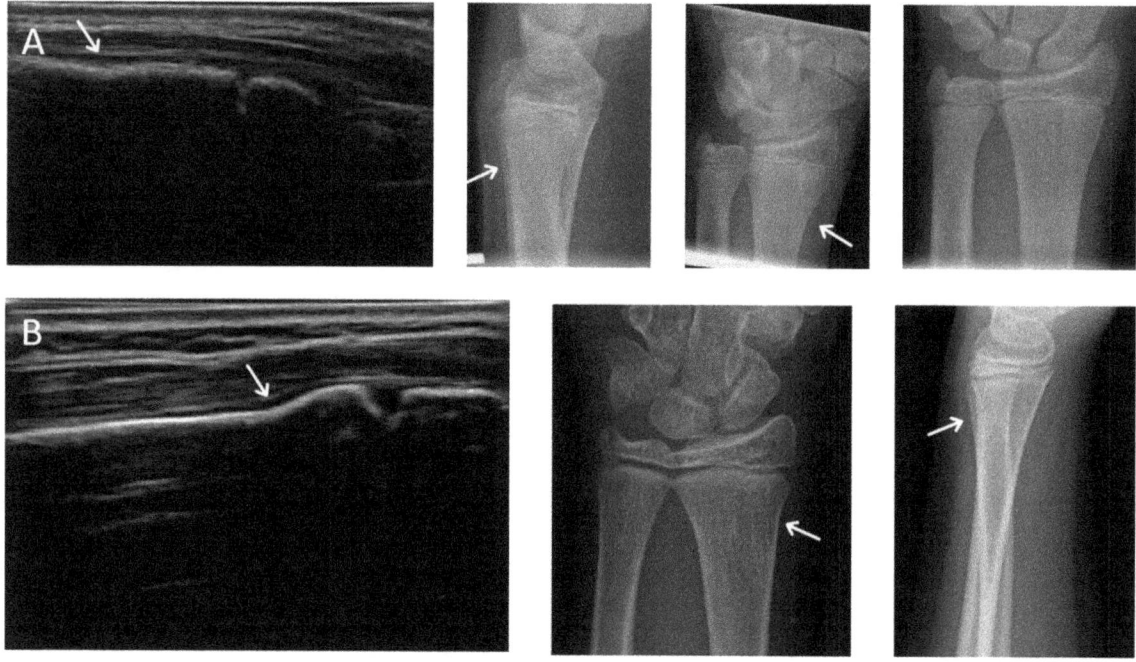

Figure 1. Possible missed fractures. (**A,B**) are dorsal longitudinal views of the distal radius of two possible X-ray false negatives. Note the excess angulation of the distal radius may represent torus fractures. The possible defect is observable on X-ray.

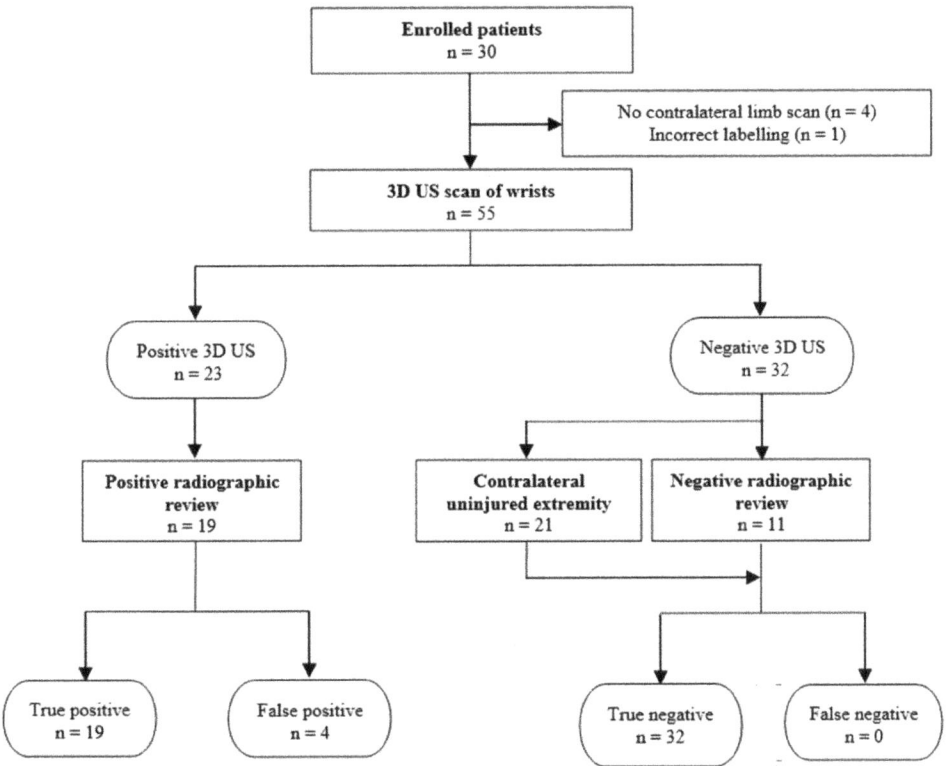

Figure 2. STARD flow diagram, showing the number of children who received the US and gold standard radiograph [15]. The US results are from combined readers.

3.2. AI Interpretation

We trained multiple CNN models using 2D images extracted from 21 wrist sweeps (~6000 images). We validated the AI prediction on 1640 image slices extracted from 72 3DUS volumes (36 volar and 36 dorsal) acquired from 36 wrists. Our technique gave accuracies of 95% and 94% per slice for images extracted from dorsal and volar views. Each 3DUS volume was analyzed slice by slice and sweeps with more than 30 slices predicted to be fractured were categorized as class 1. Our technique was 89% and 92% accurate in classifying dorsal and volar sweeps. For each patient, predictions on dorsal and volar sweeps were combined to arrive at a final AI-aided diagnosis. When compared against human assessments of the same patient, AI-aided diagnosis gave sensitivity = 100% and specificity = 89% (Table 3). Evaluation of agreement of the AI prediction with human readers gave ICC = 0.80 (CI (0.62, 0.92)) and Cohen's Kappa = 0.48–0.74.

Table 3. Diagnostic accuracy of AI evaluation on individual image slices (per slice), 3DUS sweeps (per sweep), and at the patient level (per patient) in test data not used for AI network training.

Per Image					
Image Type	Normal	Fractured	Sensitivity	Specificity	Accuracy
2D Image Volar Sagittal	504	277	98%	89%	94%
2D Image Dorsal Sagittal	486	373	99%	90%	95%
Per Sweep					
Image Type	Normal	Fractured	Sensitivity	Specificity	Accuracy
Sweep Volar Sagittal	23	13	85%	91%	89%
Sweep Dorsal Sagittal	23	13	100%	87%	92%
Per Patient					
Image Type	Normal	Fractured	Sensitivity	Specificity	Accuracy
Sweep Volar and Dorsal	23	13	100	87%	92%

4. Discussion

In this pilot study, we found that 3D ultrasound was highly accurate at detecting fractures, whether interpreted by human experts or automatically by artificial intelligence.

A recent meta-analysis of 16 studies produced pooled statistics of 97% SN, 95% SP, 20 LR+, and 0.03 LR− for usage of 2D US in pediatric distal forearm fractures [12]. Our results are comparable to previous studies and demonstrate the ability of 3DUS to be a diagnostic tool in distal radius fractures. This is the first study to show that 3DUS scans allow radiologists and trainees to diagnose pediatric distal forearm fractures, with the benefit of minimal scanning and reading training.

The radiologist achieved very high sensitivity of 100% and 95% for the other 2 readers. While our data had a small number of fractures, it suggested that a negative 3DUS in ER can effectively rule out a distal radius fracture. A rational clinical management plan would be to send children with a positive 3DUS scan for radiographs to confirm the presence of a fracture and aid in treatment planning, while children with a negative 3DUS scan by this protocol could potentially be discharged without radiographs, reducing cost to the healthcare system. Although the trainees missed 5% of positive cases, none of the three readers had previous experience reading US images of wrist fractures and their training was limited to 5 fractures and 5 normal sweeps. Thus, due to limited experience, we combined the results from all three readers to offer insight into the performance of individuals if they had more training and experience. A larger study with more data for training and testing could improve overall performance. In addition, future studies investigating the ability of ultrasound in identification of the fracture pattern and treatment planning can further expand the clinical role of ultrasound. Future research involving ED physicians interpreting the wrist sweeps would determine whether these scans are useful in clinical practice.

Reviewing the discordant cases, there were several individual reader false positives, with the false-positive rate reduced by using the combined reading values, further suggesting the need for more training. Another reason for false positives was US artifacts, including double or interrupted cortical margins, likely caused by motion artifact and side-lobe artifact. The 3DUS obtained hundreds of images per sweep, and some of these images included artifacts that might not be identified as frequently on 2DUS. Adding 5 min of user training specifically demonstrating examples of these artifacts could help users avoid misinterpretation. Users who identify these artifacts at the time of scanning would be encouraged to perform repeat scans, subject to time constraints in the clinical department.

A benefit of 3DUS was that unlike in previous studies of 2DUS, 3DUS allowed retrospective review of the scans. Scans in previous studies were performed by emergency physicians or residents as part of the patient care team [7,10,16]. The history and physical exam alongside the US likely augmented the overall clinical picture and improved the SN and SP of those studies [10]. The 3D sweep allowed for a simple scanning protocol which reduced the training that medical students with limited clinical knowledge required to just 1 h. Training in previous studies focused on anatomy, identification of fracture, and viewing method [10,16]. We expect that ED physicians with point-of-care US training can readily employ this technique to evaluate patients and make decisions on additional imaging. Furthermore, while US images are considered highly user-dependent [9,17], by capturing a sweep of the fracture and allowing for retrospective review, user dependency can be reduced and allow any healthcare practitioner to obtain a useful scan, and ED physicians can review the scan at their convenience. This also allows radiologists to aid in the interpretation of the study if there are any concerns. With minimal user training, we replicated the high reported sensitivity of 2DUS using 3DUS. Our specificity with 3DUS was somewhat lower than the best reported 2DUS results, but on review of images, this could be rectified in the future by a few extra minutes of reader training. The value added by 3DUS was not in increasing the already high accuracy of well-performed 2DUS, but in allowing scans to be performed by users with less training, generating comprehensive saved images that can be reviewed more reliably.

There were 2 possible radiographic false negatives out of 10 negative radiographs, as the US revealed subtle cortical irregularities that could represent undisplaced fractures. Retrospective review of two X-rays in light of ultrasound findings showed subtle cortical contour irregularities that might have represented the fractures identified on US (Figure 3). Previous studies had also reported the possibility that ultrasound may identify subtle fractures not seen on radiographs [7]. The clinical significance of these possible undisplaced fractures is unknown. Future study could potentially perform limited MRI in this small subset of patients with discrepant ultrasound/X-ray findings to clarify vs. an external gold standard.

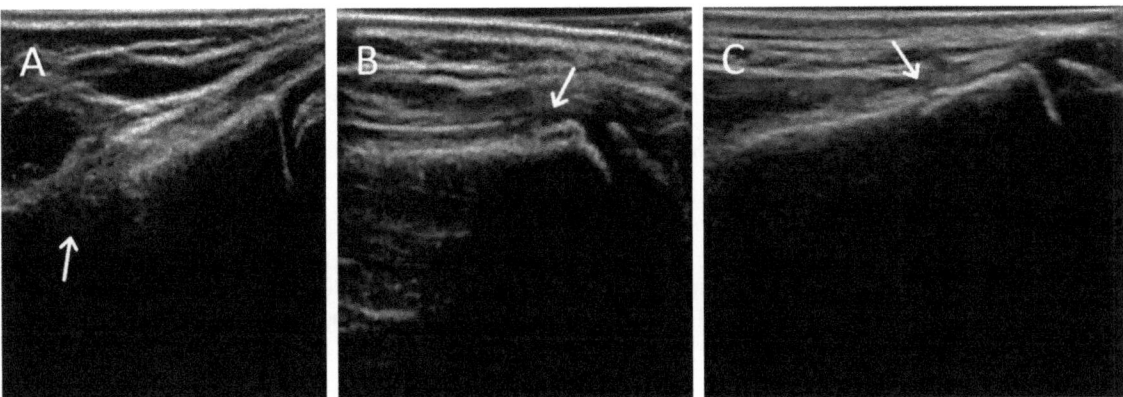

Figure 3. Examples of 3DUS scanning artifacts. (**A**) Edge effects, (**B**) double cortex from motion, (**C**) overlapping cortex.

Another key benefit of 3DUS was that the 'sweep' images obtained gave a comprehensive dataset, showing the full anatomy of the distal radius and ulna, suitable for automated reconstruction using artificial intelligence (AI), and eventually, automated diagnosis of wrist fractures [17].

The 3DUS probe used in this study was costly but not necessary. We used 3DUS to ensure the sweeps produced were as consistent as possible for accurate training of the AI algorithm. Readily available conventional 2DUS probes can produce a cine '2D sweep' video when the user moves any 2DUS probe manually across the arm. Our future research will include testing whether 2DUS manual 'sweep' videos can be interpreted with the same diagnostic accuracy as 3DUS sweeps. Ultimately, a package combining cine ultrasound acquisition by a minimally trained user using a portable handheld probe with automated

AI analysis of the obtained images could be a rapid diagnostic aid to efficiently rule out or detect wrist fractures at the point of care.

4.1. AI Interpretation

A CNN-based technique was developed to automatically detect fractures by combining the information in volar and dorsal sagittal scans. It correctly detected all fractures, corresponding to expert-level sensitivity of 100% in 3D sweeps. One of 13 fractures was missed in the volar scans but correctly detected in the corresponding dorsal scan. This is expected as not all fractures involve the volar cortex. The model also showed high agreement with human interpretation in terms of ICC and kappa. Given that 3/13 fractures were missed by at least one human reader, the sensitivity of the AI technique (100%) is particularly high.

AI-aided analysis of 3DUS eliminates inter-observer variability and saves expert time. The end-to-end execution time of AI models on V100 NVIDIA GPU was <2 seconds per sweep, which is well-suited for real-time applications. The AI models can be accessed from emergency departments and the interpretation can be obtained along with the scan report.

4.2. Limitations

This study had limitations. We had a small sample size and limited the current study to the distal radius. Less common but important fractures of the distal ulna or scaphoid could potentially also be detected by 3DUS, and this requires further study. Due to ethical restrictions on radiation dose in children, we were unable to obtain radiographs of contralateral limbs. It was presumed that no acute fractures were present in these 30 limbs, all of which were asymptomatic (nontender and moved freely by the children during ultrasound examination). Furthermore, there was no external reference standard such as MRI available, for logistical reasons.

Although we were pleasantly surprised by the success of our AI approach even on this small training dataset, a limitation of our AI is that it is not fully explainable. The image features that contributed to the diagnosis had not been identified. As future work, we plan to use explainable AI techniques such as a Deep Taylor decomposition to identify regions in the ultrasound image that contributed to a particular diagnosis [18].

5. Conclusions

Our data suggests that 3DUS, whether interpreted by human experts or artificial intelligence, is comparable to X-ray in diagnosing pediatric distal radius fractures, with nearly 100% sensitivity, i.e., a negative 3DUS can rule out fracture. 3DUS, particularly when combined with AI, could reduce the need for radiographs for forearm fractures in the emergency department.

Author Contributions: Conceptualization, J.J.; Data curation, J.Z.; Formal analysis, S.M., A.R.H. and J.J.; Methodology, J.Z., N.B. and J.J.; Writing—original draft, J.Z.; Writing—review and editing, J.Z., N.B., S.M., A.R.H. and J.J. All authors have read and agreed to the published version of the manuscript.

Funding: This work was funded in part by the David and Beatrice Reidford Research Scholarship and in part by the University of Alberta Department of Radiology and Diagnostic Imaging Endowment.

Institutional Review Board Statement: The study was conducted according to the guidelines of the Declaration of Helsinki, and approved by the Institutional Review Board of University of Alberta (Pro00077093 Dec 2017).

Informed Consent Statement: Informed consent was obtained from all subjects involved in the study.

Data Availability Statement: The data presented in this study are available upon request from the corresponding author. The data are not publicly available due to patient privacy requirements of clinical data.

Acknowledgments: We would like to thank Bill Sevcik and Andrew Dixon for their assistance in making the study possible to perform in Stollery Children's Hospital Emergency Department.

Conflicts of Interest: J.J. is a co-founder of MEDO.ai, a startup investigating AI analysis of ultrasound images. MEDO had no role in this study. The authors declare no other potential conflict of interest. The funders had no role in the design of the study; in the collection, analyses, or interpretation of data; in the writing of the manuscript, or in the decision to publish the results.

References

1. Connors, C.; Millar, W.J. Changes in Children's Hospital Use. *Health Rep.* **1999**, *11*, 9–20. [PubMed]
2. Nellans, K.W.; Kowalski, E.; Chung, K.C. The Epidemiology of Distal Radius Fractures. *Hand Clin.* **2012**, *28*, 113–125. [CrossRef] [PubMed]
3. Bae, D.S. Pediatric Distal Radius and Forearm Fractures. *J. Hand Surg. Am.* **2008**, *33*, 1911–1923. [CrossRef] [PubMed]
4. Slaar, A.; Bentohami, A.; Kessels, J.; Bijlsma, T.S.; van Dijkman, B.A.; Maas, M.; Wilde, J.C.H.; Goslings, J.C.; Schep, N.W.L. The Role of Plain Radiography in Paediatric Wrist Trauma. *Insights Imaging* **2012**, *3*, 513–517. [CrossRef] [PubMed]
5. Ryan, L.M.; Teach, S.J.; Searcy, K.; Singer, S.A.; Wood, R.; Wright, J.L.; Chamberlain, J.M. Epidemiology of Pediatric Forearm Fractures in Washington, DC. *J. Trauma Acute Care Surg.* **2010**, *69*, S200–S205. [CrossRef] [PubMed]
6. Chen, L.; Kim, Y.; Moore, C.L. Diagnosis and Guided Reduction of Forearm Fractures in Children Using Bedside Ultrasound. *Pediatr. Emerg. Care* **2007**, *23*, 528–531. [CrossRef] [PubMed]
7. Rowlands, R.; Rippey, J.; Tie, S.; Flynn, J. Bedside Ultrasound vs X-Ray for the Diagnosis of Forearm Fractures in Children. *J. Emerg. Med.* **2017**, *52*, 208–215. [CrossRef] [PubMed]
8. Lee, S.H.; Yun, S.J. Diagnostic Performance of Ultrasonography for Detection of Pediatric Elbow Fracture: A Meta-Analysis. *Ann. Emerg. Med.* **2019**, *74*, 493–502. [CrossRef] [PubMed]
9. Hedelin, H.; Tingström, C.; Hebelka, H.; Karlsson, J. Minimal Training Sufficient to Diagnose Pediatric Wrist Fractures with Ultrasound. *Crit. Ultrasound J.* **2017**, *9*, 11. [CrossRef]
10. Epema, A.C.; Spanjer, M.J.B.; Ras, L.; Kelder, J.C.; Sanders, M. Point-of-Care Ultrasound Compared with Conventional Radiographic Evaluation in Children with Suspected Distal Forearm Fractures in the Netherlands: A Diagnostic Accuracy Study. *Emerg. Med. J.* **2019**, *36*, 613–616. [CrossRef] [PubMed]
11. Galletebeitia Laka, I.; Samson, F.; Gorostiza, I.; Gonzalez, A.; Gonzalez, C. The Utility of Clinical Ultrasonography in Identifying Distal Forearm Fractures in the Pediatric Emergency Department. *Eur. J. Emerg. Med.* **2019**, *26*, 118–122. [CrossRef] [PubMed]
12. Douma-Den Hamer, D.; Blanker, M.H.; Edens, M.A.; Buijteweg, L.N.; Boomsma, M.F.; Van Helden, S.H.; Mauritz, G.J. Ultrasound for Distal Forearm Fracture: A Systematic Review and Diagnostic Meta-Analysis. *PLoS ONE* **2016**, *11*, 1–16. [CrossRef]
13. Yamashita, R.; Nishio, M.; Do, R.K.G.; Togashi, K. Convolutional Neural Networks: An Overview and Application in Radiology. *Insights Imaging* **2018**, *9*, 611–629. [CrossRef] [PubMed]
14. McHugh, M.L. Interrater Reliability: The Kappa Statistic. *Biochem. Med.* **2012**, *22*, 276–282. [CrossRef]
15. Bossuyt, P.M.; Reitsma, J.B.; Bruns, D.E.; Gatsonis, C.A.; Glaziou, P.P.; Irwig, L.; Lijmer, J.G.; Moher, D.; Rennie, D.; de Vet, H.C.W.; et al. STARD 2015: An Updated List of Essential Items for Reporting Diagnostic Accuracy Studies. *BMJ* **2015**, *351*, h5527. [CrossRef]
16. Herren, C.; Sobottke, R.; Ringe, M.J.; Visel, D.; Graf, M.; Müller, D.; Siewe, J. Ultrasound-Guided Diagnosis of Fractures of the Distal Forearm in Children. *Orthop. Traumatol. Surg. Res.* **2015**, *101*, 501–505. [CrossRef]
17. Nicholson, J.A.; Tsang, S.T.J.; MacGillivray, T.J.; Perks, F.; Simpson, A.H.R.W. What Is the Role of Ultrasound in Fracture Management? *Bone Jt. Res.* **2019**, *8*, 304–312. [CrossRef] [PubMed]
18. Montavon, G.; Samek, W.; Müller, K.-R. Methods for Interpreting and Understanding Deep Neural Networks. *Digit. Signal Process.* **2018**, *73*, 1–15. [CrossRef]

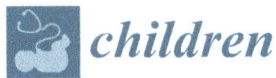

Article

Apophyseal Avulsion of the Rectus Femoris Tendon Origin in Adolescent Soccer Players

Hanneke Weel [1], A. J. Peter Joosten [2] and Christiaan J. A. van Bergen [2,*]

1 Bergman Clinics, Department of Orthopedics Arnhem, Mr. E.N. van Kleffensstraat 14, 6842 CV Arnhem, The Netherlands; h.weel@bergmanclinics.nl
2 Department of Orthopedic Surgery, Amphia Hospital, 4800 RK Breda, The Netherlands; ajoosten@amphia.nl
* Correspondence: cvanbergen@amphia.nl; Tel.: +31-76-5955000

Abstract: Apophyseal avulsions of the rectus femorus tendon (RFT) at the anterior inferior iliac spine (AIIS) can occur in adolescents, often while performing soccer. Patient-reported outcomes (PROMs) and time to return to sport of these patients are relatively unknown. Therefore, the aim of this study was to assess the PROMs and return to sports of patients with AIIS avulsions and compare the results with those reported in the literature. This is a case series of seven consecutive patients presenting at our hospital between 2018 and 2020 with an apophyseal avulsion of the RFT from the AIIS. The patients were assessed with use of the WOMAC and Tegner scores and return to sports was evaluated. All patients were male soccer players (median age 13 years; range, 12–17). They were all initially treated non-operatively. One of the patients subsequently needed excision surgery of a heterotopic ossification because of non-transient hip impingement. All other patients recovered after a period of relative rest. Median time to return to sports was 2.5 months (range, 2–3). At a median follow-up of 33 months (range, 18–45), the WOMAC (median, 100; range, 91–100) and Tegner scores (median, 9; range, 5–9) were high. In accordance with the existing literature, most patients with apophyseal avulsions of the AIIS recover well with non-operative treatment. However, the avulsion can lead to hip impingement due to heterotopic ossifications possibly needing surgical excision. Sport resumption is achievable after 2–3 months, and patient-reported outcomes are highly satisfactory in the long term.

Keywords: apophysial avulsion; rectus femoris tendon; adolescent; sport

Citation: Weel, H.; Joosten, A.J.P.; van Bergen, C.J.A. Apophyseal Avulsion of the Rectus Femoris Tendon Origin in Adolescent Soccer Players. *Children* 2022, 9, 1016. https://doi.org/10.3390/children9071016

Academic Editor: Angelo Gabriele Aulisa

Received: 31 May 2022
Accepted: 6 July 2022
Published: 8 July 2022

Publisher's Note: MDPI stays neutral with regard to jurisdictional claims in published maps and institutional affiliations.

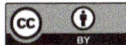

Copyright: © 2022 by the authors. Licensee MDPI, Basel, Switzerland. This article is an open access article distributed under the terms and conditions of the Creative Commons Attribution (CC BY) license (https://creativecommons.org/licenses/by/4.0/).

1. Introduction

In the paediatric pelvis, the apophyseal plate is a biomechanical weak spot [1] because the cartilaginous growth plate fails in tension before the musculotendinous unit does [2]. Apophyses are at risk to avulsion fractures in adolescents, especially in athletes due to strong contraction forces of the attached muscles. Pelvic avulsions are often seen in adolescent athletes, with the avulsion at the anterior inferior iliac spine (AIIS) counting for 22–49% of the pelvic avulsions, followed by the anterior superior iliac spine with 20–30% [3–6]. The direct head of the rectus femoris tendon (RFT) originates from the AIIS, proximal to the hip joint, whereas the reflected head originates from the anterior acetabular ridge and anterior hip joint capsule, which is rarely affected by avulsion injuries. The apophysis is especially at risk of injury between formation of the secondary growth centre and its closure. For the AIIS, this period lays between ages 13.6 and 16.3 years in boys and between 14 and 14.9 in girls [2]. Avulsion injury of the AIIS typically occurs with eccentric force at the hip, such as seen in sprinting and kicking a ball. Boys are more often affected than girls [4], with up to 70% of the affected adolescents performing ball sports [3], but also track and field [3,4] and rarely skiing [7].

Patients with AIIS injuries may describe feeling or hearing a "pop" at the time of injury. This is reported to be present in 33% [5]. Swelling and ecchymosis may be present.

According to Müller et al. physical examination demonstrates tenderness at the AIIS on palpation (in 98%), weakness of muscles (85%), pain during motion (47%), and sometimes a notable limping (23%) [5]. Pain and weakness with hip flexion, knee extension, or a resisted straight leg raise also may be present [5].

Displacement of the apophysis is thought to be restricted by a relatively thick periosteum. When the avulsion is not more than 15 [3] or 20 mm [8] displaced, the treatment of choice is conservative. Conservative treatment mostly starts with rest, builds up with progressively regaining motion until allowance of weight bearing, then starting training muscle strength until return to sports, as first described in detail by Metzmaker and Pappas [9]. Although non-surgical treatment usually leads to high success rates in the short term [3,4,8–10], patients with AIIS avulsions are 4.5 times more likely to experience future hip pain beyond 3 months compared with other pelvic avulsions [4]. Complication rates are reported to be high (64%) and similarly distributed over both nonoperative and operative treatments, with non-union and heterotopic ossifications mostly reported [3]. However, return to sports and long-term patient-reported outcomes are rarely reported in the literature. Therefore, the aim of this study was to assess return to sports and long-term patient-reported outcomes of adolescents with avulsion fractures of the AIIS.

2. Materials and Methods

2.1. Patients

This retrospective case series included all consecutive patients presenting to the authors' outpatient clinic of the orthopaedic department of a large teaching hospital (Amphia Hospital, Breda, the Netherlands) from January 2018 until the end of 2020. Inclusion criteria were adolescents, defined by the World Health Organisation (WHO) as patients between 10 and 19 years of age, minimum follow-up of 1 year, and confirmation of the diagnosis on radiography of the pelvis. There were no exclusion criteria.

2.2. Assessment

Collected injury data included: side of injury, type and level of sports, trauma mechanism (if applicable), age, gender, any signs of prodromal symptoms, previous treatment, and underlying illnesses/previous medical history. At a minimum of 12 months after presentation, patients were contacted. After informed consent of patient and caretaker was obtained, they completed two patient-reported outcome measures (PROMs). Because of the retrospective design of the study, consisting of data without burden for the involved subjects, the approval of a medical ethics committee was not required.

2.3. WOMAC

The Western Ontario and McMaster Universities Osteoarthritis Index (WOMAC) was used to assess the patients at follow-up. The WOMAC evaluates three dimensions: pain, stiffness, and physical function with 5, 2, and 17 questions, respectively. The Likert version of the WOMAC is rated on an ordinal scale of 0–4, with lower scores indicating lower levels of symptoms or physical disability. Each subscale is summated to a maximum score of 20, 8, and 68, respectively. There is also an index score or global score, which is most commonly calculated by summating the scores for the three subscales. The questionnaire has been validated in Dutch [11], self-administered and takes 5–10 min to complete [12]. It is the only anatomic-specific paediatric sports PROM of the hip available, validated in a Dutch population aged 12–35 years [13].

2.4. Tegner Score

The Tegner score is an activity score, filled out by the patient. It rates the physical intensity of performed work and/or sports, scoring from 0 to 10. A higher score corresponds with a higher activity level [14].

2.5. Data Analysis

The data were processed descriptively. Patient demographics were summarised. Because of the small number of patients, median and range were used to describe the continuous data. Data analysis was performed using IBM SPSS Statistics Version 26.0 (IBM, Armonk, NY, USA).

3. Results

Seven patients met the inclusion criteria (Table 1), and six could be included at the final follow-up (Table 2). All patients were adolescent, with a median age of 13 years (range, 12–17). They were all male and soccer players. All were without relevant medical history, without signs of hyperlaxity and with a negative family history for orthopaedic problems. The median displacement of the apophysis from the AIIS as measured on the radiographs was 8 mm (range, 0–15 mm).

Table 1. Patient characteristics at presentation.

Case	Age	Gender	Side	Previous Symptoms	Trauma Mechanism	Diagnosis	Displacement from AIIS	Time to RtS (Months)
1	12	Male	R	None	Kicking a ball	X	5 mm	NA
2	13	Male	R	None	Kicking a ball	X/CT	15 mm	3
3	13	Male	R	None	Kicking a ball	X/US	0 mm	2
4	13	Male	L + R	Yes	No trauma	X	0 mm	Unknown *
5	15	Male	R	None	Kicking a ball	X	8 mm	2
6	16	Male	L	None	Fall on knee	X/MRI	10 mm	3
7	17	Male	L	Yes	Jump	X/CT	10 mm	3

AIIS: anterior inferior iliac spine; CT: computed tomography; L: left; MRI: magnetic resonance imaging; NA: not applicable (quit soccer because lost interest); R: right; RtS: return to sport; US: ultrasound; X: X-ray; * already recovered from injury at presentation.

Table 2. Patient-reported outcomes at final follow-up.

Case	WOMAC Pain	WOMAC Joint	WOMAC ph.F	WOMAC Total	Tegner Score	FU (m)
1	100	100	100	100	6	45
2	95	100	88	91	9	18
3	100	100	100	100	9	43
4	100	100	100	100	9	34
6	100	100	100	100	9	20
7	100	100	100	100	5	31

WOMAC: Western Ontario and McMaster Universities Osteoarthritis Index; ph.F: physical functioning; FU (m): follow-up (months).

3.1. Treatment

Initially, all patients were treated conservatively. The treatment consisted of relative rest for 6 weeks, followed by a personalised program with support of a physiotherapist, containing gradual progress of activity until return to sports.

One patient required surgery, after initial conservative treatment failed (case 7 in Tables 1 and 2). Despite intensifying physiotherapy, no progression was seen. When 2.5 months passed by after presentation, he still had symptoms, consisting of pain and limitations of the hip, which worsened over time. New radiographs and a computed tomography (CT) scan were made and showed an ossified non-union avulsion of the rectus femoris tendon (RFT) from the AIIS with heterotopic ossification (Figures 1 and 2). The heterotopic ossification caused mechanical symptoms during sports and his work as a plumber. Therefore, surgery was performed to remove the ossification.

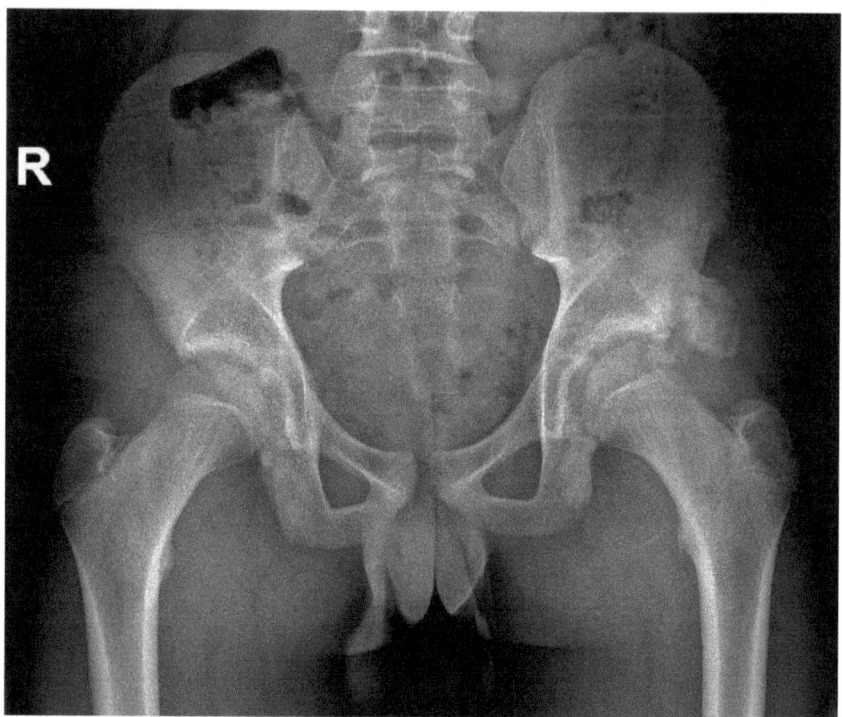

Figure 1. X-ray of the pelvis 2 months after an avulsion of the origin of the left rectus femoris tendon, showing a big osseous calcification on the anterior inferior iliac spine. (Only relevant findings are described).

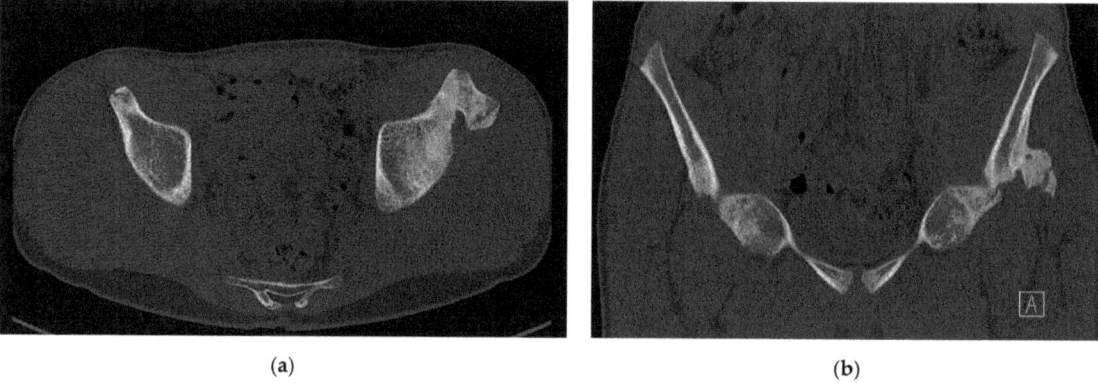

(a) (b)

Figure 2. Computed tomography scan with an axial (**a**) and a coronal (**b**) view of the osseous calcification on the left anterior inferior iliac spine, showing a heterotopic ossification of the origin of the rectus femoris tendon.

During surgery, the ossification was removed using the Smith–Petersen approach. Through the interval between the tensor fascia lata and the sartorius muscles, the RFT was split and the ossification removed with an osteotome. The 3.5 by 2 by 2 cm ossification was sent to the pathologist for analysis. Then, the hip was taken through range of motion, showing no impingement. The RFT split and the fascia were closed, leaving the lateral femoral cutaneous nerve intact.

Postoperatively, the patient was allowed to partially bear weight with crutches for 4 weeks and started training with a physiotherapist. The first 2 weeks he was prescribed NSAIDs to prevent recurrence of the ossification. No peak load or kicking was allowed for 10 weeks. The pathological exam showed a benign calcification. At 6 and 12 weeks, the patient was pain free and had a full range of motion of the hip. Radiography at 6 weeks postoperatively did not show a remnant or recurrence (Figure 3). At 12 weeks, the patient was running and working as a plumber again without symptoms. No complications were observed. At final follow up after 31 months, he had quit soccer due to loss of interest, but was still without any complains.

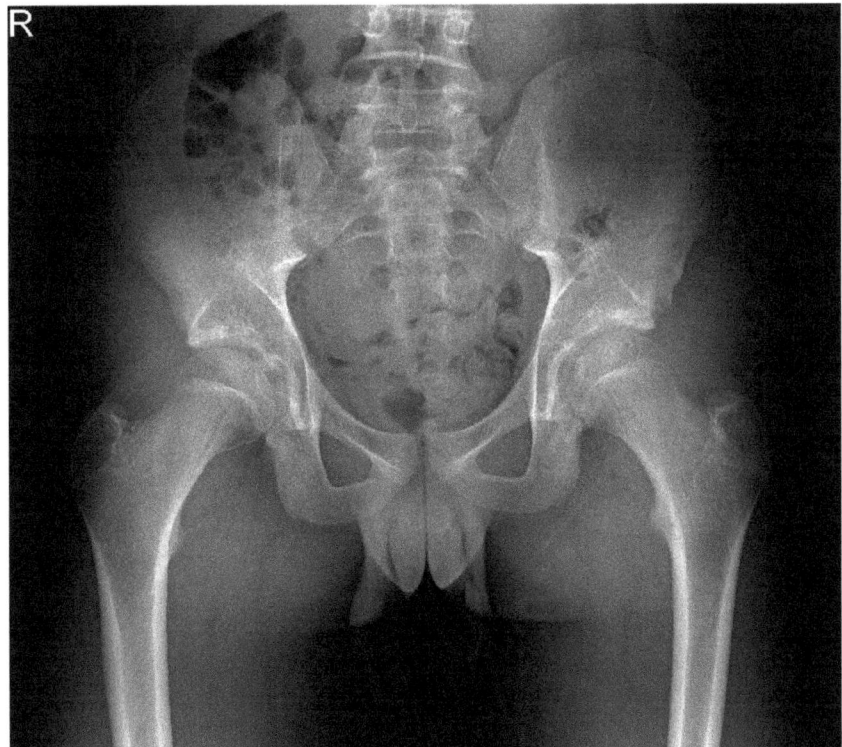

Figure 3. Plain pelvic radiograph 6 weeks after surgical removal of the heterotopic ossification.

3.2. Outcomes

All patients returned to soccer, except for one who lost interest (see Table 1). The median time to return to sports was 2.5 (range, 2–3) months (see Table 1).

In total, 6 out of 7 patients were included at the final follow-up of a median 33 months (range, 18–45). In all patients, including the one who was treated surgically, WOMAC-scores were high to perfect, with a median of 100 (range, 91–100). Likewise, Tegner scores were high, with a median of 9 (range, 5–9), indicating competitive soccer (Table 2).

4. Discussion

In this case series, we present seven soccer players with an AIIS avulsion. Six of them could be successfully treated with a conservative physiotherapy program. In one of them, conservative treatment failed because of mechanical impingement due to a heterotopic ossification. This patient was successfully treated with surgical resection of the ossification.

To our knowledge, we were the first to assess long-term PROMs in adolescents with avulsion fractures of the AIIS. In all patients, all domains of the WOMAC score as well as the total WOMAC score were high, indicating good and pain-free hip function. The Tegner scores, representing level of sports and physical work activities, were also reported to be high.

In the literature, only limited reported cases of surgically treated AIIS avulsions are reported [15,16], most likely due to high success rates with conservative treatment, being reported between 75 and 100% [4,9]. Nevertheless, the AIIS avulsion are described to be 4.47 times more likely to experience future hip pain beyond 3 months compared with other pelvic avulsions [4]. A variety of reasons for these ongoing symptoms are named, such as non-union, hip impingement, heterotopic ossifications, re-fractures, and tendinopathies. It has also been suggested that there may be an association between avulsion of the reflected head of the RFT and labral injuries; in a retrospective study, 2 out of 9 RFT avulsions had labral lesions on magnetic resonance (MR) arthrogram [17].

In our series, one of the patients required surgery, because of impingement and obstructive symptoms due to heterotopic ossification. Lambrechts et al. also reported that secondary surgery can be needed in case of a heterotopic ossification [18]. Other cases show that swelling and pain of an AIIS avulsion can sometimes be mistaken for malignancies, resulting into excision surgery [19–22]. The local tenderness combined with an exostosis on imaging studies may mimic a (pseudo-) tumour.

Recently, it was suggested that adolescent sport players are at risk of rectus femoris avulsion fractures at the AIIS when there is a lack of abdominal muscle strength [23]. We do not have data on this hypothesis, but 2 out of 7 patients reported to have experienced symptoms, previous to the injury. One of them even had an avulsion at both sides. Theoretically, this could be a very cautious suggestion of too much stress on the apophysis in the growing skeleton. From other apophysitis, for example, the little league elbow, we do know that overload is a substantial risk factor [24].

All patients returned to soccer, except for one who lost interest, with a median time to return to sports being 2.5 (range, 2–3) months. In all patients, including the one who was treated surgically, WOMAC-scores were high to perfect, with a median of 100 (range, 91–100). Likewise, Tegner scores were high, with a median of 9 (range, 5–9). A review by Caderazzi [25] evaluated the return to sport rate in 86 patients; 90% of the conservative group and 95% of the surgical patients returned to sports at follow-up, being comparable to our series. The complication rate in the conservative group of Caderazzi et al. was 18%, compared to 22% in the surgical group. The rate of non-unions was lower in the surgical group (0%) than in the conservative group (2.5%), whereas there were more heterotopic ossifications in patients treated surgically (9% vs. 1.8%). In our case series, only one patient required secondary surgery. There were no further complications detected in the patients treated conservatively, nor in the surgically treated patient.

Plain radiographs are included in the initial diagnostic workup, with anteroposterior and frog-leg lateral views of the pelvis and hip. When negative, but with persistent suspicion of an avulsion, CT or MR may assist if the diagnosis is unclear on initial radiographic evaluation [26]. These additional images can also visualise more clearly the amount of displacement, possibly influencing choice of treatment. In our series, 4 out of 7 needed additional work-up, mostly to more precisely measure displacement and determine treatment.

This study has limitations. The major limitation is the relatively small series, and non-standard follow-up times. There was one missing respondent in the long-term follow-up evaluation.

5. Conclusions

In adolescent soccer players, pain in the groin region should be taken seriously, because the apophyseal plate is a biomechanical weak spot. In this case series, we presented seven cases, of whom six had good results with physiotherapy-guided conservative treatment. One patient required surgical removal of a heterotopic ossification. Sports were resumed after 2–3 months. Long-term follow-up showed high scores on WOMAC and Tegner, in both the surgically and conservatively treated patients, indicating good and pain-free functioning of the hip and high levels of physical activity.

Author Contributions: Conceptualisation, H.W. and A.J.P.J.; methodology, H.W.; software, H.W.; validation, H.W., C.J.A.v.B. and A.J.P.J.; formal analysis, H.W.; investigation, H.W. and A.J.P.J.; resources, H.W., A.J.P.J. and C.J.A.v.B.; data curation, H.W.; writing—original draft preparation, H.W.; writing—review and editing, H.W. and C.J.A.v.B.; visualisation, H.W.; supervision, C.J.A.v.B.; project administration, H.W. and C.J.A.v.B.; funding acquisition, not applicable. All authors have read and agreed to the published version of the manuscript.

Funding: This research received no external funding.

Institutional Review Board Statement: Ethical review and approval were waived for this study due to the retrospective design of the study, consisting of data without burden for the involved subjects.

Informed Consent Statement: Informed consent was obtained from all subjects involved in the study.

Data Availability Statement: Not applicable.

Conflicts of Interest: The authors declare no conflict of interest.

References

1. Vandervliet, E.J.M.; Vanhoenacker, F.M.; Snoeckx, A.; Gielen, J.L.; Van Dyck, P.; Parizel, P.M. Sports-related acute and chronic avulsion injuries in children and adolescents with special emphasis on tennis. *Br. J. Sports Med.* **2007**, *41*, 827–831. [CrossRef] [PubMed]
2. Parvaresh, K.C.; Upasani, V.V.; Bomar, J.D.; Pennock, A.T. Secondary Ossification Center Appearance and Closure in the Pelvis and Proximal Femur. *J. Pediatr. Orthop.* **2018**, *38*, 418–423. [CrossRef] [PubMed]
3. Eberbach, H.; Hohloch, L.; Feucht, M.J.; Konstantinidis, L.; Südkamp, N.P.; Zwingmann, J. Operative versus conservative treatment of apophyseal avulsion fractures of the pelvis in the adolescents: A systematical review with meta-analysis of clinical outcome and return to sports. *BMC Musculoskelet. Disord.* **2017**, *18*, 162. [CrossRef] [PubMed]
4. Schuett, D.J.; Bomar, J.D.; Pennock, A.T. Pelvic Apophyseal Avulsion Fractures: A Retrospective Review of 228 Cases. *J. Pediatr. Orthop.* **2015**, *35*, 617–623. [CrossRef] [PubMed]
5. Moeller, J.L.; Galasso, L. Pelvic Region Avulsion Fractures in Adolescent Athletes: A Series of 242 Cases. *Clin. J. Sport Med.* **2020**, *22*, e23–e29. [CrossRef]
6. Rossi, F.; Dragoni, S. Acute avulsion fractures of the pelvis in adolescent competitive athletes: Prevalence, location and sports distribution of 203 cases collected. *Skelet. Radiol.* **2001**, *30*, 127–131. [CrossRef]
7. Oldenburg, F.P.; Smith, M.V.; Thompson, G.H. Simultaneous Ipsilateral Avulsion of the Anterior Superior and Anterior Inferior Iliac Spines in an Adolescent. *J. Pediatr. Orthop.* **2009**, *29*, 29–30. [CrossRef]
8. McKinney, B.I.; Nelson, C.; Carrion, W. Apophyseal Avulsion Fractures of the Hip and Pelvis. *Orthopedics* **2009**, *32*, 42. [CrossRef]
9. Metzmaker, J.N.; Pappas, A.M. Avulsion fractures of the pelvis. *Am. J. Sports Med.* **1985**, *13*, 349–358. [CrossRef]
10. Serbest, S.; Tosun, H.B.; Tiftikçi, U.; Oktas, B.; Kesgin, E. Anterior Inferior Iliac Spine Avulsion Fracture: A Series of 5 Cases. *Medicine* **2015**, *94*, e562. [CrossRef]
11. Roorda, L.D.; Jones, C.A.; Waltz, M.; Lankhorst, G.J.; Bouter, L.M.; Van Der Eijken, J.W.; Willems, W.J.; Heyligers, I.C.; Voaklander, D.C.; Kelly, K.D.; et al. Satisfactory cross cultural equivalence of the Dutch WOMAC in patients with hip osteoarthritis waiting for arthroplasty. *Ann. Rheum. Dis.* **2004**, *63*, 36–42. [CrossRef] [PubMed]
12. McConnell, S.; Kolopack, P.; Davis, A. The Western Ontario and McMaster Universities Osteoarthritis Index (WOMAC): A review of its utility and measurement properties. *Arthritis Care Res.* **2001**, *45*, 453–461. [CrossRef]
13. Suryavanshi, J.R.; Goto, R.; Jivanelli, B.; PRiSM Outcomes Measures Research Interest Group; Aberdeen, J.; Duer, T.; Lam, K.C.; Franklin, C.C.; Macdonald, J.; Shea, K.G.; et al. Age-Appropriate Pediatric Sports Patient-Reported Outcome Measures and Their Psychometric Properties: A Systematic Review. *Am. J. Sports Med.* **2019**, *47*, 3270–3276. [CrossRef] [PubMed]
14. Tegner, Y.; Lysholm, J. Rating systems in the evaluation of knee ligament injuries. *Clin. Orthop. Relat. Res.* **1985**, *198*, 43–49. [CrossRef]
15. Carr, J.B., 2nd; Conte, E.; Rajadhyaksha, E.A.; Laroche, K.A.; Gwathmey, F.W.; Carson, E.W. Operative Fixation of an Anterior Inferior Iliac Spine Apophyseal Avulsion Fracture Nonunion in an Adolescent Soccer Player: A Case Report. *JBJS Case Connect.* **2017**, *7*, e29. [CrossRef]
16. Sinikumpu, J.-J.; Hetsroni, I.; Schilders, E.; Lempainen, L.; Serlo, W.; Orava, S. Operative treatment of pelvic apophyseal avulsions in adolescent and young adult athletes: A follow-up study. *Eur. J. Orthop. Surg. Traumatol.* **2017**, *28*, 423–429. [CrossRef] [PubMed]

17. Foote, C.J.; Maizlin, Z.V.; Shrouder, J.; Grant, M.M.; Bedi, A.; Ayeni, O.R. The Association Between Avulsions of the Reflected Head of the Rectus Femoris and Labral Tears: A retrospective study. *J. Pediatr. Orthop.* **2013**, *33*, 227–231. [CrossRef] [PubMed]
18. Lambrechts, M.J.; Gray, A.D.; Hoernschemeyer, D.G.; Gupta, S.K. Hip Impingement after Anterior Inferior Iliac Spine Avulsion Fractures: A Case Report with Review of the Literature. *Case Rep. Orthop.* **2020**, *2020*, 8893062. [CrossRef]
19. Resnick, J.M.; Carrasco, C.H.; Edeiken, J.; Yasko, A.W.; Ro, J.Y.; Ayala, A.G. Avulsion fracture of the anterior inferior iliac spine with abundant reactive ossification in the soft tissue. *Skelet. Radiol.* **1996**, *25*, 580–584. [CrossRef]
20. Karakas, H.M.; Alicioglu, B.; Erdem, G. Bilateral Anterior Inferior Iliac Spine Avulsion in an Adolescent Soccer Player: A Typical Imitator of Malignant Bone Lesions. *South. Med. J.* **2009**, *102*, 758–760. [CrossRef]
21. Knobloch, K.; Krämer, R.; Sommer, K.; Gänsslen, A.; Vogt, P.M. Avulsion injuries of the anterior inferior iliac spine among soccer players—A differential diagnosis to neoplasm decades following the trauma. *Sportverletz. Sportschaden* **2007**, *21*, 152–156. [CrossRef]
22. Incedayi, M.; Ozyurek, S.; Aribal, S.; Keklikci, K.; Sonmez, G. Avulsion Fracture of the Anterior Inferior Iliac Spine Mimicking a Bone Tumor: A Case Report. *Oman Med. J.* **2014**, *29*, 220–222. [CrossRef] [PubMed]
23. Lasky-McFarlin, C.; Thomas, M.; Newman, J.; Thorpe, D. Lack of Abdominal Stability and Control as a Possible Contributor to Rectus Femoris Avulsion Fracture in the Adolescent Soccer Player: A Case Report. *Pediatr. Phys. Ther.* **2020**, *33*, E15–E22. [CrossRef] [PubMed]
24. Delgado, J.; Jaramillo, D.; Chauvin, N.A. Imaging the Injured Pediatric Athlete: Upper Extremity. *RadioGraphics* **2016**, *36*, 1672–1687. [CrossRef] [PubMed]
25. Calderazzi, F.; Nosenzo, A.; Galavotti, C.; Menozzi, M.; Pogliacomi, F.; Ceccarelli, F. Apophyseal avulsion fractures of the pelvis. A review. *Acta Biomed.* **2018**, *89*, 470–476. [CrossRef] [PubMed]
26. Yeager, K.C.; Silva, S.R.; Richter, D.L. Pelvic Avulsion Injuries in the Adolescent Athlete. *Clin. Sports Med.* **2021**, *40*, 375–384. [CrossRef] [PubMed]

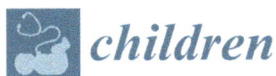

Article

A Prospective Cohort Study on Quality of Life among the Pediatric Population after Surgery for Recurrent Patellar Dislocation

Alexandru Herdea [1], Vlad Pencea [1], Claudiu N. Lungu [2], Adham Charkaoui [3,*] and Alexandru Ulici [1]

1 Pediatric Orthopedics "Grigore Alexandrescu" Children's Emergency Hospital, 011743 Bucharest, Romania; alexherdea@yahoo.com (A.H.); vladpencea@gmail.com (V.P.); alexandru.ulici@umfcd.ro (A.U.)
2 Department of Surgery, Country Emergency Hospital Braila, 810249 Brăila, Romania; lunguclaudiu5555@gmail.com
3 Morphological and Functional Sciences Department, Faculty of Medicine and Pharmacy, University of Galați, 800008 Galati, Romania
* Correspondence: adham.charkaoui@ugal.ro; Tel.: +40-740-510-556

Abstract: Patellofemoral instability is a frequent cause of knee pathology affecting quality of life among the pediatric population. Here, we present a prospective cohort study which included patients who had undergone surgical management using the lateral release and medial imbrication approach (LRMI) or medial patellofemoral ligament reconstruction (MPFL-R). The object of this study was to assess the quality of life among children that have undergone surgical treatment for patellar dislocation. Quality of life was assessed before and after surgery using the Pediatric International Knee Documentation Committee form (Pedi-IKDC), a questionnaire that aims to quantify knee functionality. Postoperative scarring was evaluated using The Stony Brook Scar Evaluation Scale. One hundred and eight patients were selected and grouped according to the type of procedure. Before surgery, the two groups had similar mean Pedi-IKDC scores (41,4 MPFL-R vs. 39,4 LRMI $p = 0.314$). Improvements were observed in the postoperative scores. The MPFL-R technique showed promising outcomes. When comparing the two surgical groups, there was a significant difference in favor of MPFL-R group (MPFL-R 77.71 points vs. LRMI 59.74 points, $p < 0.0001$–95% CI (11.22–24.72)). Using the Stony Brook Scar Evaluation Scale, a significant difference in scar quality in favor of MPFL-R was observed (4,5 MPFL-R vs. 2,77 LRMI $p = 0.002$). In conclusion, this study provides objective evidence-based outcome assessments that support the medial patellofemoral ligament reconstruction technique as the gold standard for patellofemoral instability.

Keywords: recurrent patellar dislocation; knee injury; medial patellofemoral ligament reconstruction

Citation: Herdea, A.; Pencea, V.; Lungu, C.N.; Charkaoui, A.; Ulici, A. A Prospective Cohort Study on Quality of Life among the Pediatric Population after Surgery for Recurrent Patellar Dislocation. *Children* 2021, *8*, 830. https://doi.org/10.3390/children8100830

Academic Editor: Christiaan J. A. van Bergen

Received: 15 August 2021
Accepted: 18 September 2021
Published: 22 September 2021

Publisher's Note: MDPI stays neutral with regard to jurisdictional claims in published maps and institutional affiliations.

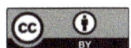

Copyright: © 2021 by the authors. Licensee MDPI, Basel, Switzerland. This article is an open access article distributed under the terms and conditions of the Creative Commons Attribution (CC BY) license (https://creativecommons.org/licenses/by/4.0/).

1. Introduction

Patellofemoral instability is a frequent cause of knee injury that occurs in the pediatric population [1,2]. The incidence rate is 29–43 per 100,000 individuals. The incidence of chronic instability is exceptionally high among girls between 10 and 17 [3]. The dynamics of the patellofemoral joint depends on both bony and soft tissue structures [4]. Therefore, developmental anomalies, traumatic disruption of static restraints, and weak dynamic stabilizers can lead to symptomatic instability [5,6]. Osteochondral fractures are an infrequent accompanying injury which can be successfully managed with the Steadman technique [7]. Some patients may benefit from platelet-rich plasma (PRP) injections in order to reduce the pain caused by injury to other structures of the knee such as the meniscus [8].

Clinical diagnosis is mainly based on the medical history of patellar dislocation and the extent of the hemarthrosis that must be evacuated to reduce pain [9]. In order to correctly assess a patellofemoral instability, clinical examination, conventional X-rays, and C.T. or MRI are needed [10]. However, in most severe cases, computed tomography followed by 3D reconstruction and 3D printing can help the orthopedic surgeon to plan the safest and the most effective surgical approach [11].

Conservative treatment usually consists of cast or splint immobilization, resulting in longer rehabilitation periods as well as a recurrence rate of up to 44% [6,8]. Surgical treatment is the next recommended step if conservative management fails to improve the symptoms significantly. Surgery is recommended in the case of recurrent dislocation [12].

Two popular surgical treatments are lateral release with medial imbrication (LRMI) and medial patellofemoral ligament reconstruction (MPFL-R). Lateral release is sometimes also performed along with MPFL-R to reduce the pull of the lateral retinaculum in order to decrease the stress placed on the medial retinaculum, and is an especially useful technique in pediatric patients [13]. However, there is conflicting information in the literature regarding LRMI, with several recent studies demonstrating good outcomes following application of the technique. In contrast, other studies have shown a high failure rate and a high occurrence of complications [14,15]. MPFL-R aims to restore the normal anatomy of the knee joint with either a autograft or a synthetic graft. Because the MPFL is the main restraint to lateral dislocation in the first 30° of flexion, proper reconstruction will prevent the recurrence of dislocation and prevent undue stress on the knee caused by an abnormal anatomy [16].

The International Knee Documentation Committee Pediatric (IKDC-Pedi) questionnaire has been shown to be relevant is assessments of patient QoL in a variety of knee injuries, including patellar dislocation [17].

2. Materials and Methods

The purpose of the study was to assess the QoL of patients that suffered from episodic patellar dislocation and were treated using LRMI or MPFL-R with a double bundle synthetic graft. The average patient age at diagnosis of patellar dislocation was 13.3 years ± 2 years; see Figure 1 Most patients (96%) had at least two more luxation episodes between diagnosis and surgery.

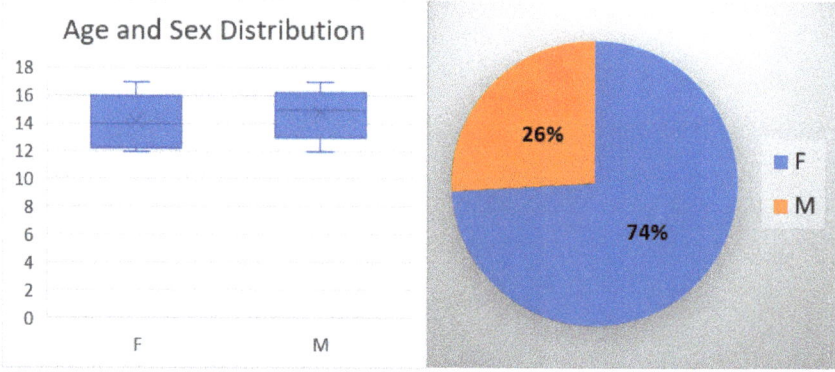

Figure 1. Age and sex distribution.

The study was carried out on 108 pediatric patients (aged 10–18) that had undergone either LRMI or MPFL-R between 2013–2018. The diagnosis was established based on clinical findings, radiologic exams, and magnetic resonance imaging scans, using the following inclusion criteria: history of multiple locked dislocations or locked dislocation present at admission, presence of hemarthrosis, positive apprehension test, painful medial parapatellar structures, and femoral epicondyle, as well as a minimum follow-up of 24 months. Exclusion criteria were: avulsion fracture or femoral condyle osteochondral fracture, lack of preoperative and postoperative knee radiographs, or lack of informed consent. Knee radiographs performed in the anteroposterior and lateral view were used to identify complications. Magnetic resonance imaging (MRI) was used to evaluate soft tissue lesions and to determine the treatment plan by examining the growth plate and assessing whether additional procedures were needed, such as trochleoplasty or patellar tendon realignment. Both surgeries have similar indications, namely, recurrent patellar dislocation with severe trochlear dysplasia. Postop complications that would affect patient outcomes include recurrent dislocation or pain due to the altered knee anatomy; however, the latter occurs mainly in LRMI. LRMI also presents a risk of overly reducing lateral forces on the patella, thus inducing medial dislocation, worsening the patient's QoL and requiring further corrective surgery [18].

Patients were randomly assigned to a surgical group in the following manner: those diagnosed on an even date were assigned to LRMI while those diagnosed on an uneven date were assigned to MPFL-R. Following the randomization, 80 patients were assigned to the LRMI group and 28 to the MPFL-R group. The mean age at surgery was 14.2 years ± 2 years in the LRMI group and 14.5 years ± 2 years in the MPFL-R group. There were no statistically significant differences in age ($p = 0.091$) or sex ($p = 0.07$); see Figure 1.

The postoperative rehabilitation protocol consisted of 1 week of avoiding weight-bearing movements on the operated knee, with subsequent physiotherapy with the purpose of increasing knee stability and proprioception.

Quality of life was evaluated before and after surgery using the Pediatric International Knee Documentation Committee (IKDC-Pedi) form. The postoperative evaluation of the quality of life was conducted after 24 months of follow-up. The average interval from surgery to follow-up was 30 months (25–50 months). Postoperative scarring was also assessed using The Stony Brook Scar Evaluation Scale (SBSES). Patients filled out the questionnaires under parental guidance in the presence of the attending physician.

For statistical analysis, we assumed a null hypothesis of equal efficacy of MPFL-R and LRMI. We set the significance level at 5% (0.05). We modeled the frequency by running a Shapiro-Wilk Test. As the data went through normal distribution, the independent Student-T test was used to compare IKDC-Pedi scores between patients who had undergone LRMI surgery and those who experienced MPFL-R. The response to the athletic ability-related question on the Pedi-IKDC form could not be used to express a normal distribution, so a Mann-Whitney U test was run to check for statistical significance. As the scar evaluation data was not equally distributed, a Mann-Whitney U test was also needed. Standard deviation (S.D.) was calculated, and a confidence interval (CI) of 95% was used.

The acquired and statistically analyzed data comprised the following variables: age, sex, type of surgery, date of surgery, athletic level, preoperative IKDC-Pedi score, postoperative IKDC-Pedi score, postoperative The Stony Brook Scar Evaluation Scale.

3. Results

A total number of 130 patients were operated on for episodic patellar dislocation in the selected time interval. Five of them were excluded from the study due to a lack of adequate postoperative radiographs. Twelve more were excluded because they underwent other, subsequent surgical techniques. Five patients did not consent to take part in the study. One hundred and eight recreational athletes fulfilled the inclusion and exclusion criteria, completed the questionnaires, and presented at follow-up (see flow chart below-Figure 2).

Preoperatively, the Pedi-IKDC scores were similar between the two surgical groups (MPFL-R 41.4 points vs. LRMI 39.4 points), and the difference was not statistically significant ($p = 0.314$). We found significant improvement following both surgical approaches, with the MPFL-R group scoring better than LRMI in postoperative IKDC-Pedi forms compared to preoperative assessment (MPFL-R + 36.36 points-95% CI (27.76–44.97) vs. LRMI +20 points-95% CI (15.11–25.53), $p < 0.0001$). A statistically significant difference in the postoperative IKDC-Pedi score between the two groups (MPFL-R 77.71 points vs. LRMI 59.74 points, $p < 0.0001$-95% CI (11.22–24.72)) was observed (see Figure 3).

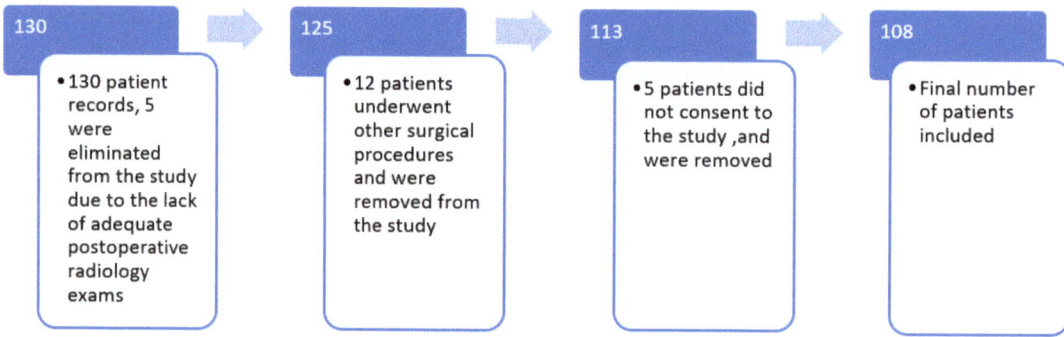

Figure 2. Flow diagram of the patients included in the study. After inclusion and exclusion criteria were applied, 108 patients remained in the study.

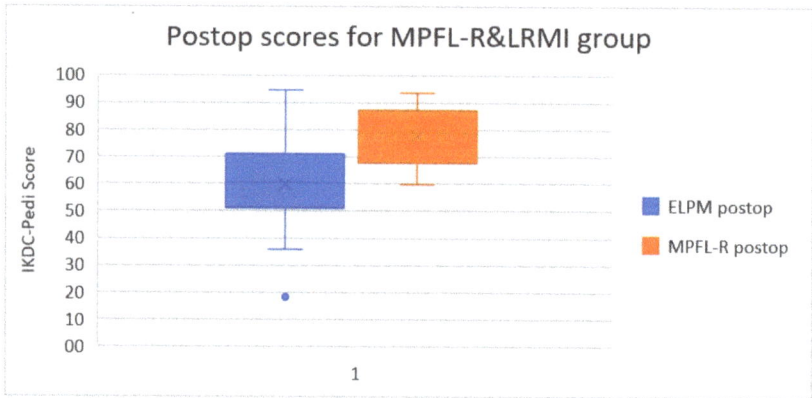

Figure 3. Postoperative scores for MPFL-R and LRMI group. The *p* values are represented in the label for each group.

There was also a statistically significant difference regarding the pain related questions of the Pedi-IKDC questionnaire, favoring MPFL-R (MPFL-R 15.8 points vs. LRMI 12.3 points $p = 0.00175$ 95% CI (1.36–6.21).

4. Discussion

The patients from the MPFL-R group had significantly better IKDC-Pedi scores as well as significantly better scar quality. The different Pedi-IKDC scores were primarily tied to patient ability to improve or return to their previous activity level. The questions related to athletic ability showed the most significant differences in favor of MPFL-R. One possible explanation may be the faster mobilization postsurgery, which would protect against the muscular atrophy caused by immobilization [19].

IKDC-Pedi was chosen as the QoL measurement because it had better responsiveness than KOOS-Child. In addition, as a shorter questionnaire makes, it is more likely to be fully completed in a clinical setting [20].

The Stony Brook Scar Evaluation Scale (SBSES) was selected for the same reasons: the short time required for its completion and its good clinical relevancy [21].

This is because MPFL-R restores the normal anatomy of the knee, thus facilitating regular joint reaction forces [18]. However, in LRMI, the increased joint forces could cause unpleasant sensations like pressure or pain in the knee joint [22].

The postoperative score for the MPFL-R group correlated with data from other studies found in literature, indicating good surgical technique and rehabilitation programs [23]. The LRMI group had fewer reported redislocations than most studies using a similar surgical technique, yet the IKDC-Pedi score was lower than expected [24,25].

The cosmetic differences between the two procedures are also undeniable. MPFL-R is far less invasive and results in a significantly better-looking postsurgical scar. The SBSES does not consider scar length, and it should be mentioned that the MPFL-R group has two short scars while the LRMI has one long scar. As observed in our study, this is a cause of distress for patients even if the scar itself has healed without abnormal pigmentation, elevation, or depression.

One significant factor in this patient group is tibial and femoral physis [26]. While the surgical technique used for MPFL-R in this study does not usually affect the growth plate, there is still a slight risk. In contrast, the LRMI procedure only involves the soft tissues surrounding the knee, eliminating any risk of damage to the growth plate.

Lateral release on its own has yielded unsatisfactory outcomes in the history of pa-llar dislocation treatment [27], and release of a normal lateral retinaculum may increase lateral patellar translation and cause even more instability due to the role of the lateral retinaculum in resisting lateral patellar translation [28]. In one study which compared MPFL-R without lateral release and MPFL-R with a lateral release, the groups had similar outcomes, thus showing that lateral release is not mandatory [29].

The follow-up period was clinically relevant because most redislocations (70%) occur within 24 months postoperatively [30]. However, it is insufficient to determine whether differences in joint anatomy that result after surgery remotely affect the incidence of osteoarthritis. This would require a lengthy, hard-to-manage longitudinal study. However, when considering the fact that patellar instability very often leads to unfavorable outcomes in adults, either surgery is desirable compared to nonsurgical treatment [31].

The strengths in our study were the homogeneity of the surgical techniques that were identical for all patients and the homogeneity of the study groups concerning risk factors for patellar dislocation. The limitations were the unequal treatment groups as well as differences in follow-up period.

5. Conclusions

MPFL-R increased patient quality of life more than LRMI. MPFL-R interventions are minimally invasive, reduce postoperative recovery time and increase quality of life. This study provides further evidence for the recommendation of MPFL-R as the gold standard for patellofemoral instability. However, further studies are needed to observe the long-term stability and side effects of MPFL-R.

Author Contributions: Conceptualization, produced the results, discussion and conclusions, and assembled the paper, A.H., V.P., C.N.L., A.C. and A.U. All authors have read and agreed to the published version of the manuscript.

Funding: This research received no external funding.

Institutional Review Board Statement: The study was conducted according to the guidelines of the Declaration of Helsinki and approved by the Ethics Committee of "Grigore Alexandrescu" Children's Emergency Clinical Hospital of Bucharest on the 1 March 2013. The study code is 7/01.03.2013.

Informed Consent Statement: Informed consent was obtained from the parents of all subjects involved in the study.

Data Availability Statement: The datasets used and analyzed during the current study are available from the corresponding author on reasonable request.

Conflicts of Interest: The authors declare no conflict of interest.

Abbreviations

LRMI	Lateral Release and Medial Imbrication approach
MPFL-R	Medial Patellofemoral Ligament Reconstruction
Pedi-IKDC	Pediatric International Knee Documentation Committee form
MPFL	The medial patellofemoral ligament
QoL	The quality of life
SBSES	The Stony Brook Scar Evaluation Scale
SD	Standard deviation
CI	Confidence interval
PRP	Platelet-Rich Plasma

References

1. Fithian, D.C.; Paxton, E.W.; Stone, M.L.; Silva, P.; Davis, D.K.; Elias, D.A.; White, L. Epidemiology and Natural History of Acute Patellar Dislocation. *Am. J. Sports Med.* **2004**, *32*, 1114–1121. [CrossRef] [PubMed]
2. Hennrikus, W.; Pylawka, T. Patellofemoral instability in skeletally immature athletes. *J. Bone Jt. Surg. Am.* **2013**, *95*, 176–183.
3. Atkin, D.; Fithian, D.; Marangi, K.; Stone, M.; Dobson, B.; Mendelsohn, C. Characteristics of patients with primary acute lateral patelar dislocation and their recovery within the first 6 months. *Am. J. Sports Med.* **2000**, *28*, 472–479. [CrossRef]
4. Steense, R.N.; Bentley, J.C.; Trinh, T.O.; Backes, J.R.; Wiltfong, R.E. The prevalence and combined prevalences of an-atomic factors associated with recurrent patellar dislocaton: A magnetic resonance imaging study. *Am. J. Sports Med.* **2015**, *43*, 921–927. [CrossRef]
5. Ries, Z.; Bollier, M. Patellofemoral Instability in Active Adolescents. *J. Knee Surg.* **2015**, *28*, 265–278. [CrossRef]
6. Arendt, J.A.; Moore, A. First time patella dislocations: Characterizing their readiness for return to activity. *Br. J. Sports Med.* **2011**, *45*, 335–336. [CrossRef]
7. Pellegrino, M.; Trinchese, E.; Bisaccia, M.; Rinonapoli, G.; Meccariello, L.; Falzarano, G.; Medici, A.; Piscitelli, L.; Ferrara, P.; Caraffa, A. Long term outcome of grade III and IV chondral injuries of the knee treat with Steadman microfracture technique. *Clin. Case Miner. Bone Metab.* **2016**, *13*, 237–240.
8. Popescu, M.B.; Carp, M.; Tevanov, I.; Nahoi, C.A.; Stratila, M.A.; Haram, O.M.; Ulici, A. Isolated Meniscus Tears in Adolescent Patients Treated with Platelet-Rich Plasma Intra-articular Injections: 3-Month Clinical Outcome. *BioMed Res. Int.* **2020**, *2020*, 1–5. [CrossRef] [PubMed]
9. Sisk, D.; Fredericson, M. Update of Risk Factors, Diagnosis, and Management of Patellofemoral Pain. *Curr. Rev. Musculoskelet. Med.* **2019**, *12*, 534–541. [CrossRef]
10. Clark, D.; Metcalfe, A.; Wogan, C.; Mandalia, V.; Eldridge, J. Adolescent patellar instability. *Bone Jt. J.* **2017**, *99-B*, 159–170. [CrossRef] [PubMed]
11. Tevanov, I.; Liciu, E.; Chirila, M.; Dusca, A.; Ulici, A. The use of 3D printing in impoving patient-doctor relationship and malpractice prevention. *Rom. Soc. Leg. Med.* **2017**, *25*, 279–282. [CrossRef]
12. Vellios, E.E.; Trivellas, M.; Arshi, A.; Beck, J.J. Recurrent Patellofemoral Instability in the Pediatric Patient: Manage-ment and Pitfalls. *Curr. Rev. Musculoskelet. Med.* **2020**, *13*, 58–68. [CrossRef]
13. Roger, J.; Viste, A.; Cievet-Bonfils, M.; Pracros, J.-P.; Raux, S.; Chotel, F. Axial patellar engagement index and patellar tilt after medial patello-femoral ligament reconstruction in children and adolescents. *Orthop. Traumatol. Surg. Res.* **2019**, *105*, 133–138. [CrossRef]
14. Lee, J.-J.; Lee, S.-J.; Won, Y.-G.; Choi, C.-H. Lateral release and medial plication for recurrent patella dislocation. *Knee Surg. Sports Traumatol. Arthrosc.* **2012**, *20*, 2438–2444. [CrossRef] [PubMed]
15. Elkousy, H. Complications in Brief: Arthroscopic Lateral Release. *Clin. Orthop. Relat. Res.* **2012**, *470*, 2949–2953. [CrossRef] [PubMed]
16. Vavken, P.; Wimmer, M.D.; Camathias, C.; Quidde, J.; Valderrabano, V.; Pagenstert, G. Treating Patella Instability in Skeletally Immature Patients. *Arthrosc. J. Arthrosc. Relat. Surg.* **2013**, *29*, 1410–1422. [CrossRef] [PubMed]
17. Dietvorst, M.; Reijman, M.; Van Groningen, B.; Van Der Steen, M.C.; Janssen, R. PROMs in paediatric knee ligament injury: Use the Pedi-IKDC and avoid using adult PROMs. *Knee Surg. Sports Traumatol. Arthrosc.* **2017**, *27*, 1965–1973. [CrossRef] [PubMed]
18. Edmonds, E.W.; Glaser, D.A. Adolescent Patella Instability Extensor Mechanics. *J. Pediatr. Orthop.* **2016**, *36*, 262–267. [CrossRef]
19. Appel, H. Muscular atrophy following immobilisation. *Sports Med.* **1990**, *10*, 42–58. [CrossRef]
20. van der Velden, C.A.; van der Steen, M.C.; Leenders, J.; Florens, Q.; van Douveren, M.P.; Janssen, R.P.; Reijman, M. Pedi-IKDC or KOOS-child: Which questionnaire should be used in children with knee disorders? *BMC Musculoskelet. Disord.* **2019**, *20*, 1–8. [CrossRef]
21. Singer, A.J.; Arora, B.; Dagum, A.; Valentine, S.; Hollander, J. Development and Validation of a Novel Scar Evalua-tion Score. *Plast. Reconstr. Surg.* **2007**, *120*, 1892–1897. [CrossRef]
22. Schneider, D.K.; Grawe, B.; Magnussen, R.A.; Ceasar, A.; Parikh, S.N.; Wall, E.J.; Colosimo, A.J.; Kaeding, C.C.; Myer, G.D. Outcomes after isolated medial patellofemoral ligament recon-struction for the treatment of recurrent lateral patellar dislocations: A systematic review and meta-analysis. *Am. J. Sports Med.* **2016**, *44*, 2993–3005. [CrossRef]

23. Longo, U.G.; Rizzello, G.; Ciuffreda, M.; Loppini, M.; Baldari, A.; Maffulli, N.; Denaro, V. Elmslie-Trillat, Maquet, Fulkerson, Roux Goldthwait, and Other Distal Realignment Procedures for the Management of Patellar Dislocation: Systematic Review and Quantitative Synthesis of the Literature. *Arthrosc J. Arthrosc. Relat.* **2016**, *32*, 929–943. [CrossRef]
24. Nwachukwu, B.U.; So, C.; Schairer, W.; Green, D.W.; Dodwell, E. Surgical versus conservative management of acute patellar dislocation in children and adolescents: A systematic review. *Knee Surg. Sports Traumatol. Arthrosc.* **2016**, *24*, 760–767. [CrossRef]
25. Ostermeier, S.; Holst, M.; Hurschler, C.; Windhagen, H.; Stukenborg-Colsman, C. Dynamic measurement of patello-femoral kinematics and contact pressure after lateral retinacular. *Knee Surg. Sports Traumatol. Arthrosc.* **2007**, *15*, 547–554. [CrossRef]
26. Desio, S.M.; Burks, R.T.; Bachus, K.N. Soft Tissue Restraints to Lateral Patellar Translation in the Human Knee. *Am. J. Sports Med.* **1998**, *26*, 59–65. [CrossRef]
27. Malatray, M.; Magnussen, R.; Lustig, S. and Servien, E. Lateral retinacular release is not recommended in association to MPFL reconstruction in recurrent patellar dislocation. *Knee Surg. Sports Traumatol. Arthrosc.* **2019**, *27*, 2659–2664. [CrossRef]
28. McCarthy, M.A.; Bollier, M.J. Medial Patella Subluxation: Diagnosis and Treatment. *Iowa Orthop. J.* **2015**, *35*, 26–33. [PubMed]
29. Studer, K.; Vacariu, A.; Rutz, E.; Camathias, C. High failure rate 10.8 years after vastus medialis transfer and lateral release (Green's quadricepsplasty) for recurrent dislocation of the patella. *Arch. Orthop. Trauma Surg.* **2020**, *140*, 1349–1357.
30. Apostolovic, M.; Vukomanovic, B.; Slavkovic, N.; Vuckovic, V.; Djuricic, G.; Kocev, N. Acute patellar dislocation in ado-lescents: Operative versus nonoperative treatment. *Int. Orthopaedics.* **2011**, *35*, 1483–1487. [CrossRef] [PubMed]
31. Bisaccia, M.; Caraffa, A.; Meccariello, L.; Ripani, U.; Bisaccia, O.; Gomez-Garrido, D.; Carrado-Gomez, M.; Pace, V.; Rollo, G.; Giaracuni, M.; et al. Displaced patella fractures: Percutaneous cerclage wiring and second arthroscopic look. *Clin. Cases Min. Bone Metab.* **2019**, *16*, 48–52.

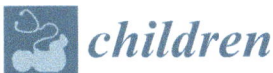

Article

Elastic Stable Intramedullary Nailing for Treatment of Pediatric Tibial Fractures: A 20-Year Single Center Experience of 132 Cases

Zenon Pogorelić [1,2,*,†], Viktor Vegan [2,†], Miro Jukić [1,2], Carlos Martin Llorente Muñoz [3] and Dubravko Furlan [1]

[1] Department of Pediatric Surgery, University Hospital of Split, 21000 Split, Croatia; mirojukic.mefst@gmail.com (M.J.); dfurlan@inet.hr (D.F.)
[2] Department of Surgery, School of Medicine, University of Split, 21000 Split, Croatia; vv11398@gmail.com
[3] Surgical Clinic Medix-Muñoz, 28 000 Madrid, Spain; llorentecm@gmail.com
* Correspondence: zpogorelic@gmail.com; Tel.: +385-21-556654
† These authors contributed equally to this work.

Abstract: Objective: The aim of this study was to analyze the outcomes and complications in children treated with elastic stable intramedullary nailing (ESIN) for tibial fractures. Methods: The study included 132 patients (92 males) with a median age of 11 years (IQR 10, 15) treated with ESIN for displaced tibial shaft fractures or dia-metaphyseal distal tibial fractures from March 2002 to March 2022. The median follow-up was 118.5 months (IQR 74.5, 170). The primary outcome was success rate, while secondary outcomes were the time of bone healing, length of hospital stay, and associated injuries. Demographic data, type and nature of fracture, indication for surgery, healing time, operative time, complications of treatment, and time to implant removal were recorded. Results: Complete radiographic healing was achieved at a median of 7 weeks (IQR 6, 9). Most of the patients (n = 111; 84.1%) had fractures localized in the shaft of the tibia. The most common injuries were acquired by road traffic accidents (n = 42) and by a fall in the same level (n = 29), followed by injuries from sport activities (n = 21) or motorbike accidents (n = 18). Associated injuries were reported in 37 (28%) children. Fractures were closed in the majority of the children (n = 100; 76%), while 32 (24%) children presented with an open fracture. Children with open fractures were significantly older than children with closed fractures (13.5 years (IQR 10, 15) vs. 11 years (IQR 8.5, 14.5); p = 0.031). Furthermore, children with open fractures had a significantly longer hospital stay (7 days (IQR 5, 9) vs. 3 days (IQR 3, 6); p = 0.001), a higher rate of associated injuries (n = 14 (43.7%) vs. n = 23 (23%); p = 0.022), and a higher rate of postoperative complications (n = 7 (21.9%) vs. n = 8 (8%); p = 0.031). No intraoperative complications were recorded. A total of 15 (11.4%) postoperative complications were recorded. Most complications (60%) were minor complications, mostly related to the wound at the nail insertion site and were managed conservatively. A total of six (4.5%) patients required reoperation due to angulation of the fragments (n = 5) or refracture (n = 1). Conclusion: ESIN is a minimally invasive bone surgery technique and is a highly effective treatment for pediatric tibial unstable fractures with a low rate of complications. Based on the given results, surgical stabilization of the tibial fractures using titanium intramedullary nailing can be safely performed without casting with early physiotherapy.

Keywords: titanium elastic nails; tibial fracture; children; elastic stable intramedullary nailing (ESIN)

Citation: Pogorelić, Z.; Vegan, V.; Jukić, M.; Llorente Muñoz, C.M.; Furlan, D. Elastic Stable Intramedullary Nailing for Treatment of Pediatric Tibial Fractures: A 20-Year Single Center Experience of 132 Cases. *Children* **2022**, *9*, 845. https://doi.org/10.3390/children9060845

Academic Editor: Christiaan J. A. van Bergen

Received: 30 April 2022
Accepted: 7 June 2022
Published: 7 June 2022

Publisher's Note: MDPI stays neutral with regard to jurisdictional claims in published maps and institutional affiliations.

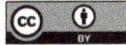

Copyright: © 2022 by the authors. Licensee MDPI, Basel, Switzerland. This article is an open access article distributed under the terms and conditions of the Creative Commons Attribution (CC BY) license (https://creativecommons.org/licenses/by/4.0/).

1. Introduction

Lower leg fractures in children are the third most common location after forearm and femur fractures [1,2]. Among all the lower leg fractures, isolated tibial fractures are the most frequent and account for about 70% of the fractures. Both bones are broken in 30% of patients, and isolated fibular fractures are rare [3]. According to the type, the transverse or short oblique fractures of the tibia are most commonly seen [4,5]. The tibia is most susceptible to trauma in the area of transition from the middle to the distal third due to anatomical changes in the cross-section of the bone from triangular to round in shape [6]. The choice of the treatment method depends on the bone age, body weight and general condition of the patient, and the type, angle, and the location of the fracture. In the earliest and preschool age, fractures are usually treated conservatively because short-term immobilization is sufficient to stabilize fractures with periosteal callus and the high potential for remodeling corrects almost all deformities. In older children, bone healing is slower, and the required stability of the fragments over time is difficult to achieve with immobilization. In total, only 10% of all fractures in children require surgical treatment [7]. Several recent studies pointed out that pediatric tibial fractures have been increasingly treated by a surgical approach [8,9]. According to good medical practice and guidelines, surgery should be undertaken only in cases of severe dislocation that could not be reduced, fracture instability, open fractures, compartment syndrome, neurovascular dysfunction, failed non-operative management, or in cases of polytrauma [10]. Surgical techniques for the treatment of tibial fractures in children include elastic stable intramedullary osteosynthesis with titanium nails (ESIN), Kirschner wires, osteosynthetic plate placement, and external fixation [11,12]. The use of elastic stable intramedullary nails has almost become a routine treatment method for pediatric diaphyseal fractures of long bones in the last few years. There is much evidence that proves this method has the benefits of early immediate stability to the involved bone segment, which permits early mobilization and return to normal activities of the patients without immobilization, with very low complication rates [13–16]. The benefits of ESIN, compared to other surgical techniques, include shorter surgical time, minimal soft-tissue dissection, improved cosmesis, less pain, early mobilization, and relatively easy implant removal [13–16]. Although many authors recommend immobilization in the postoperative period, our previous study clearly showed that immobilization is not necessary and that there is no increased number of complications if immobilization did not occur [13,15,17–19]. The aim of this retrospective analysis was to evaluate the outcomes of treatment and complication rates of tibial fractures treated with ESIN in children and adolescents in a representative cohort of 132 patients in order to underline the safeness and efficiency of this technique. Moreover, our goal was to present that immobilization is not required after ESIN osteosynthesis.

2. Materials and Methods

2.1. Patients

A retrospective search of 132 children (92 males) who underwent ESIN for tibial fractures, from March 2002 to March 2022 in a Clinic of Pediatric Surgery at University Hospital of Split, Croatia, was performed. The median follow-up was 118.5 (IQR 74.5, 170) months, while the median age was 12 (IQR 10, 15) years. Inclusion criteria were the diagnosis of displaced tibial shaft or dia-metaphyseal distal tibial fractures in patients of both genders, between 3 and 17 years of age treated with ESIN, followed up for a minimum of three months. Exclusion criteria were patients outside the predetermined age range, patients with conservative treatment of fractures or treated operatively with other methods (expert tibial nail, external fixation, plating), patients with proximal tibial fractures, patients with epiphyseal injuries, patients with closed physis or body weight > 70 kg, patients with follow-up shorter than three months, and patients with incomplete data. For the purpose of this study, the patients were subdivided in two subgroups regarding the localization of the fracture. The patients from the first subgroup had a tibial shaft fracture, while the patients from the second group had a distal tibial fracture. The outcomes of treatment were compared between the groups.

The Institutional Review Board (IRB) of our hospital approved the study (IRB reference, 500-03-/22-01/16, date of approval 3 March 2022).

2.2. Outcomes of the Study and Hypothesis

The primary outcome of the study was the success rate of the ESIN method in the treatment of lower leg fractures, which is presented as a number of postoperative complications. Postoperative complications included wound complications, bleeding, fragment angulation, and refracture. Secondary outcomes were the time of bone healing, length of hospital stay, and associated injuries.

Hypothesis (H1). The ESIN is an effective method of treating lower leg fractures in children with excellent healing results and a low complication rate.

2.3. Study Design

This study was designed as a retrospective cross-sectional cohort study. According to the structure, this study was categorized as qualitative research, while according to the intervention and data processing, it was of a descriptive type. The source of data were electronic case records of the patients. All patients underwent emergency surgery, using the ESIN method, due to lower leg fractures. The age, gender, type of fracture, indication for surgery, fracture mechanism, lateralization, associated injuries, healing time, operative time, complications of treatment, and time to nail removal were analyzed for each patient.

2.4. Radiographic Assessments and Indications for Surgery

All children underwent full-length anteroposterior (AP) and lateral (LL) radiographs of the lower leg. Displacement was assessed on mentioned radiographs.

The indications for surgery were open fractures, polytrauma, loss of reduction after conservative treatment, compartment syndrome, or initially severely displaced and unstable fractures (displacement for more than two-thirds of the diameter and/or angulation > 30° after manipulation). In regard to type of fracture, the most commonly severely displaced mild oblique, transverse, and spiral fractures were selected for surgery. Age limit was not strictly selected but the patients with closed physis and body weight > 70 kg were treated using an expert tibial nail.

2.5. Surgical Procedure

The surgery was performed under general anesthesia in the supine position. Titanium intramedullary nails (TEN; Synthes® GmbH, Oberdorf, Switzerland) were used in all patients. The diameter and length of the nails were selected according to the bone length and child's age (two nails must fill at least two-thirds of the medulla at the narrowest part of the bone). After preparation of the surgical field, the fracture site and proximal tibial epiphysis were marked under fluoroscopy. Two mini longitudinal incisions were made on the medial and lateral side at the level of the tibial metaphysis, proximal to the desired bony entrance. The starting point for nail insertion was located 1.5–2 cm distal to the bone epiphysis below the tibial tubercles. The cortical bone was shown by blunt dissection of soft tissues. Before the insertion, the nails were manually bent into a slight "C" shape that allowed fixation of the nail at three points. A drill was used to pierce the bone cortex which made it easier for the nail to enter the intramedullary canal. Both nails were then introduced into the intramedullary canal through the input incisions anteromedially and anterolaterally to the level of the fracture. Under fluoroscopic supervision, the fracture was reduced in both planes. After fluoroscopic confirmation, the first nail continued to advance toward the distal metaphysis of the tibia. If AP and LL X-rays confirmed that the distal position of the first intramedullary nail was correct, the second nail was inserted. Both titanium nails were pushed through the intramedullary canal towards the distal until their tips reached just above the distal tibial epiphysis, with special attention paid to not crossing the distal tibial physis, and at the end of the procedure, shortened at subcutaneous level. The surgical incisions were sutured using non-absorbable nylon sutures. After surgery, there was no casting in any of the age groups and physical therapy was started on the second or third postoperative day, depending on the patient's condition and/or associated injuries.

2.6. Pain Management, Physical Therapy, and Follow-Up

All the patients were kept in hospital after the surgery. Most children with tibial fractures have the strongest pain within the first 48 h after the injury and use analgesia mostly for three days after injury. Our protocol includes fentanyl in a dose of 1.5 µg/kg immediately after surgery. After that period, Ibuprofen in a dose of 10 mg/kg and paracetamol in a dose of 15 mg/kg, individually or in combination, are the analgesics most commonly used, with no clear superiority.

On the first postoperative day, strict rest is required, mostly due to pain control. From the second or third postoperative day (individually, depending on age and other factors, such as general condition of the patient or associated injuries), physical therapy and getting out of bed with crutches begins. After the patient learns to walk stably using crutches, if the other parameters are satisfactory, the patient is discharged to home care, continued with ambulatory physical therapy after discharge. For the first three or four weeks, the patient does not step on the operated leg, and then, after radiological verification of the fracture, begins gradual weight bearing. For the first few days, the bearing is approximately one-seventh of the body weight, after which the bearing gradually increases. On average, after 8 to 10 weeks of osteosynthesis, after radiologically verifying a good callus, a crutch-free gait begins. Each patient underwent an intraoperative X-ray after repositioning the bone fragments and placing of titanium elastic nails. Control X-rays were taken seven days after the procedure, and after one, three, and six months, or until healing of the bone was completed (Figure 1). Radiological evaluation was carried out using standard AP and LL radiographs at each visit to evaluate the consolidation of the fracture and identify complications such as secondary displacement, shortening, nail migration, delayed union, nonunion or malunion, and re-fracture (Figure 2). Nonunion was defined as the lack of appropriate healing within six months from index surgery. Malunion was defined as angular deformity of greater than 5–10° (depending on patient's age) in the coronal or sagittal plane. Limb length inequality >1 cm was considered as limb shortening. All nails were removed under general anesthesia when the radiological healing was evident at the median of six months.

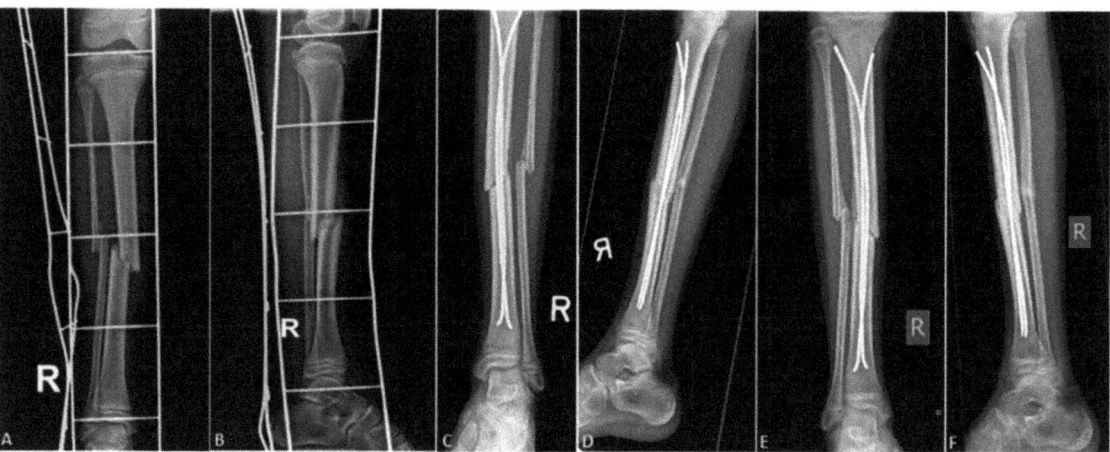

Figure 1. Displaced tibial shaft fracture in 11-year-old female patient: (**A**) preoperative AP radiograph; (**B**) preoperative LL radiograph; (**C**) AP radiograph one month after surgery; (**D**) LL radiograph one month after surgery; (**E**) AP radiograph three months after surgery; (**F**) LL radiograph three months after surgery.

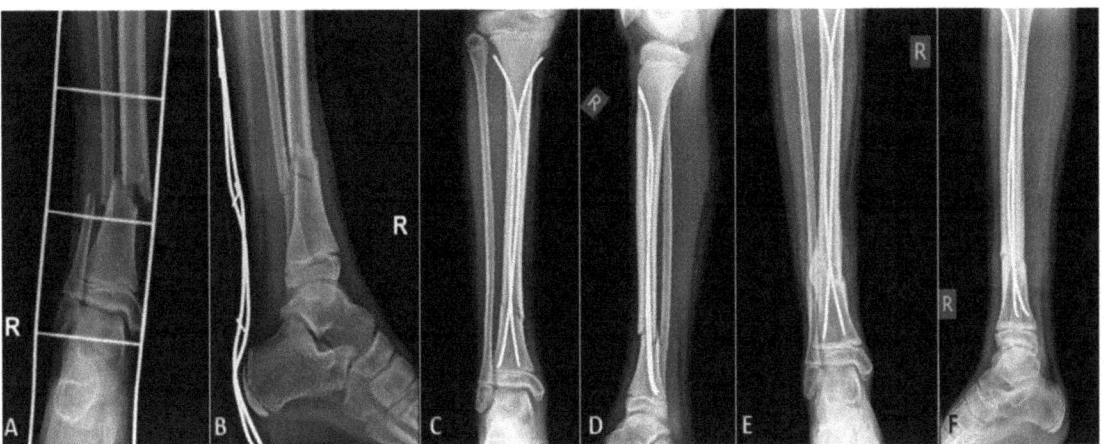

Figure 2. Displaced distal tibial fracture in 9-year-old male patient: (**A**) preoperative AP radiograph; (**B**) preoperative LL radiograph; (**C**) AP radiograph one month after surgery; (**D**) LL radiograph one month after surgery; (**E**) AP radiograph three months after surgery; (**F**) LL radiograph three months after surgery.

2.7. Statistical Analysis

The data were analyzed using Microsoft Excel for Windows Version 16.0 (Microsoft Corporation, Redmond, WA, USA), and Statistical Package for Social Sciences, version 19.0 (IBM SPSS Corp, Armonk, NY, USA) software programs. Distributions of quantitative data were described by medians and interquartile range (IQR), while categorical variables were expressed in absolute numbers and percentages. Differences in median values of quantitative variables between the examined groups were tested by the Mann–Whitney U-test. A comparison of different categories of variations was performed by the Chi-square test. In cases where the frequency rate of individual variants was low, Fisher's exact test was used. All values of $p < 0.05$ were considered statistically significant.

3. Results

In the selected study period, which included 132 children operated on using ESIN for tibial fractures, there were 92 (69.7%) boys and 40 (30.3%) girls. The median age was 12 (IQR 10, 15) years. There were 100 (75.8%) closed and 32 (24.2%) open fractures. Median duration of hospital stay was 4.5 (IQR 2, 5) days. Most of the patients ($n = 111$ (84.1%)) had a fracture localized in the shaft of the tibia, while the other 21 (15.9%) had a fracture localized in the distal part of the bone (Table 1). A total of 32 complicated fractures were recorded. Using Gustilo - Anderson classification a total of 16 fractures (50%) were categorized as grade 1, 13 (40.6%) as a grade 2 and 3 (9.4%) as a grade 3. Most common mechanism of injury was traffic accident (31.8%) and the most common type of fracture was complicated fracture (24.2%) (Table 2).

Statistical comparison of data between patients who had open and closed fractures showed that children with open fractures were significantly older than children with closed fractures (13.5 years (IQR 10, 15) vs. 11 years (IQR 8.5, 14.5); $p = 0.031$). Furthermore, children with open fractures had a significantly longer hospital stay (7 days (IQR 5, 9) vs. 3 days (IQR 3, 6); $p = 0.001$), a higher rate of associated injuries ($n = 14$ (43.7%) vs. $n = 23$ (23%); $p = 0.022$), and a higher rate of postoperative complications ($n = 7$ (21.9%) vs. $n = 8$ (8%); $p = 0.031$). No statistically significant difference was found between the examined groups in relation to the sex of the patient ($p = 0.308$), duration of surgery ($p = 0.301$), and lateralization of the fracture ($p = 0.758$).

Table 1. Demographic data of the patients and clinical characteristics of fractures.

Patient Characteristics	All Fractures (n = 132)	Open Fractures (n = 32)	Closed Fractures (n = 100)	p	Distal Fractures (n = 21)	Diaphyseal Fractures (n = 111)	p
Age	12	13.5	11	0.031 *	12	12	0.499 *
Median; years (IQR)	(10, 15)	(10, 15)	(8.5, 14.5)		(10, 15)	(9, 15)	
Sex; n (%) Male	92 (69.7)	20 (62.5)	72 (72)	0.308 †	15 (71.4)	77 (69.4)	0.850 †
Female	40 (30.3)	12 (37.5)	28 (28)		6 (28.6)	34 (30.6)	
Lateralization; n (%)							
Left	67 (50.8)	17 (53.1)	50 (50)	0.758 †	11 (52.4)	56 (50.5)	0.871 †
Right	65 (49.2)	15 (46.9)	50 (50)		10 (47.6)	55 (49.5)	
Time of healing	7	10	7	0.015 *	6.5	7.5	0.374 *
Median; weeks (IQR)	(6, 9)	(10, 12)	(6, 9)		(6, 7)	(6, 9)	
Hospital stay	4.5	7	3	0.001 *	4.5	3.5	0.354 *
Median; days (IQR)	(2, 5)	(5, 9)	(3, 6)		(3, 6)	(3, 5)	
Duration of surgery	54	56	53	0.301 *	58	56	0.411 *
Median; min (IQR)	(47, 66)	(49, 70)	(48, 64)		(46, 67)	(49, 59)	
Associated injuries; n (%)	37 (28)	14 (43.7)	23 (23)	0.022 †	3 (14.3)	34 (30.6)	0.185 ‡
Complications; n (%)	15 (11.4)	7 (21.9)	8 (8)	0.031 †	3 (14.3)	12 (10.8)	0.645 ‡

* Mann–Whitney U test; † Chi-square test; ‡ Fisher's exact test; IQR—interquartile range.

Table 2. Distribution of the patients according to fracture type and mechanism of injury.

Mechanism of Injury	Distal Fracture (n = 17)	Oblique Fracture (n = 25)	Comminuted Fracture (n = 14)	Complicated Fracture (n = 32)	Transverse Fracture (n = 18)	Spiral Fracture (n = 26)
Fall from height (n = 9)	1	2	1	2	1	2
Fall in same level (n = 29)	5	5	3	4	4	8
Road traffic accident (n = 42)	5	9	1	21	1	5
Sport (n = 21)	1	5	1	2	6	6
Bicycle riding (n = 10)	2	2	2	0	3	1
Motorbike (n = 18)	1	2	5	3	3	4
Electric scooter (n = 3)	2	0	1	0	0	0

Associated injuries were reported in 37 (28%) children with tibial fractures. Their incidence and severity were directly related to the mechanism of injury. Most of the associated injuries have been reported in children with complicated tibial fractures who have been exposed to high kinetic energies. There was a total of 60 different associated injuries reported (Table 3).

An appropriate fragment position was achieved by closed reduction in 116 (87.9%) patients and 16 (12.1%) patients required open reduction due to repositioning difficulties or soft tissue interposition. No intraoperative complications were recorded. Postoperative complications were reported in 15 (11.4%) patients (Table 4). Most complications (n = 9; 60%) were minor complications, mostly related to the wound at the nail insertion site, which were managed conservatively. Six (4.5%) patients required reoperation due to angulation of the fragments or refracture. In distal fractures of the tibia, the rate of postoperative complications was slightly higher (14.3%) compared to the fractures localized in the tibial shaft (10.8%).

Complete radiographic healing was achieved in the majority of the patients at a median of 7 (IQR 6, 9) weeks. The implants were removed under general anesthesia after healing without any complications at the median time of 6 (IQR 5, 8) months. After removal of the intramedullary nails, all patients regained full limb function and all complications were successfully resolved. All patients were followed until the end of this study and the median follow-up time was 118.5 (IQR 74.5, 170) months.

Table 3. Associated injuries of children who underwent ESIN due to tibial fracture.

Associated Injuries	n	%
Excoriations and wounds	24	40
Epiphysiolysis and fractures of long bones	13	21.7
Soft tissue hematomas	9	15
Parenchymal organ injuries	4	6.6
Fractures of short bones	3	5
Teeth injuries	2	3.3
Nerve injuries	2	3.3
Serial rib fracture and pneumothorax	1	1.7
Fracture of pelvis	1	1.7
Subarachnoid hemorrhage	1	1.7
Total	60	100

Table 4. Postoperative complications.

Complication	n	%
Angulation of the fragments	5	33.3
Entry skin irritations	4	26.7
Protrusions of the nails	2	13.3
Blisters	2	13.3
Pseudoaneurysm	1	6.7
Refracture	1	6.7
Total	15	100.0

4. Discussion

Pediatric fractures of the tibia can generally be managed by a non-operative approach [20–22]. However, this conservative type of treatment requires prolonged immobilization, careful follow-up, and complications such as secondary displacement, angulations, muscle atrophy, and refractures are not rare [23]. In younger children, up to four years of age, most of the lower leg fractures occur from falls or torsional forces, causing spiral and oblique tibial fractures. The fibula is usually intact in these fractures, preventing shortening but risking varus deformity. Older children usually suffer from indirect sporting injuries or direct injury from motor vehicle trauma, where both bones are usually involved. The cases with isolated tibial fracture usually are stable, not severely displaced or shortened, and may be usually treated conservatively with closed reduction and casting. Contrary to the above, the cases with both bones involved are usually displaced and require reduction and surgical treatment due to instability or shortening [3,4,13,22].

In recent years, the number of surgical procedures and indications for surgical treatment has significantly increased [8]. The ESIN method is currently a gold standard for the treatment of diaphyseal fractures in the pediatric population and adolescents [16]. Invention of the ESIN method gave an opportunity to children who sustained a fracture of a long bone that their time of hospitalization and immobilization can be significantly shorter. Moreover, this method became very popular because it is highly effective, complications are usually minor, and potential damage to the epiphyseal growth plate is minimized [21,22]. Intramedullary titanium nails provide stable and elastic fixation of the bone fragments, which allows controlled motion at the fracture site and provides quicker healing [24]. ESIN for the treatment of pediatric tibial fractures results in reliable healing for a majority of patients, but at the same time poses risks for angular deformities and delayed healing. Open fractures and compartment syndrome were associated with adverse radiographic outcomes [25].

The results obtained from the present study clearly showed that ESIN is a safe and effective method for treatment of tibial shaft and dia-metaphyseal distal tibial fractures with a low number of complications and relatively short length of hospital stay. Most of the complications were graded as minor (entry skin irritation, inflammation of the wound), while severe complications such as angulation of the fragments or refracture were rarely reported. Most of the authors recommend casting for a few weeks after surgery, probably due to fear of displacement of fragments or angulation [21,26–28]. In this study, we clearly showed that titanium intramedullary nailing may be safely performed without casting and one of the most important benefits of this method is early physiotherapy. Several previous reports on upper and lower extremities support this constancy [13,15,17–19].

Swindells and Rajan performed a systematic review of seven different retrospective studies regarding tibial ESIN with outcomes of 210 patients [29]. The authors of those studies described several indications for use of ESIN in pediatric patients, but most of them stated that the main indication was unstable fractures. The longest mean healing time in those studies was 20.7 weeks, reported by Srivastava et al. [21], and the shortest was 7 weeks, reported by Kubiak et al. [24]. Reported complication rates were similar, ranging from 12% to 35%. The most commonly reported complications were delayed union, malunion, nonunion, leg length discrepancy, and infections. All seven studies concluded that ESIN is an effective and safe method for treatment of unstable fractures of the tibial shaft in children and adolescents. They also concluded that most of the pediatric tibial fractures can be treated by a non-operative approach, but in cases where the surgery cannot be avoided, ESIN provides an acceptable and valuable option.

Griffet et al. reported that all 86 children included in their study were able to have unrestricted physical activity six months after the treatment with the ESIN method for tibial fractures [30]. They showed that the fixation of pediatric diaphyseal tibial fractures using ESIN is an effective method of treatment in pediatric patients and adolescents.

Uludağ et al. published a study which included 20 children. The mean time of radiographic healing was 11 weeks and there were six (30%) instances of irritation and infections at the nail entry site [31]. Furthermore, they reported that three of six patients with an open fracture had infections of the wound. All their patients gained full range of motion of the ankle and knee joints. They concluded that intramedullary fixation with ESIN provides favorable outcomes in the treatment of unstable pediatric tibial shaft fractures that cannot be reduced with conservative treatment modalities.

Onta et al. reported that their 18 patients had a mean hospitalization time of 5.7 days and that all children achieved radiographic healing at the mean time of 13.3 weeks [32]. All of their patients had excellent final results and all of them had full range of movement at the knee joint. Four children had minor complications (nail protrusion and skin irritation), which were managed non-operatively. They concluded that ESIN had benefits of low blood loss compared to plating, and they also reported easier nursing care, early ambulation, and no complications of prolonged immobilization.

Shen et al. published a study with 21 children that went under the surgery procedure with the ESIN method due to severely displaced dia-metaphyseal distal tibial fractures. They reported a mean hospitalization time of 3.9 days, and the mean time of the nail removal was 7.1 months [33]. A total of 19 patients achieved radiographic healing at the mean time of 9.6 weeks and two patients had delayed healing 10 months after the surgery. Their study showed good functional and radiological results in the pediatric population who had severely displaced DTDMJ (distal tibial diaphyseal metaphyseal junction) fractures that could not be casted.

Kc et al. reported that in their study, which included 45 children treated with the ESIN method due to fracture of tibia, that they had a mean healing time of 11.17 weeks [34]. They recorded 20 postoperative complications which included 2 malunions, 4 delayed unions, 3 limb shortening, 2 limb lengthening, 6 nail prominences and skin irritations, 2 superficial infections on the nail entry site, and 1 refracture. However, none of their patients required secondary surgical intervention due to those complications. They concluded that ESIN is a simple, easy, reliable, and effective method for management of pediatric tibial fractures with shorter operative time, lesser blood loss, shorter length of hospital stay, and adequate time for bone healing.

Pennock et al. in their study compared 44 patients who underwent ESIN with 26 patients who received open reduction with internal fixation (ORIF) for tribal shaft fractures [28]. Patients that underwent ORIF had a longer mean surgical time and their mean casting time was seven weeks; minor complications were recorded in 10 (38%) patients and major ones were recorded in 3 (12%) patients. Patients that underwent ESIN had a shorter surgical time, and their mean casting time was 10.5 weeks; minor complications were recorded in 12 (27%) cases, while major complications were recorded in 8 (18%) cases. They concluded that patients treated with ORIF tend to heal and mobilize a few weeks faster, they have slightly more anatomic reductions at final healing, and they are less likely to require implant removal. Moreover, they pointed out that both ESIN and ORIF treatments contribute to a faster return to activities and that potential advantages of ORIF must be balanced with the potential increased risk of wound complications.

There is no exact consensus among the authors which age or height should be set as a limit for ESIN. Many authors used ESIN for treatment of pediatric and adolescent tibial fractures without any limits [13,22,33,35]. In previous studies, the rate of delayed healing was shown to vary by around 10% [13,22,33]. Gordon et al. in their study reported that patients with delayed union were older and they concluded the lack of stability may be the key factor behind the delayed healing [22]. Although there is a wide age (height) range in the majority of the studies, age of the patients ranges between 10 and 12 years of age [13,22,23,26,33,35,36]. A recent study showed that patients with tibial fractures who weigh 50 kg or less and with proximal tibial growth plates wide open can be treated with elastic stable intramedullary nailing, while more mature adolescents benefit from rigid intramedullary nailing as rigid nailing allows more precise fracture alignment without increased risk of growth disturbance [36]. Similar findings were observed in another recent study [37]. Hanf-Osetek et al. in their study compared children weighing less than 50 kg or more than 50 kg and found that the use of ESIN in displaced tibial shaft fractures in growing children weighing 50 kg or more is acceptable and safe [38]. A recent study performed by Thabet et al. compared adolescents treated for tibial shaft fractures using ESIN, interlocking nails, plates, and screws or external fixators and showed that open fractures had higher complication rates but no statistically significant differences in complication rates between the fixation methods was observed [39]. In general, the good results using the ESIN method may be obtained when the surgeon has a good knowledge of the method, respects and understands indications for surgery, and the main principles of the correction of the fracture and its stability [40].

In our study, of the sample of 132 children, the mean time of radiographic healing was seven weeks. We recorded complications in fifteen (11.36%) patients, which included five angulations of the fragments, four entry site irritations, two protrusions of the nails, two skin blisters, one pseudoaneurysm, and one refracture. Six (4.5%) of our patients needed a reoperation due to angulations of the fragment and refracture. The median of surgical time was 56 min. These results are similar to previous reports. Although most of the previously mentioned studies reported usage of a postoperative cast or a slab, our department policy is that after the surgical procedure with ESIN, no type of immobilization is needed. According to our positive results of this study, which included 132 patients, we proved that cast immobilization is not needed after the surgery procedure with the ESIN method due to tibia fracture.

The results of this study must be interpreted within the context of several limitations. First, this was a single-center study, and the data were collected retrospectively. Furthermore, sample size was relatively small (although significantly higher than in most of the published reports). Next, there was a lack of a comparison group because a very low number of the patients were treated with other surgical techniques (such as plating, external fixation, or expert tibial nail). The majority of pediatric tibial fractures can be successfully treated conservatively by non-operative management and only the patients who fail conservative treatment (or are open/polytrauma/initially unable to reduce) are selected for surgery (most commonly ESIN). Accordingly, we were not able to design an adequate control group. Moreover, as this was a retrospective study, we could not find the data regarding functional outcome for the majority of the patients, especially for those operated on in earlier years. Prospective, multicenter studies with a larger sample size need to be conducted in the future before any definite conclusions in this regard should be drawn.

5. Conclusions

ESIN fulfills all criteria of minimally invasive bone surgery and is a highly effective treatment for pediatric tibial unstable fractures with a low rate of complications. Furthermore, the results of this study clearly showed that titanium intramedullary nailing may be safely performed without casting, and one of the most important benefits of this method is early physiotherapy.

Author Contributions: Conceptualization, Z.P. and D.F.; Formal analysis, V.V. and Z.P.; Writing—original draft preparation, M.J., V.V. and C.M.L.M.; Writing—review and editing, Z.P., C.M.L.M. and D.F. All authors have read and agreed to the published version of the manuscript.

Funding: This research received no external funding.

Institutional Review Board Statement: The study was conducted according to the guidelines of the Declaration of Helsinki and approved by the Institutional Review Board of the University Hospital of Split (IRB reference, 500-03-/22-01/16, date of approval 3 March 2022).

Informed Consent Statement: Not applicable.

Data Availability Statement: The data presented in this study are available upon request of the respective author.

Conflicts of Interest: The authors declare no conflict of interest.

References

1. Metaizeau, J.D.; Denis, D. Update on leg fractures in paediatric patients. *Orthop. Traumatol. Surg. Res.* **2019**, *105*, 143–151. [CrossRef]
2. Palmu, S.A.; Auro, S.; Lohman, M.; Paukku, R.T.; Peltonen, J.I.; Nietosvaara, Y. Tibial fractures in children. A retrospective 27-year follow-up study. *Acta Orthop.* **2014**, *85*, 513–517. [CrossRef]
3. Martus, J.E. Operative fixation versus cast immobilization: Tibial shaft fractures in adolescents. *J. Pediatr. Orthop.* **2021**, *41*, 33–38. [CrossRef]
4. Joeris, A.; Lutz, N.; Wicki, B.; Slongo, T.; Audigé, L. An epidemiological evaluation of pediatric long bone fractures—A retrospective cohort study of 2716 patients from two Swiss tertiary pediatric hospitals. *BMC Pediatr.* **2014**, *14*, 314. [CrossRef]
5. Weber, B.; Kalbitz, M.; Baur, M.; Braun, C.K.; Zwingmann, J.; Pressmar, J. Lower leg fractures in children and adolescents-comparison of conservative vs. ECMES Treatment. *Front. Pediatr.* **2021**, *9*, 597870. [CrossRef]
6. Fox, J.; Enriquez, B.; Bompadre, V.; Carlin, K.; Dales, M. Observation Versus Cast Treatment of Toddler's Fractures. *J. Pediatr. Orthop.* **2022**, *42*, e480–e485. [CrossRef]
7. Patel, N.K.; Horstman, J.; Kuester, V.; Sambandam, S.; Mounasamy, V. Pediatric tibial shaft fractures. *Indian J. Orthop.* **2018**, *52*, 522–528. [CrossRef]
8. Stenroos, A.; Laaksonen, T.; Nietosvaara, N.; Jalkanen, J.; Nietosvaara, Y. One in three of pediatric tibia shaft fractures is currently treated operatively: A 6-year epidemiological study in two university hospitals in Finland treatment of pediatric tibia shaft fractures. *Scand. J. Surg.* **2018**, *107*, 269–274. [CrossRef]
9. Kleiner, J.E.; Raducha, J.E.; Cruz, A.I., Jr. Increasing rates of surgical treatment for paediatric tibial shaft fractures: A national database study from between 2000 and 2012. *J. Child. Orthop.* **2019**, *13*, 213–219. [CrossRef]
10. Cruz, A.I., Jr.; Raducha, J.E.; Swarup, I.; Schachne, J.M.; Fabricant, P.D. Evidence-based update on the surgical treatment of pediatric tibial shaft fractures. *Curr. Opin. Pediatr.* **2019**, *31*, 92–102. [CrossRef]
11. Mashru, R.P.; Herman, M.J.; Pizzutillo, P.D. Tibial shaft fractures in children and adolescents. *J. Am. Acad. Orthop. Surg.* **2005**, *13*, 345–352. [CrossRef] [PubMed]
12. Hogue, G.D.; Wilkins, K.E.; Kim, I.S. Management of pediatric tibial shaft fractures. *J. Am. Acad. Orthop. Surg.* **2019**, *27*, 769–778. [CrossRef]

13. Furlan, D.; Pogorelić, Z.; Biočić, M.; Jurić, I.; Budimir, D.; Todorić, J.; Šušnjar, T.; Todorić, D.; Meštrović, J. Elastic stable intramedullary nailing for pediatric long bone fractures: Experience with 175 fractures. *Scand. J. Surg.* **2011**, *100*, 208–215. [CrossRef]
14. Egger, A.; Murphy, J.; Johnson, M.; Hosseinzadeh, P.; Louer, C. Elastic stable intramedullary nailing of pediatric tibial fractures. *JBJS Essent. Surg. Tech.* **2020**, *10*, e19.00063. [CrossRef]
15. Pogorelić, Z.; Gulin, M.; Jukić, M.; Biliškov, A.N.; Furlan, D. Elastic stable intramedullary nailing for treatment of pediatric forearm fractures: A 15-year single centre retrospective study of 173 cases. *Acta Orthop. Traumatol. Turc.* **2020**, *54*, 378–384. [CrossRef]
16. Cosma, D.; Vasilescu, D.E. Elastic stable intramedullary nailing for fractures in children—Specific applications. *Clujul Med.* **2014**, *87*, 147–151. [CrossRef]
17. Pogorelić, Z.; Vodopić, T.; Jukić, M.; Furlan, D. Elastic stable intramedullary nailing for treatment of pediatric femoral fractures; A 15-year single centre experience. *Bull. Emerg. Trauma.* **2019**, *7*, 169–175. [CrossRef]
18. Pogorelić, Z.; Kadić, S.; Milunović, K.P.; Pintarić, I.; Jukić, M.; Furlan, D. Flexible intramedullary nailing for treatment of proximal humeral and humeral shaft fractures in children: A retrospective series of 118 cases. *Orthop. Traumatol. Surg. Res.* **2017**, *103*, 765–770. [CrossRef]
19. Pogorelić, Z.; Capitain, A.; Jukić, M.; Žufić, V.; Furlan, D. Flexible intramedullary nailing for radial neck fractures in children. *Acta Orthop. Traumatol. Turc.* **2020**, *54*, 618–622. [CrossRef]
20. Goodwin, R.C.; Gaynor, T.; Mahar, A.; Oka, R.; Lalonde, F.D. Intramedullary flexible nail fixation of unstable pediatric tibial diaphyseal fractures. *J. Pediatr. Orthop.* **2005**, *25*, 570–576. [CrossRef]
21. Srivastava, A.K.; Mehlman, C.T.; Wall, E.J.; Do, T.T. Elastic stable intramedullary nailing of tibial shaft fractures in children. *J. Pediatr. Orthop.* **2008**, *28*, 152–158. [CrossRef]
22. Gordon, J.E.; Gregush, R.V.; Schoenecker, P.L.; Dobbs, M.B.; Luhmann, S.J. Complications after titanium elastic nailing of pediatric tibial fractures. *J. Pediatr. Orthop.* **2007**, *27*, 442–446. [CrossRef] [PubMed]
23. O'Brien, T.; Weisman, D.S.; Ronchetti, P.; Piller, C.P.; Maloney, M. Flexible titanium nailing for the treatment of the unstable pediatric tibial fracture. *J. Pediatr. Orthop.* **2004**, *24*, 601–609. [CrossRef]
24. Kubiak, E.N.; Egol, K.A.; Scher, D.; Wasserman, B.; Feldman, D.; Koval, K.J. Operative treatment of tibial fractures in children: Are elastic stable intramedullary nails an improvement over external fixation? *J. Bone Jt. Surg. Am.* **2005**, *87*, 1761–1768. [CrossRef]
25. Pennock, A.T.; Huang, S.G.; Pedowitz, J.M.; Pandya, N.K.; McLaughlin, D.C.; Bastrom, T.P.; Ellis, H.B. Risk factors for adverse radiographic outcomes after elastic stable intramedullary nailing of unstable diaphyseal tibia fractures in children. *J. Pediatr. Orthop.* **2020**, *40*, 481–486. [CrossRef]
26. Sankar, W.N.; Jones, K.J.; David Horn, B.; Wells, L. Titanium elastic nails for pediatric tibial shaft fractures. *J. Child. Orthop.* **2007**, *1*, 281–286. [CrossRef] [PubMed]
27. Vallamshetla, V.R.; De Silva, U.; Bache, C.E.; Gibbons, P.J. Flexible intramedullary nails for unstable fractures of the tibia in children. An eight-year experience. *J. Bone Jt. Surg. Br.* **2006**, *88*, 536–540. [CrossRef] [PubMed]
28. Pennock, A.T.; Bastrom, T.P.; Upasani, V.V. Elastic Intramedullary Nailing Versus Open Reduction Internal Fixation of Pediatric Tibial Shaft Fractures. *J. Pediatr. Orthop.* **2017**, *37*, e403–e408. [CrossRef]
29. Swindells, M.G.; Rajan, R.A. Elastic intramedullary nailing in unstable fractures of the paediatric tibial diaphysis: A systematic review. *J. Child. Orthop.* **2010**, *4*, 45–51. [CrossRef]
30. Griffet, J.; Leroux, J.; Boudjouraf, N.; Abou-Daher, A.; El Hayek, T. Elastic stable intramedullary nailing of tibial shaft fractures in children. *J. Child. Orthop.* **2011**, *5*, 297–304. [CrossRef]
31. Uludağ, A.; Tosun, H.B. Treatment of unstable pediatric tibial shaft fractures with titanium elastic nails. *Medicina* **2019**, *55*, 266. [CrossRef] [PubMed]
32. Onta, P.R.; Thapa, P.; Sapkota, K.; Ranjeet, N.; Kishore, A.; Gupta, M. Outcome of diaphyseal fracture of tibia treated with flexible intramedullary nailing in pediatrics age group; A prospective study. *Am. J. Public Health* **2015**, *3*, 65–68.
33. Shen, K.; Cai, H.; Wang, Z.; Xu, Y. Elastic stable intramedullary nailing for severely displaced distal tibial fractures in children. *Medicine* **2016**, *95*, e4980. [CrossRef]
34. Kc, K.M.; Acharya, P.; Sigdel, A. Titanium Elastic Nailing System (TENS) for tibia fractures in children: Functional outcomes and complications. *JNMA J. Nepal. Med. Assoc.* **2016**, *55*, 55–60. [CrossRef] [PubMed]
35. Aslani, H.; Tabrizi, A.; Sadighi, A.; Mirblok, A.R. Treatment of open pediatric tibial fractures by external fixation versus flexible intramedullary nailing: A comparative study. *Arch. Trauma Res.* **2013**, *2*, 108–112. [CrossRef]
36. Widbom-Kolhanen, S.; Helenius, I. Intramedullary nailing of paediatric tibial fractures: Comparison between flexible and rigid nails. *Scand. J. Surg.* **2021**, *110*, 265–270. [CrossRef]
37. Williams, K.A.; Thier, Z.T.; Mathews, C.G.; Locke, M.D. Physeal-Sparing Rigid Intramedullary Nailing in Adolescent Tibial Shaft Fractures: A Pilot Study. *Cureus* **2021**, *13*, e13893. [CrossRef]
38. Hanf-Osetek, D.; Bilski, P.; Łabądź, D.; Snela, S. Tibial shaft fractures in children: Flexible intramedullary nailing in growing children especially weighing 50 kg (110 lbs) or more. *J. Pediatr. Orthop. B* **2022**. [CrossRef]

39. Thabet, A.M.; Craft, M.; Pisquiy, J.; Jeon, S.; Abdelgawad, A.; Azzam, W. Tibial shaft fractures in the adolescents: Treatment outcomes and the risk factors for complications. *Injury* **2022**, *53*, 706–712. [CrossRef] [PubMed]
40. Lascombes, P.; Haumont, T.; Journeau, P. Use and abuse of flexible intramedullary nailing in children and adolescents. *J. Pediatr. Orthop.* **2006**, *26*, 827–834. [CrossRef]

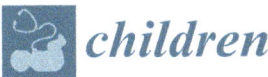

Review

NSAID Use and Effects on Pediatric Bone Healing: A Review of Current Literature

Stephanie Choo and Julia A. V. Nuelle *

Department of Orthopaedic Surgery, Missouri Orthopaedic Institute, University of Missouri, Columbia, MO 65212, USA; slcdn4@health.missouri.edu
* Correspondence: julia.nuelle@health.missouri.edu

Abstract: This systematic review evaluates and synthesizes the available peer-reviewed evidence regarding the impact of non-steroidal anti-inflammatory drugs (NSAIDs) on fracture healing in skeletally immature patients. Evidence supports the use of NSAIDs in this patient population for adequate pain control without increasing the risk of nonunion, particularly in long bone fractures and pseudoarthrosis after spine fusion. However, further clinical studies are needed to fill remaining gaps in knowledge, specifically with respect to the spectrum of available NSAIDs, dosage, and duration of use, in order to make broad evidence-based recommendations regarding the optimal use of NSAIDs during bone healing in skeletally immature patients.

Keywords: NSAIDs; ibuprofen; fracture healing; pediatrics; evidence-based recommendations

Citation: Choo, S.; Nuelle, J.A.V. NSAID Use and Effects on Pediatric Bone Healing: A Review of Current Literature. *Children* 2021, *8*, 821. https://doi.org/10.3390/children 8090821

Academic Editor: Christiaan J. A. van Bergen

Received: 7 July 2021
Accepted: 12 September 2021
Published: 18 September 2021

Publisher's Note: MDPI stays neutral with regard to jurisdictional claims in published maps and institutional affiliations.

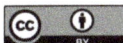

Copyright: © 2021 by the authors. Licensee MDPI, Basel, Switzerland. This article is an open access article distributed under the terms and conditions of the Creative Commons Attribution (CC BY) license (https:// creativecommons.org/licenses/by/ 4.0/).

1. Introduction

Nonsteroidal anti-inflammatory drugs (NSAIDs) have consistently been some of the most widely used medications for decades, based on their anti-inflammatory and analgesic mechanisms of action, in conjunction with their safety profiles and non-addictive characteristics [1]. The opioid epidemic has generated a strong impetus for the use of multimodal pain regimens, aimed at effectively managing pain with less reliance on opioids and the associated risks of misuse, abuse, addiction, morbidity, and mortality [2–4]. Decreased reliance on opioids also mitigates the known side effects of this class of medication, including nausea, vomiting, dizziness, and constipation. As such, NSAIDs provide an attractive choice as a mainstay of multimodal pain management protocols. There is hesitancy, however, to prescribe NSAIDs within the period following a fracture, arising from concern around delayed healing or non-union, given the potential blockade of the required inflammatory phase of bone healing.

Fracture nonunions are painful, can negatively impact the patient's quality of life, and are costly to the healthcare system [5]. In general, the incidence of fracture nonunion has been reported to range from 5% to 10% in the skeletally mature patient population, with even higher rates associated with at-risk patients and fractures of the scaphoid (15.5%), tibia and fibula (14%), and femur (13.9%) [6,7]. Pseudoarthrosis in the pediatric population is substantially less, at a rate of <1% [8]. Several animal models and retrospective cohort studies have demonstrated the potential for NSAIDs to increase the risk of non-union in the skeletally mature population [6,9,10]. However, recent prospective studies have shown that NSAIDs do not increase the risk of nonunion, while improving pain control with a potential opioid-sparing effect [11–13]. In addition to these contrasting results in skeletally mature population studies, evidence-based recommendations regarding the use of NSAIDs for pain management after fractures in the pediatric, skeletally immature population have similarly not been conclusive to date.

Fracture risk in pediatric patients is high, however, the incidence for nonunion is relatively low [8]. Still, while NSAIDs are highly desirable for effective pain management with a reduction in opioid use in this patient population, there has been an apparent hesitancy in prescribing NSAIDs to pediatric patients with fractures due to physicians' concerns for non-unions based on some of the published data for adults. The concerns, based on anecdotal extrapolation to the pediatric population, does not have a sound physiologic basis in light of distinct differences in bone healing between patients that are skeletally immature and skeletally mature [14], and may unnecessarily inhibit best practice. Therefore, the purpose of this study was to (1) systematically review available evidence regarding skeletally immature fracture healing patterns based on exposure to NSAIDs to synthesize recommendations on NSAID use for pain control post-injury, and (2) determine critical gaps in knowledge towards establishing evidence-based care for analgesia after fractures in the pediatric population.

2. Materials and Methods

Using PRISMA guidelines, two electronic databases—PUBMED and Cochrane—were systematically searched using combinations of the keywords "NSAIDS", "ibuprofen", "non-steroidal", "anti-inflammatory drugs", "naproxen", "ketorolac", "bone healing", "fracture healing", "bone fractures", "bone union", "non union", "children", "pediatric", "child", and "skeletally immature" as terms, title words, and abstract words. Reference lists from identified articles were also reviewed for inclusion. Studies in the English language and published between the years 2000–2021 were considered for inclusion. Studies were included when they assessed NSAID effects on bone healing in individuals who are skeletally immature and/or evaluated pediatric outcomes after NSAIDs use in association with fracture management. The exclusion criteria, included fracture or bone healing following orthopaedic surgical intervention not included as a study outcome, as well as studies of patients who are skeletally mature. The title and abstract of each qualifying article were screened and full-text manuscripts were retrieved in cases of uncertainty for inclusion. The following data from included studies were then extracted: Date of publication, number of patients, number of males and females, mean age, the incidence of nonunion or pseudoarthrosis, length of follow-up, type and amount of medication used, and the study type/level of evidence. An independent reviewer determined the final eligibility of studies included for systematic review. The synthesis of included articles followed the PICO (Population, Intervention, Comparison, Outcome) reporting methodology. The Cochrane Risk of Bias Tool was also utilized to assess and report bias risk.

3. Results

The database search produced a total of 37 studies for review. A reference lists review produced an additional 4 relevant studies. Based on a full review of these 41 articles, 8 met inclusion criteria for systematic review (Figure 1).

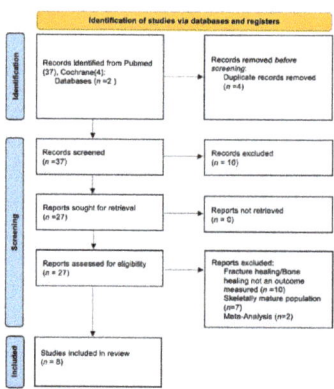

Figure 1. PRISMA 2020 flow diagram for new systematic reviews which included searches of databases and registers only.

From these 10 studies, 6 were retrospective cohort studies, 2 were prospective randomized control trials, and 2 were meta-analysis. The meta-analysis studies were excluded from this analysis as the 4 retrospective pediatric studies, cited in this literature, are also included in this current review. Demographic data for each study are included in Table 1. Qualitative synthesis, including risk of bias assessment for these 10 studies, were reported in Table 2.

Table 1. Demographics.

Study Year	Author	Number of Patients	Male/Female	Mean Age (Not Exposed/Exposed)	Mean Follow Up (Not Exposed/Exposed)
2018	Zura et al. [8]	237,033 fractures	146,234 fractures/ 90,790 fractures	0–18 years	12 months
2008	Sucato et al. [13]	319 total (158 exposed)	50/269	14.2 years	39 months
2003	Vitale et al. [15]	208 total (60 exposed)	59/149	13.4 years	67 months
2010	Kay et al. [16]	221 total (169 exposed)	142/79	6.7 years (5.5 years/7.1 years)	6.2 months (6.7 months/ 6.9 months)
2011	Kay et al. [17]	327 total (299 exposed)	181/136	(8.4 years/9.2 years)	(38 months/ 44 months)
2016	DePeter et al. [18]	808 total (338 exposed)	508/300	7 years (7 years/7 years)	–
2009	Drendel et al. [19]	336 total (169 exposed)	126/210	(8.2 years/7.4 years)	4 years
2020	Nuelle et al. [20]	95 total (49 exposed)	58/37	7.6 years	6 months

Table 2. Synthesis of Examined Studies Evaluating Effect of NSAIDs on Bone Healing in Skeletally Immature Patients.

Study	Fracture Locations	NSAID Used	Clinical Relevance/Findings	LOE/Study Type	Risk for Bias
Drendel et al. [19]	Upper extremity fractures	Ibuprofen	Primary outcome: Ibuprofen was at least as effective as acetaminophen with codeine as outpatient analgesia for children with arm fractures Secondary outcome: No nonunions reported with use of ibuprofen or acetaminophen with codeine	I—RCT	Low risk
Nuelle et al. [20]	Long bone fractures	Ibuprofen and Ketorolac	Ibuprofen does not impair clinical or radiographic long bone fracture healing in skeletally immature patients	I—RCT	Low risk

Table 2. Cont.

Study	Fracture Locations	NSAID Used	Clinical Relevance/Findings	LOE/Study Type	Risk for Bias
Zura et al. [8]	Metacarpal, radius, ankle, patella, radius and ulna, fibula, pelvis, clavicle, humerus, femur, tibia, ulna, metatarsal, tarsal, tibia and fibula, scaphoid	Did not specify	NSAIDs alone did not increase risk of pediatric nonunion Risk factors for pediatric nonunion are similar to adult nonunion risk factors [increasing age, male gender, high body-mass index, severe fracture (e.g., open fracture, multiple fractures), and tobacco smoking] Opioids should be used cautiously in pediatric patients, as they are associated with a significant and substantial elevation of nonunion risk	II—Prognostic Retrospective Study	Moderate risk
DePeter et al. [18]	Tibia, femur, humerus, scaphoid, or fifth metatarsus	Ibuprofen	There was no statistically significant association between ibuprofen exposure and the development of a bone healing complications in the tibia, femur, humerus, scaphoid, or fifth metatarsal	III—Retrospective Comparative Study	Moderate risk
Sucato et al. [13]	Vertebrae	Ketorolac	Ketorolac does not increase the incidence of developing a pseudoarthrosis when used as an adjunct for postoperative analgesia following a PSFI for AIS using segmental spinal instrumentation and iliac crest bone graft.	III—Retrospective Comparative Study	Moderate risk
Kay et al. [16]	Supracondylar, forearm, lateral condyle, femur, tibia, or ankle fractures	Ketorolac and ibuprofen	Perioperative ketorolac use does not increase the risk of complications after operative fracture care of supracondylar, forearm, lateral condyle, femur, tibia, or ankle fractures in children	III—Retrospective Comparative Study	Moderate risk

Table 2. Cont.

Study	Fracture Locations	NSAID Used	Clinical Relevance/Findings	LOE/Study Type	Risk for Bias
Kay et al. [17]	Lower extremity osteotomies	Ketorolac	Perioperative ketorolac is safe for children having lower extremity osteotomies as there is no significant difference in the rate of either osseous or soft tissue complications between ketorolac provided and no ketorolac patients	III—Retrospective Comparative Study	Moderate risk
Vitale et al. [15]	Vertebrae	Ketorolac	Degree of spine curvature is significant in predicting reoperation; treatment with ketorolac is not a significant independent predictor for nonunion/reoperation	III—Retrospective Comparative Study	Moderate risk

LOE = Level of Evidence; RCT = Randomized Controlled Trial.

3.1. Retrospective Cohort Studies

Vitale et al. [15] conducted a retrospective study to determine whether an association exists between the use of ketorolac and postoperative complications in children undergoing spinal fusion surgery for scoliosis. Ketorolac was shown to be an effective alternative to opioid medications for analgesia [21]. This study investigated potentially related complications, including bony fusion failure and the requirement for revision surgery due to pseudoarthrosis, as well as infected hardware, hardware failure, and bleeding risk represented by need for transfusion. Based on the review of 10 years of medical records, a total of 208 children who had undergone corrective spinal fusion surgery for scoliosis were included. Sixty patients (29%) received ketorolac postoperatively and the remaining 148 (71%) did not. The group of patients that were given ketorolac in the post-operative period was composed primarily of complicated patients (typically a greater degree of curvature) as determined by the operative surgeon. They reported an average dose of ketorolac to be 0.5 mg/kg intravenous (IV), every 6 h for 2–3 days, starting 24 to 48 h postoperatively. Patients were followed through clinical and radiographic assessments for an average of 62 months (ketorolac group) and 69 months (no ketorolac group). Analyses from this study produced no statistically significant differences between ketorolac versus no ketorolac for fusion rate, pseudarthrosis, or other potentially related complications. The only independent variable that was significantly associated with the need for revision surgery, due to pseudoarthrosis, hardware failure, or hardware infection was the degree of curvature of the spine prior to intervention.

The study by Sucato et al. [13] referenced a study by Glassman and colleagues, which demonstrated the significant inhibitory effects of ketorolac on spinal fusion when used as an adjunct for postoperative pain in adult patients [22], and served as the impetus for the former authors' similar study in a pediatric population. This retrospective study compared patients who had postoperative ketorolac and those who did not, following posterior spinal fusion and instrumentation for adolescent idiopathic scoliosis (AIS). Overall, 161 patients did not receive ketorolac postoperatively and 158 did. Pseudoarthrosis was defined by surgical exploration and confirmation in the patients who presented with ongoing symptoms after initial fixation. This study noted the average number of ketorolac doses was 6.7 for a duration of 48 h after surgery. Patients in the ketorolac group augmented their medical pain management with an additional 5.8 doses of ibuprofen after surgery on average in comparison to the non-ketorolac group's average of 0.7 doses. Mean follow-up for both groups was 39 months after fixation and the overall incidence of pseudoarthrosis during this time was 2.5% (8 of 319 patients) with no statistically significant difference between the ketorolac and non-ketorolac groups (1.9% vs 3.1%). The data from this study led the investigators to conclude that pseudoarthrosis risks are similar for AIS patients, regardless of ketorolac use, a finding consistent with those of Vitale et al. [15].

Kay et al. [16] performed a retrospective review of 221 children who sustained fractures (supracondylar humerus (42%), lateral condyle (12%), forearm (10%), femur (18%), tibia (7%), or ankle (7%)) requiring operative fixation. Of the 221 patients, 169 were treated with ketorolac postoperatively and 52 were not. The decision to use ketorolac for treatment was based on the preference of the anesthesiologist or the pain management team. The ketorolac group received weight-based dosing every 6 h while in the hospital, and the non-ketorolac group was treated with ibuprofen. These patients, on average, stayed 2.5 days in the hospital, discharged with ibuprofen, and followed for an average of 6.2 ± 7.5 months after fixation. No complications related to ketorolac or ibuprofen administration were reported, and there were no cases of delayed union or malunion in this pediatric fracture cohort.

In their 2011 study, Kay et al. [17] performed a retrospective review of 327 children undergoing lower extremity osteotomy surgery, of which 299 patients received ketorolac perioperatively and 28 patients did not. Delayed union occurred in 5 of 682 osteotomies (0.7%), which included 0.6% in the ketorolac group and 1.8% in the non-ketorolac group ($p = 0.893$). No nonunions were documented. The data in this study led the investigators to conclude that perioperative ketorolac is acceptable for pain management in patients who are skeletally immature and undergoing lower extremity osteotomies without significant risks regarding bone healing.

Zura et al. [8] performed a retrospective cohort study of 237,033 fractures in pediatric patients to identify risk factors for nonunion. Data were acquired from Truven Health Analytics health claims in a single calendar year (1 January 2011—31 December, 2012). The study population maintained a low nonunion rate until age 11 where a strong inflection point occurred such that a significant increase in nonunion rate was noted for each fracture location analyzed ($p < 0.001$), with tibia, fibula, femoral neck, and scaphoid having >5% nonunion risk after age 11. Interestingly, this study reported that pediatric fracture patients that used NSAIDs with opioids ($p < 0.01$; OR = 2.52) or opioids alone ($p < 0.01$; OR = 2.47) had a nearly 2.5 times increased risk of non-union, while patients (age 0 to 18 years) who consumed NSAIDs alone did not show a statistically significant increase in risk. This study did not specify which NSAIDs were used, or the dosage and duration of use. This data led the authors to conclude that NSAID use is appropriate for pain management during bone healing in pediatric patients, but should not be used in conjunction with opioids, especially after age 11.

DePeter et al. [18] performed a retrospective study in children aged 6 months to 17 years, assessing patients with common fractures that have been reported to have a higher incidence of healing complications, including in the tibia, femur, humerus, scaphoid, and fifth metatarsal fractures. A total of 808 patients were included in this study, of which a total of 27 (3%) showed bone healing complications, 1% from nonunion, 0.4% delayed union, and 2% loss of reduction. Of the 338 patients (42%) exposed to ibuprofen, 10 patients (3%) went on to non-union, which was not significantly ($p = 0.61$) different from patients not consuming ibuprofen. These data led the authors to conclude that there was no significant association between ibuprofen use and the development of bone healing complications in this pediatric high-risk fracture population.

3.2. Prospective Randomized Studies

Nuelle et al. [20] performed a randomized, parallel, single-blinded clinical trial to assess the impact of NSAIDs on acute-phase bone healing in patients who are skeletally immature with a variety of long bone fractures. This study assessed 97 fractures in pediatric patients, randomized to control ($n = 47$) or NSAID ($n = 50$) cohorts. The control group was provided weight-based acetaminophen for pain control and oxycodone for breakthrough pain. If a patient was in the emergency department, weight-based fentanyl was available for administration. Patients in the NSAID group were prescribed weight-based ibuprofen for pain control, as well as oxycodone for breakthrough pain. NSAID patients in the emergency department were permitted to have ketorolac for pain control if needed. Clinical visits involving radiographs of the fractured extremity occurred at 1–2 weeks, 6 weeks, 10–12 weeks, and 6 months after injury. Fracture healing was determined by clinical examination, absence of tenderness to palpation at fracture site, and radiographs demonstrating callus formation bridging in 3 cortices. As a secondary outcome measure, pain control was assessed by the patient's caregiver recording the patient's visual analog scale pain score, as well as the amount and type of pain medication used, for a total of 3 weeks after the injury. This study demonstrated that, by 6 weeks following initial fracture treatment, 82% of the control group had united fractures and 92% of the NSAID group had healed fractures, with no significant difference ($p = 0.22$) between both groups. By the 10–12 week appointment, 98% of control and 100% of NSAID patients had healed fractures, and the 6-month follow-up demonstrated 100% healed fractures for both cohorts. Of note, pain scores were similar for both groups with acetaminophen used for 3.9 days on average versus ibuprofen use for 4.3 days on average. Oxycodone was used for breakthrough pain for a mean of 2.4 days in the control cohort and 1.9 days in the NSAID cohort. These data led the authors to conclude that ibuprofen can be used to effectively manage pain in pediatric patients during the acute post-treatment period following long bone fractures without impairing fracture healing.

Drendel et al. [19] performed a randomized, double-blind, clinical trial assessing ibuprofen versus acetaminophen with codeine in pediatric patients treated for upper extremity fractures. In contrast to Nuelle et al. [20], the primary outcome measure for this study was pain control, with fracture healing as a secondary outcome measure. Pain was assessed using the visual Bieri Faces Pain Scale and caregivers were also asked to keep a diary documenting the patient's tolerability of the medication. Non-unions were assessed by reviewing medical records for 1 year following treatment, with a follow-up phone call to the patient's caregiver for verification when an adverse event related to fracture healing was noted. The study enrolled 336 children, and 169 patients were randomized to the ibuprofen group and 167 to the acetaminophen with codeine group. Of the 244 patients that met the criteria and were analyzed, the proportion of "treatment failures" and the need for rescue IV pain medication was lower in the ibuprofen group than the acetaminophen with codeine group (20.3% vs 31.0%, respectively). However, this difference was not statistically significant. Pain scores were similar between the two groups. However, medication-related adverse effects reported during the first 3 days of treatment were significantly higher for the acetaminophen with codeine group at 50.9% versus the ibuprofen group at 29.5% (% difference 21.4, confidence interval (CI) 9.1 to 33.7). Chart review and telephone calls determined that four (1.6%) of the children sustained re-fracture within 1 year of the original fracture, and of those, three (75%) received acetaminophen with codeine. There were no reports of nonunion in either group. These data led the authors to conclude that ibuprofen was as effective as an acetaminophen with codeine in providing analgesia for children with upper extremity fractures. The drug was associated with less medication-related adverse effects and was not associated with re-fracture or nonunion in this patient population.

4. Discussion

This systematic review of available evidence regarding NSAID exposure, and bone healing in patients who are skeletally immature, produced six retrospective studies and two prospective clinical trials for inclusion. The qualitative synthesis of these studies suggested that the best current evidence supports the use of two NSAIDs, ibuprofen and ketorolac, as safe and effective medications for pain management. These medications did not show an increased risk of pseudoarthrosis after spinal fusions or nonunion after fractures of the upper and lower extremity, scaphoid, or metatarsals in the pediatric population.

Concerns regarding the use of NSAIDs in the acute phase of bone healing have been based on animal studies and clinical assessments of patients that are skeletally mature. To date, there have been no studies demonstrating that NSAID use in the acute phases of bone healing result in higher rates of nonunion.

Bone healing involves a complex cascade of events with the end-goal being the formation of bridging vascularized woven bone capable of functional remodeling over time [23]. Studies have indicated that prostaglandins, which are important in the regulation of osteoclastic bone resorption and osteoblastic bone formation, required for bone healing, are released at the time of fracture via cyclooxygenase enzyme activity (COX-2) [8]. As COX inhibitors, NSAIDs can arrest the cell cycle and increase cytotoxicity and apoptosis of osteoblasts, leading to ineffective mineralization of newly formed extracellular bone matrix [24]. In studies of skeletally mature animals [25–28], non-selective NSAIDs were shown to delay long bone healing without any detrimental effects on long-term outcomes. Whereas selective NSAIDs were associated with detrimental long-term effects on material and structural properties of healing bone. Research that focused on dose and time effects suggested avoiding NSAID treatment during the initial weeks of fracture healing, in order to avoid these negative effects on fracture callus [7]. However, the physiology of the skeletally immature system is distinct from the skeletally mature. Some contributors to this unique physiology, which may make skeletally immature patients less prone to pseudoarthrosis, include thicker periosteum, greater subperiosteal hematoma, active physes, and enhanced metabolic activity. Capello et al. explored the effects of NSAID administration during the acute phase of fracture healing in skeletally immature animals, and found no significant difference in strength, stiffness, or histologic characteristics of fracture callus. These finds support the view that the bone healing physiology of the skeletally immature is not perturbed by NSAID administration at physiologic doses [29].

A large inceptive cohort study by Zura et al. demonstrated the combination of NSAIDs and opioids (multivariate odds ratio (OR), 1.84; 95% CI, 1.73–1.95) is a risk factor for nonunion. However, this study found no significant association of NSAIDs alone with nonunion (multivariate OR, 0.98, 95% CI, 0.89–1.07, $p = 06$), but found opioids alone to be a moderately strong positive risk factor for nonunion (multivariate OR, 1.43, 95% CI, 1.34–1.52, $p \leq 0.001$) [6]. Zura et al. expanded on this original study to isolate pediatric patient risk factors for nonunion and found similar results, further supporting the finding that NSAIDs are not significant contributors to fracture nonunion, but NSAIDs combined with opioids, lead to significant risks [8].

This analysis is limited by the number of studies available, as well as heterogeneity of the bone healing types included in the reviewed studies, including fractures treated operatively compared with those treated by closed means, osteotomies, as well as spinal fusions. As with all reviews, this review is an analysis of the best available published data. Certainly, future studies on the potential multicenter participation and non-inferiority designs, examining each of these bone healing types, are warranted. More robust data are needed to assess the impact of NSAID use on bone healing in the skeletally immature population.

5. Conclusions

Clinical data investigating the effects of NSAIDS on bone healing in the pediatric population is sparse. The retrospective studies of pediatric patients who used NSAID following posterior spinal fusion did not demonstrate inhibition of bone healing [13,15]. Two studies by Kay et al. found no cases of nonunion in pediatric patients who received ketorolac around the time of operative fixation of common pediatric fractures or lower extremity osteotomy [16,17]. DePeter et al. similarly found no healing complications arose for the pediatric population exposed to ibuprofen during fracture healing. The two prospective studies by Nuelle et al. [20] and Drendel et al. [19] support the use of ibuprofen for long bone fractures in the acute healing period for adequate pain control without compromising bone healing. In conclusion, based on the current available evidence, NSAID use in the acute phase of bone healing in skeletally immature patients is not associated with a higher rate of pseudoarthrosis.

Funding: This research received no external funding.

Institutional Review Board Statement: Ethical review and approval were waived for this study, due to this study being a literature review.

Informed Consent Statement: Patient consent was waived due to this study being a literature review.

Acknowledgments: The authors would like to thank Adelina Colbert for her assistance with the review and submission of this manuscript.

Conflicts of Interest: J.A.V.N. receives research support from the Henry M. Jackson Foundation. She serves on the Editorial Board for Arthroscopy: The Journal of Arthroscopic and Related Surgery. These entities had no role in the design of the study; in the collection, analyses, or interpretation of data; in the writing of the manuscript, or in the decision to publish the results.

References

1. Ong, C.K.S.; Lirk, P.; Tan, C.H.; Seymour, R.A. An evidence-based update on nonsteroidal anti-inflammatory drugs. *Clin. Med. Res.* **2007**, *5*, 19–34. [CrossRef] [PubMed]
2. CDC. Identifying Increases in Opioid Overdoses [Internet]. Centers for Disease Control and Prevention, 2018. Available online: https://www.cdc.gov/vitalsigns/opioid-overdoses/index.html (accessed on 1 July 2021).
3. Alam, A.; Gomes, T.; Zheng, H.; Mamdani, M.M.; Juurlink, D.N.; Bell, C.M. Long-term analgesic use after low-risk surgery: A retrospective cohort study. *Arch. Intern. Med.* **2012**, *172*, 425–430. [CrossRef]
4. Prescription Opioid Data | Drug Overdose | CDC Injury Center [Internet]. 2021. Available online: https://www.cdc.gov/drugoverdose/deaths/prescription/index.html (accessed on 1 July 2021).
5. Kanakaris, N.K.; Giannoudis, P.V. The health economics of the treatment of long-bone non-unions. *Injury* **2007**, *38* (Suppl. S2), S77–S84. [CrossRef]
6. Zura, R.; Xiong, Z.; Einhorn, T.; Watson, J.T.; Ostrum, R.F.; Prayson, M.J.; Della Rocca, G.; Samir, M.; McKinley, T.; Wang, Z.; et al. Epidemiology of Fracture Nonunion in 18 Human Bones. *JAMA Surg.* **2016**, *151*, e162775. [CrossRef] [PubMed]
7. Gaston, M.S.; Simpson, A.H.R.W. Inhibition of fracture healing. *J. Bone Joint. Surg. Br.* **2007**, *89*, 1553–1560. [CrossRef]
8. Zura, R.; Kaste, S.C.; Heffernan, M.J.; Accousti, W.K.; Gargiulo, D.; Wang, Z.; Steen, R.G. Risk factors for nonunion of bone fracture in pediatric patients: An inception cohort study of 237,033 fractures. *Medicine* **2018**, *97*, e11691. [CrossRef]
9. Cottrell, J.; O'Connor, J.P. Effect of Non-Steroidal Anti-Inflammatory Drugs on Bone Healing. *Pharmaceuticals* **2010**, *3*, 1668–1693. [CrossRef] [PubMed]
10. Giannoudis, P.V.; MacDonald, D.A.; Matthews, S.J.; Smith, R.M.; Furlong, A.J.; De Boer, P. Nonunion of the femoral diaphysis. The influence of reaming and non-steroidal anti-inflammatory drugs. *J. Bone Joint Surg Br.* **2000**, *82*, 655–658. [CrossRef]
11. Aliuskevicius, M.; Østgaard, S.E.; Rasmussen, S. No influence of ibuprofen on bone healing after Colles' fracture—A randomized controlled clinical trial. *Injury* **2019**, *50*, 1309–1317. [CrossRef]
12. Blomquist, J.; Solheim, E.; Liavaag, S.; Baste, V.; Havelin, L.I. Do nonsteroidal anti-inflammatory drugs affect the outcome of arthroscopic Bankart repair? *Scand J. Med. Sci. Sports* **2014**, *24*, e510–e514. [CrossRef]
13. Sucato, D.J.; Lovejoy, J.F.; Agrawal, S.; Elerson, E.; Nelson, T.; McClung, A. Postoperative ketorolac does not predispose to pseudoarthrosis following posterior spinal fusion and instrumentation for adolescent idiopathic scoliosis. *Spine* **2008**, *33*, 1119–1124. [CrossRef] [PubMed]
14. Boskey, A.L.; Coleman, R. Aging and bone. *J. Dent. Res.* **2010**, *89*, 1333–1348. [CrossRef]
15. Vitale, M.G.; Choe, J.C.; Hwang, M.W.; Bauer, R.M.; Hyman, J.E.; Lee, F.Y.; Roye, D. Use of ketorolac tromethamine in children undergoing scoliosis surgery. An analysis of complications. *Spine J. Off. J. N. Am. Spine Soc.* **2003**, *3*, 55–62. [CrossRef]
16. Kay, R.M.; Directo, M.P.; Leathers, M.; Myung, K.; Skaggs, D.L. Complications of ketorolac use in children undergoing operative fracture care. *J. Pediatr. Orthop.* **2010**, *30*, 655–658. [CrossRef]
17. Kay, R.M.; Leathers, M.; Directo, M.P.; Myung, K.; Skaggs, D.L. Perioperative ketorolac use in children undergoing lower extremity osteotomies. *J. Pediatr. Orthop.* **2011**, *31*, 783–786. [CrossRef]
18. DePeter, K.C.; Blumberg, S.M.; Dienstag Becker, S.; Meltzer, J.A. Does the Use of Ibuprofen in Children with Extremity Fractures Increase their Risk for Bone Healing Complications? *J. Emerg. Med.* **2017**, *52*, 426–432. [CrossRef]
19. Drendel, A.L.; Gorelick, M.H.; Weisman, S.J.; Lyon, R.; Brousseau, D.C.; Kim, M.K. A randomized clinical trial of ibuprofen versus acetaminophen with codeine for acute pediatric arm fracture pain. *Ann. Emerg. Med.* **2009**, *54*, 553–560. [CrossRef] [PubMed]

20. Nuelle, J.A.V.; Coe, K.M.; Oliver, H.A.; Cook, J.L.; Hoernschemeyer, D.G.; Gupta, S.K. Effect of NSAID Use on Bone Healing in Pediatric Fractures: A Preliminary, Prospective, Randomized, Blinded Study. *J. Pediatr. Orthop.* **2020**, *40*, e683–e689. [CrossRef]
21. Carney, D.E.; Nicolette, L.A.; Ratner, M.H.; Minerd, A.; Baesl, T.J. Ketorolac reduces postoperative narcotic requirements. *J. Pediatr. Surg.* **2001**, *36*, 76–79. [CrossRef] [PubMed]
22. Glassman, S.D.; Rose, S.M.; Dimar, J.R.; Puno, R.M.; Campbell, M.J.; Johnson, J.R. The effect of postoperative nonsteroidal anti-inflammatory drug administration on spinal fusion. *Spine* **1998**, *23*, 834–838. [CrossRef] [PubMed]
23. Pountos, I.; Georgouli, T.; Calori, G.M.; Giannoudis, P.V. Do nonsteroidal anti-inflammatory drugs affect bone healing? A critical analysis. *Sci. World J.* **2012**, *2012*, 606404. [CrossRef] [PubMed]
24. Chang, J.-K.; Wang, G.-J.; Tsai, S.-T.; Ho, M.-L. Nonsteroidal anti-inflammatory drug effects on osteoblastic cell cycle, cytotoxicity, and cell death. *Connect. Tissue Res.* **2005**, *46*, 200–210. [CrossRef] [PubMed]
25. Aspenberg, P. Drugs and fracture repair. *Acta Orthop.* **2005**, *76*, 741–748. [CrossRef] [PubMed]
26. Simon, A.M.; Manigrasso, M.B.; O'Connor, J.P. Cyclo-oxygenase 2 function is essential for bone fracture healing. *J. Bone Miner Res. Off. J. Am. Soc. Bone Miner Res.* **2002**, *17*, 963–976. [CrossRef] [PubMed]
27. Gerstenfeld, L.C.; Thiede, M.; Seibert, K.; Mielke, C.; Phippard, D.; Svagr, B.; Cullinane, D.; Einhorn, T. Differential inhibition of fracture healing by non-selective and cyclooxygenase-2 selective non-steroidal anti-inflammatory drugs. *J. Orthop. Res. Off. Publ. Orthop. Res. Soc.* **2003**, *21*, 670–675. [CrossRef]
28. Murnaghan, M.; Li, G.; Marsh, D.R. Nonsteroidal anti-inflammatory drug-induced fracture nonunion: An inhibition of angiogenesis? *J. Bone Joint. Surg. Am.* **2006**, *88* (Suppl. S3), 140–147. [CrossRef]
29. Cappello, T.; Nuelle, J.A.V.; Katsantonis, N.; Nauer, R.K.; Lauing, K.L.; Jagodzinski, J.E.; Callaci, J.J. Ketorolac Administration Does Not Delay Early Fracture Healing in a Juvenile Rat Model. *J. Pediatric Orthop.* **2013**, *33*, 415. [CrossRef]

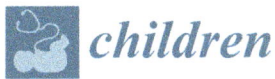

Systematic Review

The Orthopedic Effects of Electronic Cigarettes: A Systematic Review and Pediatric Case Series

Maxwell Luke Armstrong [1,*], Nicholas Smith [1], Rhiannon Tracey [2] and Heather Jackman [1]

[1] Division of Orthopedic Surgery, Janeway Children's Health and Rehabilitation Centre, Memorial University of Newfoundland, St. John's, NL A1B 3V6, Canada; nicksmith@munmed.ca (N.S.); hrjackman@gmail.com (H.J.)
[2] Division of Orthopedic Surgery, Schulich School of Medicine and Dentistry, Western University, London, ON N6A 5A5, Canada; rmt224@mun.ca
* Correspondence: mlarmstrong@mun.ca

Abstract: Electronic cigarette (EC) use is highly prevalent, especially in the adolescent population, where 29% of Canadian adolescents have used an EC in the past thirty days per national surveys. Our pediatric orthopedic referral centre observed a cluster of delayed unions of bone fractures in adolescents using ECs and present the case series here. We then asked whether electronic cigarettes impair bone healing or influence orthopedic outcomes. A PRISMA-compliant systematic review was carried out, which revealed no human clinical studies and a general paucity of evidence around ECs and musculoskeletal health. The existing experimental evidence relevant to orthopedics is summarized. The effect of ECs on the musculoskeletal system is poorly understood and is a target for further research.

Keywords: e-cigarette; vaping; adolescent health; pediatric orthopedics

Citation: Armstrong, M.L.; Smith, N.; Tracey, R.; Jackman, H. The Orthopedic Effects of Electronic Cigarettes: A Systematic Review and Pediatric Case Series. *Children* **2022**, *9*, 62. https://doi.org/10.3390/children9010062

Academic Editor: Christiaan J. A. van Bergen

Received: 9 December 2021
Accepted: 28 December 2021
Published: 4 January 2022

Publisher's Note: MDPI stays neutral with regard to jurisdictional claims in published maps and institutional affiliations.

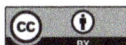

Copyright: © 2022 by the authors. Licensee MDPI, Basel, Switzerland. This article is an open access article distributed under the terms and conditions of the Creative Commons Attribution (CC BY) license (https://creativecommons.org/licenses/by/4.0/).

1. Hypothesis-Generating Cases

1.1. Ankle Fracture While Roughhousing, Eighteen Weeks in a 15-Year-Old Male

A fifteen-year-old male with no known medical history sustained a closed, minimally displaced, simple oblique trans-syndesmotic lateral malleolus fracture with no widening of the mortise. There was a remote history of occasional cigarette smoking and the patient was a current user of electronic cigarettes (EC). The fracture was reduced and splinted in a peripheral Emergency Room and referred to our centre for definitive management.

Initial treatment was circumferential casting and non-weight bearing. At one-week post-injury X-rays confirmed near-anatomic alignment. At four weeks post-injury radiographs were equivocal for callus, the patient's exam was reassuring, and a removable cast-boot was placed with progressive weight bearing. At eight weeks post-injury, there was pain at the fracture site and inability to bear full weight. The patient was counselled to discontinue EC use. Cast-boot immobilization with weight bearing as tolerated was continued. There was no clinical or radiographic change at twelve weeks post-injury (Figure 1). Delayed union was diagnosed in the absence of healing beyond the expected four to six weeks required to heal this injury [1]. At eighteen weeks post-injury the fracture was no longer symptomatic, and radiographs confirmed bony union.

1.2. Monteggia Fracture-Dislocation on a Motorcycle, Fifteen Weeks in a 14-Year-Old Male

A fourteen-year-old male presented with a closed, neurovascularly intact, displaced, and moderately comminuted diaphyseal ulnar fracture with associated posterolateral dislocation of the radial head, also known as a Monteggia fracture-dislocation. The injury occurred after ejection from an off-road motorcycle at moderate speed. There was an associated unstable C5/6 cervical spine fracture-dislocation and disc rupture with no neurological symptoms. There was no known medical history. The forearm fracture-dislocation was reduced and splinted in the trauma bay by pediatric orthopedics with near-anatomic alignment. Neurosurgery colleagues managed the spine injury with emergent anterior discectomy and fusion without complication from which he recovered well with no neurologic sequelae. There was no history of cigarette smoking, but the patient was a current user of e-cigarettes.

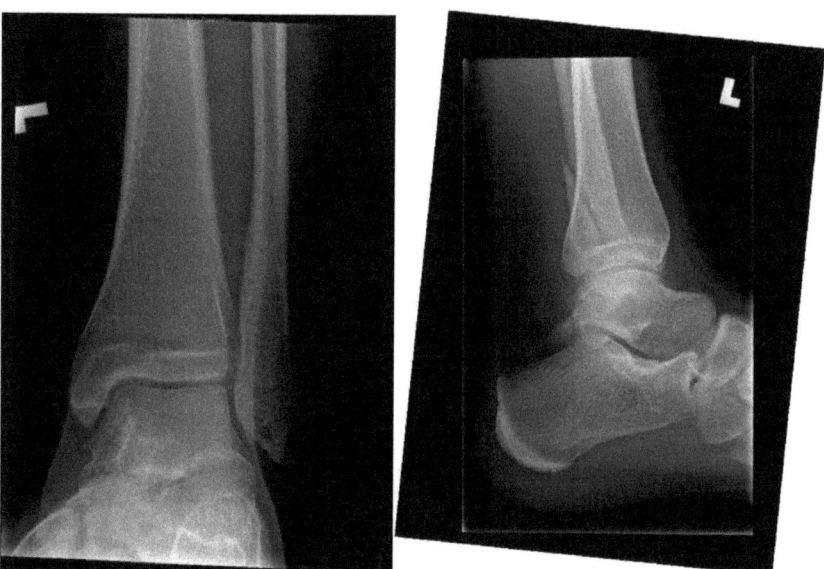

Figure 1. Twelve-week ankle radiographs demonstrating no radiographic union after fibula fracture in a pediatric electronic cigarette user.

At one-week post-injury radiographs demonstrated good alignment of the fracture and radio-capitellar joint. A long-arm circumferential cast was placed. At three weeks post-injury radiographs again demonstrated acceptable alignment and casting was continued. At seven weeks post-injury, there was no radiographic evidence of healing, and a removable cast was prescribed with instructions for twice daily non-weightbearing range of motion exercises. The patient was counselled to discontinue EC use. At eleven weeks post-injury there was continued pain at the fracture site with no radiographic evidence of healing (Figure 2). Delayed union was diagnosed as the expected healing time of a closed pediatric forearm fracture is approximately 5.5 weeks [1]. Fifteen weeks post-injury the patient had symptomatic improvement with resolution of fracture-site tenderness and radiographs showed evidence of bony union.

1.3. Forearm Fracture on a Trampoline, Eighteen Weeks in a 15-Year-Old Male

A fifteen-year-old male sustained closed, neurovascularly intact, displaced fractures of the radial and ulnar diaphyses with comminution of the radius. The mechanism of injury was a fall on an outstretched hand on a trampoline. The patient had no systemic comorbidity and no history of smoking but was a current user of electronic cigarettes. The fracture was splinted in a peripheral Emergency Room and was referred to our centre. The following day, the fractures were definitively treated without complication by open reduction internal fixation (ORIF) with plates and screws. The simple ulnar fracture was plated in compression mode, and the mildly comminuted radial fracture was approximated and plated in bridge mode.

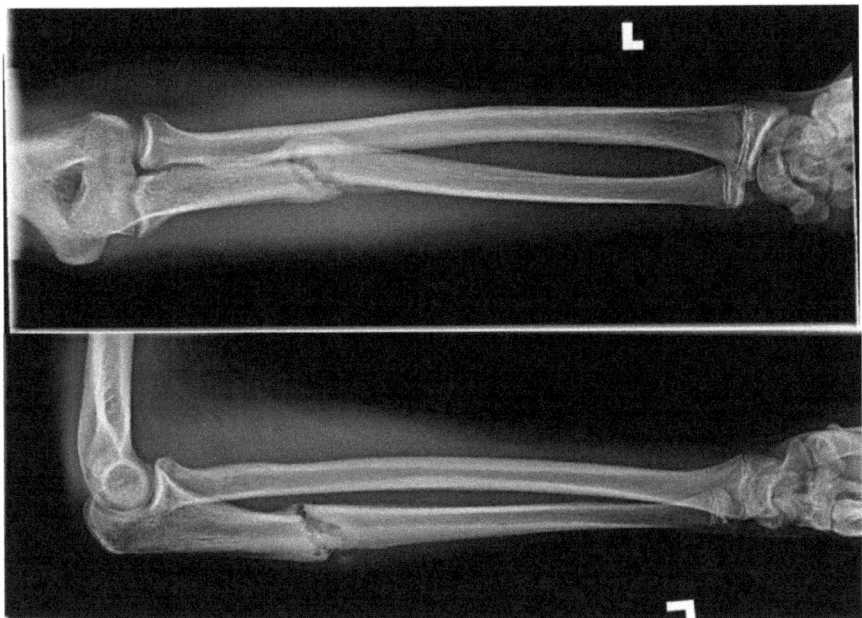

Figure 2. Eleven-week forearm radiographs demonstrating no union after Monteggia fracture-dislocation in a pediatric EC user.

Five weeks after operative treatment splint immobilization was discontinued, and a functional brace was applied. Eight weeks after ORIF, radiographs demonstrated bony union of the ulna but no union of the radius fracture despite anatomic alignment. The patient was counselled to discontinue EC use. Again, at twelve weeks, there was no union of the radius fracture and the patient had ongoing symptoms (Figure 3). Delayed union was diagnosed. Eighteen weeks after ORIF the patient had clinically improved, radiographs demonstrated bony union, and treatment was discontinued.

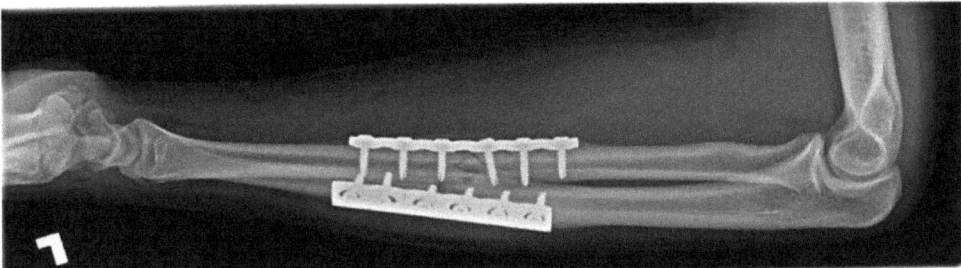

Figure 3. Twelve-week radiograph of an operatively treated both-bones forearm fracture in a pediatric electronic cigarette user. The ulna is healed, but the radius is not.

2. Background and Rationale for Review

Impaired bone healing is rare in the pediatric population. A large Scottish study found 422 fracture non-unions in 161,100 fractures diagnosed in patients aged 0–18 over five years, for an overall incidence of 0.2–0.35% per fracture [2]. Risk factors for impaired bone healing in pediatric patients include specific fracture characteristics, local bone biology, systemic host health, increasing age, and orthopedic treatment tactics. Complications of impaired bone healing may include pain, deformity, reduced mobility, and unplanned surgery [1].

During a review of the fractures treated at our pediatric orthopedic referral centre, the above cases were noted as a cluster of difficult-to-heal fractures. Retrospectively, we observed the common exposure of e-cigarette use. During the ten months in 2018–2019 when these cases were managed, 330 fractures in patients aged 12 to 18 were treated at our centre. Three of these 330 fractures had delayed union, which are the three presented above. This led us to pose the question: Do electronic cigarettes affect bone healing?

These cases are presented without any inference of an association between ECs and bone healing and serve only as a hypothesis generator. The impaired bone healing in our three cases may be attributable to a variety of factors. For example, in Case 1, patient adherence to removable cast-boot immobilization of the fibula fracture is unknown. In Case 2, a higher energy mechanism, the biology of the ulnar diaphysis, and nonoperative treatment tactics may have contributed to impaired healing. An iatrogenic fracture gap created by a bridging plate and screw fixation of a comminuted radial shaft fracture in Case 3 could be a treatment-related non-union risk factor.

Electronic cigarettes (ECs) are pocket-sized devices that combine heat and the user's inhalation to vaporize a solution to produce a cloud of vapor that mimics the experience of conventional cigarette smoking, often called 'vaping'. The solutions are proprietary but are usually composed of water, propylene glycol, and glycerine, as well as additives of flavorings and nicotine in varying concentrations [3]. A proposed danger of ECs is the ability to achieve high nicotine doses by selecting a solution with high nicotine content and vaping more frequently [3]. The long-term health effects of these products are unknown, as are the actual chemicals delivered to the bloodstream in vivo after passing the solution over a superheated coil. The characterization of the 'E-cigarette or vaping product use-associated lung injury' (EVALI) has been a recent area of intense research focus and media scrutiny [4,5]. Significant attention has also duly been given to the diagnosis and treatment of facial blast injuries from exploding devices [6].

The popularity of ECs amongst Canadian adolescents is alarming [4]. The Canadian Student Tobacco, Alcohol, and Drugs Survey (CSTADS) 2018–2019 demonstrated that 29% of students in high school were current users and had vaped in the past 30 days, a rapid increase from prior years. Daily or occasional cigarette smoking had a 3% prevalence, which was stable [7].

Complicating the issue is the marketing of ECs, which usually suggests that they are a healthier, 'cleaner' alternative to cigarettes. This appeals to consumers who perceive a healthier option with a similar experience to smoking. ECs are marketed to adults as a smoking cessation option. A range of vapour flavours and modern device styling with USB charging have likely contributed to the concerning prevalence of use in the pediatric population [7].

It is tempting to equate the health effects of conventional cigarettes and ECs as they both deliver nicotine via inhalation and the user experience is similar. However, they are chemically dissimilar products except for nicotine. While the negative effect of tobacco smoking on bone healing is unequivocal, the contribution to this effect from the chemical nicotine specifically is still under investigation [8,9].

This study asked whether electronic cigarettes had a deleterious effect on bone healing and, more broadly, on orthopedic outcomes. We conducted a PRISMA-compliant systematic review and present the results below.

3. Systematic Review

3.1. Eligibility Criteria

All publications with potential relevance to the operative or non-operative practice of orthopedics in English or French were examined (no results were found in other languages). For completeness, human, animal, and experimental studies were considered from all levels of evidence.

3.2. Search Strategy and Sources

In March 2021, the PubMed, EMBASE, and Cochrane databases were searched for relevant publications. Each of these databases were interrogated with the basic input, ((e-cigarette) OR (vaping)) AND ((orthopedics) OR (surgery)). The extended search terms from PubMed are displayed in Table 1 as an example and no limits or filters were used. To search the grey literature, the OpenGrey database (www.opengrey.eu, accessed on 22 March 2021) was searched with the same terms. This strategy yielded 608 papers for consideration after removal of duplicates.

Table 1. Detailed searching strategy.

Search: ((e-cigarette) OR (vaping)) AND ((orthopedics) OR (surgery))
("electronic nicotine delivery systems"[MeSH Terms] OR ("electronic"[All Fields] AND "nicotine"[All Fields] AND "delivery"[All Fields] AND "systems"[All Fields]) OR "electronic nicotine delivery systems"[All Fields] OR "e cigarette"[All Fields] OR ("vaped"[All Fields] OR "vaping"[MeSH Terms] OR "vaping"[All Fields] OR "vapes"[All Fields])) AND ("orthopaedic"[All Fields] OR "orthopedics"[MeSH Terms] OR "orthopedics"[All Fields] OR "orthopedic"[All Fields] OR "orthopaedical"[All Fields] OR "orthopedical"[All Fields] OR "orthopaedics"[All Fields] OR ("surgery"[MeSH Subheading] OR "surgery"[All Fields] OR "surgical procedures, operative"[MeSH Terms] OR ("surgical"[All Fields] AND "procedures"[All Fields] AND "operative"[All Fields]) OR "operative surgical procedures"[All Fields] OR "general surgery"[MeSH Terms] OR ("general"[All Fields] AND "surgery"[All Fields]) OR "general surgery"[All Fields] OR "surgery s"[All Fields] OR "surgerys"[All Fields] OR "surgeries"[All Fields]))

3.3. Study Selection and Data Colletion Process

Upon initial review of the results, it was obvious that our primary question of the effects of e-cigarettes on bone healing would not be answered by the current literature. There were no human studies of bone healing in EC users. We pursued our broader goal of collecting any literature pertaining to the effect of e-cigarettes on orthopedic outcomes. The corresponding author (M.L.A.) sorted and screened the initial 608 records for potential relevance to orthopedics based on the title and abstract. Records with titles indicating relevance exclusively to a non-orthopedic topic (i.e., smoking cessation, economics, sociology) were excluded. All potentially relevant abstracts were reviewed and excluded if there was no pertinence to the musculoskeletal system and ECs or EC vapour.

Thirty-five potentially relevant records were then retrieved for manuscript assessment. No automation tools were used. The title, abstract, and manuscript were read and assessed for pertinence to orthopedics. Further exclusions were made on the basis of no relevance to orthopedics ($n = 11$), no relevance to electronic cigarettes ($n = 1$), and for a focus only on smoking cessation ($n = 2$). Publications were grouped for their topic/purpose and quality of evidence. The systematic review workflow is summarized in Figure 4.

This review protocol was submitted for registration on the International Prospective Register of Systematic Reviews (PROSPERO identification number: 299563).

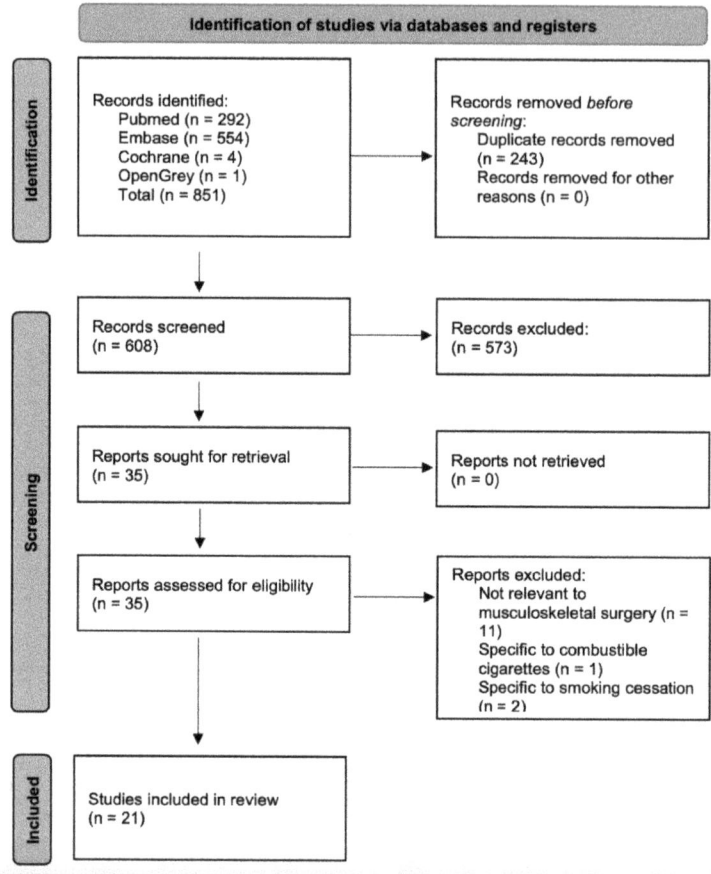

Figure 4. Systematic review flowchart.

4. Results

No Level 1 studies were found. No human clinical studies were found. Only six studies were found that were experimental, which are summarized in Table 2. In summarizing these studies, they clustered around three subtopics—basic science, musculoskeletal health, and wound healing. Data extraction was not applicable as no relevant human clinical studies on e-cigarettes were found.

Most publications were non-systematic reviews, briefs, and opinion letters. These are not discussed here but are cited in the references list per Table 2.

Table 2. Summary table of included publications.

Level 1: Meta-analyses and randomized controlled trials		
	Nil	
Level 2: Unrandomized trials, cohort studies, scientific experiments		
Basic science	Pywell et al. [10]	Nonclinical human experiment
	Romagna et al. [11]	Cell line experiment

Table 2. Cont.

MSK health	Kennedy et al. [12]	Animal experiment
	Reumann et al. [13]	Animal experiment
Dermal healing	Rau et al. [14]	Animal experiment
	Troiano et al. [15]	Animal experiment
Level 3: Expert opinion, briefs, reports		
Non-systematic review, orthopedic	Publications [16–18]	
Non-systematic review, surgery, and wounds	Publications [19–22]	
Briefs and opinion	Publications [23–30]	

5. Discussion

Our systematic review highlights the paucity of evidence about the effect of ECs on orthopedic surgery and the musculoskeletal system in general. The papers that were found pertained to basic science, musculoskeletal health, and wound healing.

Pywell et al. published a human experiment on 15 subjects that demonstrated a reduction in hand microcirculation after inhaling a 24 mg nicotine e-cigarette but not after a 0 mg e-cigarette. They concluded the consumption of nicotine causes vasoconstriction [10]. Romagna et al. exposed fibroblast cell cultures to liquified solutions of EC vapor and combustible cigarette smoke and found the liquified smoke to be significantly more cytotoxic [11].

Kennedy et al. undertook an animal experiment with rats exposed to two cigarettes daily or the nicotine equivalent of electronic cigarette vapour for four weeks. The rats had Achilles tendon transection and repair performed and then the tensile strength of the repair was measured two weeks later. The EC cohort had a significantly lower load-to-failure versus the cigarette and control cohorts, which were not significantly different [12]. Reumann et al. exposed mice to EC vapour or the nicotine equivalent of cigarette smoke daily for six months and then quantified bone strength parameters. In this study, the cigarette smoke significantly decreased bone density and bending strength compared to EC vapour and the control group, which were not significantly different [13].

In 2019, Rau et al. raised and then repaired skin flaps on a rat model exposed to low-dose EC vapour, high-dose EC vapour, or combustible cigarettes for four weeks. Five weeks after surgery flap survival was significantly decreased in the exposure groups versus the control group, but not within the three exposure groups [14]. This rat experiment was essentially repeated by Troiano et al., who also found no significant difference in flap necrosis between EC vapour- or cigarette-exposed rats but did find a significant increase in necrosis in these exposed groups versus the control [15].

Other groups have published non-systematic reviews and expert briefs of the topic, including Amaro et al. in *JBJS Reviews* in 2019. They compared and contrasted ECs with combustible cigarettes and overviewed the orthopedic issues [17]. Fiani et al. similarly overviewed the topic with a focus on the spine and molecular toxicology [18]. Nicholson et al. recently published an expert brief on the musculoskeletal biochemistry of vaping in *Bone and Joint Research* [16].

This systematic review is the most current collection of knowledge about the orthopedic effects of electronic cigarettes. This review is severely limited in its ability to draw any clinically relevant conclusions about the orthopedic effects of electronic cigarettes based on the current body of evidence. A further limitation is that a single researcher reviewed the searched publications for suitability, which may introduce bias in judgement or clerical error.

Vaping is highly prevalent, especially amongst adolescents, and its orthopedic effects are poorly understood. We presented three cases as a clinical observation that served as a hypothesis generator. We conducted a PRISMA-compliant systematic review that revealed a scarcity of evidence about vaping and musculoskeletal health. This paper serves as a starting point and a call for high-quality investigation into the orthopedic effects of electronic cigarettes.

Author Contributions: Conceptualization, H.J. and N.S.; methodology, M.L.A. and R.T.; investigation, M.L.A.; resources, H.J.; data curation, M.L.A.; writing—original draft preparation, M.L.A. and R.T.; writing—review and editing, M.L.A., N.S. and H.J.; supervision, H.J.; project administration, M.L.A. All authors have read and agreed to the published version of the manuscript.

Funding: This research received no external funding.

Institutional Review Board Statement: The study was conducted according to the guidelines of the Declaration of Helsinki and approved by the Health Research Ethics Board of Memorial University of Newfoundland (HREB # 2019.191).

Informed Consent Statement: Informed consent was obtained from all subjects involved in the study.

Data Availability Statement: No new data were created or analyzed in this study. Data sharing is not applicable to this article.

Conflicts of Interest: The authors declare no conflict of interest.

References

1. Waters, P.M.; Skaggs, D.L.; Flynn, J.M. (Eds.) *Rockwood & Wilkins' Fractures in Children*, 9th ed.; Lippincott Williams & Wilkins: Philadelphia, PA, USA, 2019.
2. Mills, L.A.; Simpson, A.H. The risk of non-union per fracture in children. *J. Child. Orthop.* **2013**, *7*, 317–322. [CrossRef] [PubMed]
3. Breland, A.B.; Spindle, T.; Weaver, M.; Eissenberg, T. Science and Electronic Cigarettes. *J. Addict. Med.* **2014**, *8*, 223–233. [CrossRef] [PubMed]
4. Perikleous, E.P.; Steiropoulos, P.; Paraskakis, E.; Constantinidis, T.C.; Nena, E. E-Cigarette Use Among Adolescents: An Overview of the Literature and Future Perspectives. *Front. Public Health* **2018**, *6*, 86. [CrossRef]
5. Bold, K.W.; Kong, G.; Camenga, D.R.; Simon, P.; Cavallo, D.A.; Morean, M.E.; Krishnan-Sarin, S. Trajectories of E-Cigarette and Conventional Cigarette Use Among Youth. *Pediatrics* **2017**, *141*, e20171832. [CrossRef] [PubMed]
6. Serror, K.; Chaouat, M.; Legrand, M.M.; Depret, F.; Haddad, J.; Malca, N.; Mimoun, M.; Boccara, D. Burns caused by electronic vaping devices (e-cigarettes): A new classification proposal based on mechanisms. *Burns* **2018**, *44*, 544–548. [CrossRef]
7. Government of Canada. *Summary of Results for the Canadian Student Tobacco, Alcohol and Drugs Survey 2016–17*; Statistics Canada: Ottawa, ON, Canada, 2018.
8. Scolaro, J.A.; Schenker, M.L.; Yannascoli, S.M.; Baldwin, K.; Mehta, S.; Ahn, J. Cigarette Smoking Increases Complications Following Fracture. *J. Bone Jt. Surg.* **2014**, *96*, 674–681. [CrossRef]
9. Argintar, E.; Triantafillou, K.; Delahay, J.; Wiesel, B. The Musculoskeletal Effects of Perioperative Smoking. *J. Am. Acad. Orthop. Surg.* **2012**, *20*, 359–363. [CrossRef]
10. Pywell, M.J.; Wordsworth, M.; Kwasnicki, R.M.; Chadha, P.; Hettiaratchy, S.; Halsey, T. The Effect of Electronic Cigarettes on Hand Microcirculation. *J. Hand Surg.* **2018**, *43*, 432–438. [CrossRef]
11. Romagna, G.; Allifranchini, E.; Bocchietto, E.; Todeschi, S.; Esposito, M.; Farsalinos, K. Cytotoxicity evaluation of electronic cigarette vapor extract on cultured mammalian fibroblasts (ClearStream-LIFE): Comparison with tobacco cigarette smoke extract. *Inhal. Toxicol.* **2013**, *25*, 354–361. [CrossRef]
12. Kennedy, P.; Saloky, K.; Yadavalli, A.; Barlow, E.; Aynardi, M.; Garner, M.; Bible, J.; Lewis, G.; Dhawan, A. Comparison of Achilles Tendon Healing After Exposure to Combusted Tobacco, Vaping, and Control in a Rat Model. *Orthop. J. Sports Med.* **2019**, *7*, 2325967119S00328. [CrossRef]
13. Reumann, M.K.; Schaefer, J.; Titz, B.; Aspera-Werz, R.H.; Wong, E.T.; Szostak, J.; Häussling, V.; Ehnert, S.; Leroy, P.; Tan, W.T.; et al. E-vapor aerosols do not compromise bone integrity relative to cigarette smoke after 6-month inhalation in an ApoE−/− mouse model. *Arch. Toxicol.* **2020**, *94*, 2163–2177. [CrossRef]
14. Rau, A.S.; Reinikovaite, V.; Schmidt, E.; Taraseviciene-Stewart, L.; Deleyiannis, F.W.-B. Electronic Cigarettes Are as Toxic to Skin Flap Survival as Tobacco Cigarettes. *Ann. Plast. Surg.* **2017**, *79*, 86–91. [CrossRef]
15. Troiano, C.; Jaleel, Z.; Spiegel, J.H. Association of Electronic Cigarette Vaping and Cigarette Smoking With Decreased Random Flap Viability in Rats. *JAMA Facial Plast. Surg.* **2019**, *21*, 5–10. [CrossRef]
16. Nicholson, T.; Scott, A.; Ede, M.N.; Jones, S.W. Do E-cigarettes and vaping have a lower risk of osteoporosis, nonunion, and infection than tobacco smoking? *Bone Jt. Res.* **2021**, *10*, 188–191. [CrossRef] [PubMed]
17. Amaro, E.J.; Shepard, N.; Moss, L.; Karamitopoulos, M.; Lajam, C. Vaping and Orthopaedic Surgery: A Review of Current Knowledge. *JBJS Rev.* **2019**, *7*, e5. [CrossRef]
18. Fiani, B.; Noblett, C.; Nanney, J.M.; Gautam, N.; Pennington, E.; Doan, T.; Nikolaidis, D. The Impact of "Vaping" Electronic Cigarettes on Spine Health. *Cureus J. Med. Sci.* **2020**, *12*, e8907. [CrossRef]

19. Fracol, M.; Dorfman, R.; Janes, L.; Kulkarni, S.; Bethke, K.; Hansen, N.; Kim, J. The Surgical Impact of E-Cigarettes: A Case Report and Review of the Current Literature. *Arch. Plast. Surg.* **2017**, *44*, 477–481. [CrossRef] [PubMed]
20. Lemay, F.; Baker, P.; McRobbie, H. Electronic cigarettes: A narrative review of the implications for the pediatric anesthesiologist. *Pediatr. Anesthesia* **2020**, *30*, 653–659. [CrossRef] [PubMed]
21. Cope, G. E-cigarettes and wound healing. *Wounds UK* **2020**, *16*, 653–659.
22. Taub, P.J.; Matarasso, A. E-Cigarettes and Potential Implications for Plastic Surgery. *Plast. Reconstr. Surg.* **2016**, *138*, 1059e–1066e. [CrossRef]
23. Farsalinos, K.; Voudris, V. It is preferable for surgical patients to use e-cigarettes rather than smoke cigarettes. *BMJ* **2014**, *348*, g1961. [CrossRef]
24. Agochukwu, N.; Liau, J.Y. Debunking the myth of e-cigarettes: A case of free flap compromise due to e-cigarette use within the first 24 hours. *J. Plast. Reconstr. Ae. Surg.* **2018**, *71*, 451–453. [CrossRef]
25. Davies, C.S.; Ismail, A. Nicotine has deleterious effects on wound healing through increased vasoconstriction. *BMJ* **2016**, *353*, i2709. [CrossRef]
26. Debusk, W.T.; Debusk, W.; Lassig, A.A.D. Implications of electronic cigarettes on postoperative wound healing. *Otolaryngol. Head Neck Surg.* **2020**, *163*, P46–P47. [CrossRef]
27. Desai, S.C. Is e-Cigarette Vaping a New Clinical Challenge to Wound Healing? *JAMA Facial Plast. Surg.* **2019**, *21*, 10–11. [CrossRef] [PubMed]
28. Holmes, W.J.M.; Southern, S.J. Detrimental effects of e-cigarettes on surgical outcomes. *BMJ* **2014**, *348*, g1156. [CrossRef] [PubMed]
29. Jeevaratnam, J.; Vijayan, R.; Blackburn, A. Hidden risks of electronic cigarettes to patients undergoing plastic surgery. *Eur. J. Plast. Surg.* **2014**, *37*, 457–458. [CrossRef]
30. Patients Should Stop e-Cigarette Use Before Plastic Surgery. *J. Calif. Dent. Assoc.* **2017**, *45*, 69. [PubMed]

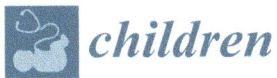

Perspective

Fractures in Osteogenesis Imperfecta: Pathogenesis, Treatment, Rehabilitation and Prevention

Wouter Nijhuis [1,*], Marjolein Verhoef [2], Christiaan van Bergen [3], Harrie Weinans [1,4] and Ralph Sakkers [1]

1. Department of Orthopedic Surgery, University Medical Center Utrecht, 3508 GA Utrecht, The Netherlands; h.h.weinans@umcutrecht.nl (H.W.); r.sakkers@umcutrecht.nl (R.S.)
2. Department of Rehabilitation, Physical Therapy Science & Sports, Brain Center Rudolf Magnus, University Medical Centre Utrecht, 3508 GA Utrecht, The Netherlands; m.verhoef-10@umcutrecht.nl
3. Department of Orthopedic Surgery, Amphia Hospital, 4818 CK Breda, The Netherlands; cvanbergen@amphia.nl
4. Department of Biomechanical Engineering, Delft University of Technology, 2600 AA Delft, The Netherlands
* Correspondence: w.h.nijhuis-2@umcutrecht.nl

Abstract: Fractures in patients with osteogenesis imperfecta (OI) are caused by a decreased strength of bone due to a decreased quality and quantity of bone matrix and architecture. Mutations in the collagen type 1 encoding genes cause the altered formation of collagen type I, one of the principal building blocks of bone tissue. Due to the complexity of the disease and the high variation of the clinical problems between patients, treatment for these patients should be individually tailored. In general, short immobilization periods with flexible casting material, use of intramedullary implants, and simultaneous deformity correction are preferred. Multidisciplinary care with a broad view of the support needed for the patient and his/her living environment is necessary for the optimal rehabilitation of these patients. Increasing bone strength with exercise, medication, and sometimes alignment surgery is generally indicated to prevent fractures.

Keywords: osteogenesis imperfecta; fracture; brittle bone disease; surgery; rehabilitation; collagen

1. Introduction

Fractures are the main characteristic in patients with osteogenesis imperfecta (OI), also called "brittle bone disease". OI is a genetic disorder with a disturbance of the production and structure of collagen type I, one of the main components of bone tissue. This rare bone disease has an incidence of 1 in 15,000–20,000 births [1]. The patients are generally clinically classified from type 1 to 5 [2], in which type 1 has the mildest symptoms and type 3 represents the most severe type compatible with life. Type 4 has a severity between type 1 and 3, and type 2 is defined as perinatal lethal. Type 5 has distinctive radial head luxation's and ossification of the interosseous membrane. In addition to the Sillence classification, several rare types have now been described in the literature [3]. Eighty-five percent of the OI population has an autosomal dominant inheritance (types 1–5,15), of which the types 1–4 have a primary collagen type 1 defect. The remainder of 15% has an autosomal recessive inheritance, and the mutations in these patients affect the metabolic pathway of bone formation in different ways. A classification based on the metabolic pathway has been proposed by Forlino et al. in 2017 [3]. The list of OI types has been increasing; these additional types are clinically more or less similar to OI type 3 in terms of severity. Clinical manifestations vary widely between the different types of OI, ranging from patients who have mild symptoms with few fractures and a normal life expectancy, to patients with frequent fractures and severe bony deformities together with severe physical impairments and reduced life expectancy [4–6].

2. Collagen and Bone Tissue Formation

Bone tissue, or matrix, is made from collagen molecules and inorganic hydroxyapatite (HA) minerals. The structure of bone matrix can be compared with reinforced concrete, where the inorganic (HA) minerals are the cement, and the collagen molecules are the steel reinforcement. Biomechanically, the inorganic HA crystals give bone matrix its stiffness, and the reinforcement with collagen type 1 fibers creates the mechanical flexibility and related toughness. Bone tensile strength and resistance to both traction and shearing forces is mainly determined by the collagen network, making up around 30% of the bone matrix [7,8].

Collagen is made intracellularly and is a protein with a triple helix structure of peptide chains that are closely packed in a characteristic quarter-staggers array to form a fibril. A collagen fiber is made from multiple fibrils in the same way as multiple small iron threads together form a steel cable see Figures 1 and 2 for more details on both normal collagen formation and collagen formation in OI [9].

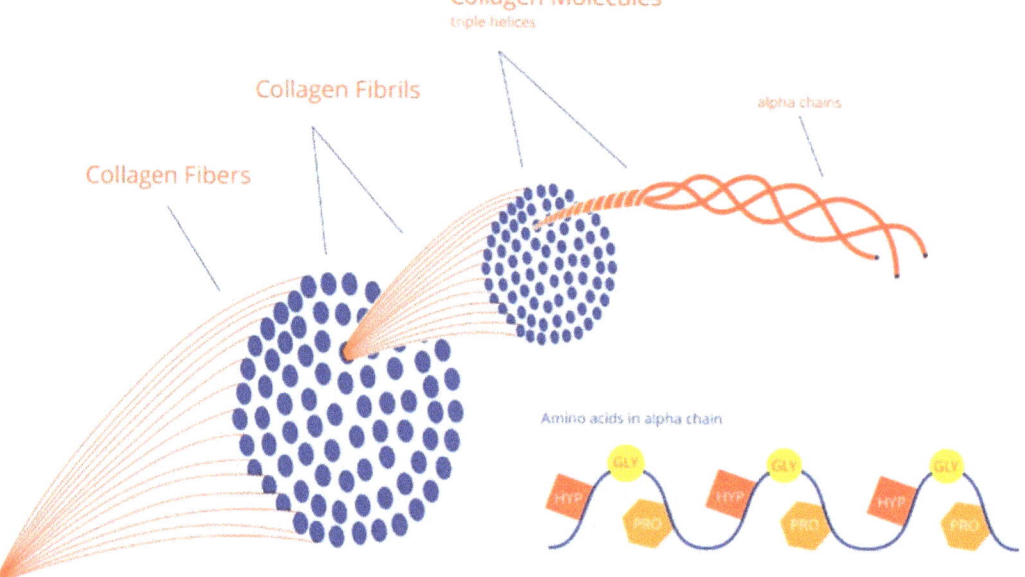

Figure 1. Multiple collagen fibrils form fibers. Reproduced with permission of Journal of Children's Orthopedics [9].

After the extrusion of collagen by the cell into the extracellular matrix, inorganic HA is deposited as crystals in and between the fibrils and fibers, resulting in increased stiffening to finally become mineralized bone matrix (see Figure 2).

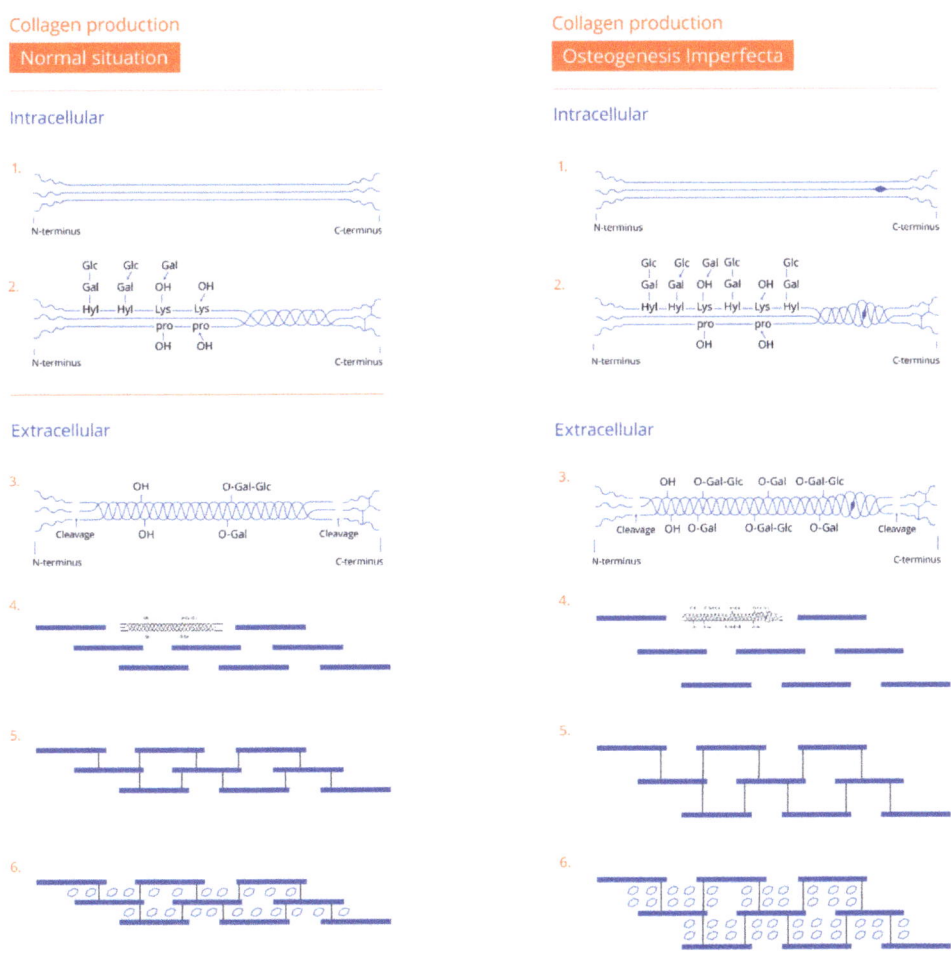

Figure 2. On the left side, a schematic view shows the formation of collagen, both intracellular and extracellular. On the right side, a similar formation is depicted, but with a mutation in one of the alpha chains, as is seen in osteogenesis imperfecta (OI). Step 1: formation of three alpha chains by ribosomes (note the bigger amino acid in one of the chains in OI). Step 2: hydroxylation and glycosylation and the triple helix formation (note the slower folding in OI with increased hydroxylation and glycosylation: Glucose (Glc), Galactose (Gal), Lysine (Lys), Hydroxylysine (Hyl), Proline (Pro)). Step 3: extracellular cleavage of the C- and N-terminus. Step 4: quarter-staggered arrays (note the increased space between the molecules in OI). Step 5: the formation of cross-links, which is unaffected in OI. Step 6: mineralization between the collagen molecules with an increased number of mineral crystals of the same size in OI. Reproduced with permission of Journal of Children's Orthopaedics [9].

3. Bone Strength and Elasticity in OI

The OI bone matrix has a lower capacity for energy absorption due to a lower strength and elasticity (Figure 3). The weaker bone matrix is susceptible to micro-damage, which causes increased activity of both osteoclasts and osteoblasts to repair these micro-damages. Increased osteoblast activity subsequently increases the osteocyte density, and thus leaves an increased porosity of bone due to osteocyte lacunae. Most likely, this increased activity at the cell level also causes an increased vascularity in the bone, which in turn adds on the increase in porosity. An increased pore percentage in OI bone has been reported at both the level of osteocyte lacunae and vascularity [10]. Next to the lower biomechanical properties of the bone matrix itself, a small rise in bone pore percentage might lead to significantly increased crack propagation through bone, in particular with repetitive loading and the accumulation of micro-damaged sites. For example, a bone pore percentage increase from 4% to 20% results in a three-fold decrease in the deformation abilities of bone before fracture [11], and thus much less energy uptake that refers to the bones brittleness (Figure 3).

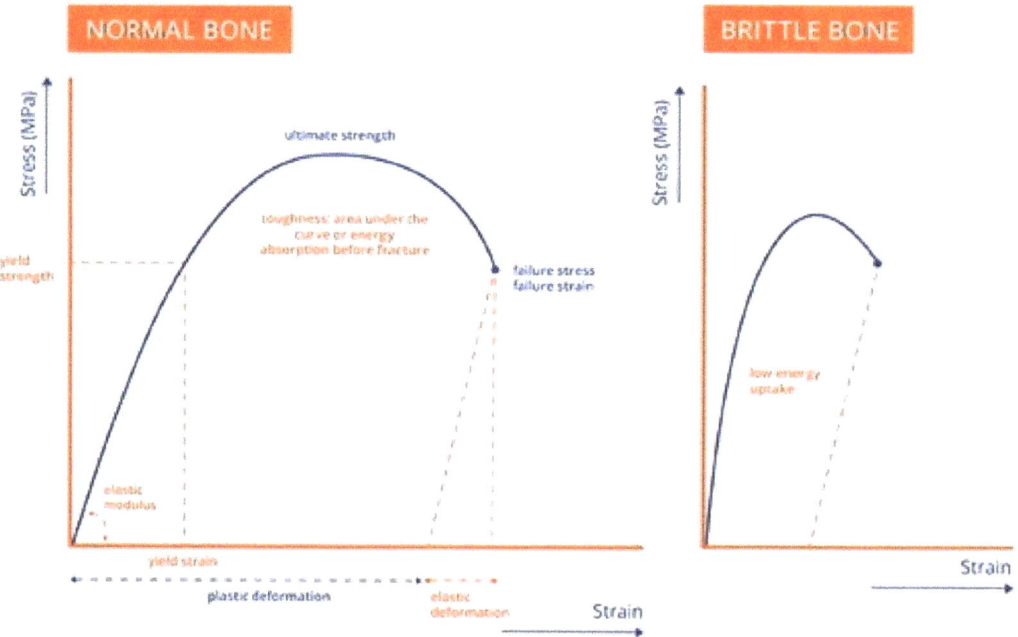

Figure 3. Brittle bone. Hypothetical stress-strain curve of bone with some of the most essential mechanical properties. For cortical bone, the deformations at yield are up to 1%, whereas for cancellous bone this can reach 5% to 10%, or even higher. Bone can absorb a substantial amount of energy and can be considered a relatively tough material (see area under the curve). Osteogenesis imperfecta bone is considered brittle, which means that it cannot absorb much energy (small area under the curve, right side). In fact, brittleness represents a combination of low strength, little plastic deformation, and lower toughness. Reproduced with permission of Journal of Children's Orthopaedics [9].

Bone strength is also decreased at the level of bone micro and macro architecture. The refinement of bone imaging technologies in recent years has especially improved the assessment of bone architecture. Measures of bone micro-architecture, bone geometry, and (volumetric) bone mass density (vBMD) can be obtained by high-resolution peripheral quantitative computed tomography (HR-pQCT) [12]. A significantly decreased cortical thickness was found in tibiae of type 1 OI patients using HR-pQCT but normal to increased cortical thickness in OI types 3 and 4 [13]. Both histomorphometric and HR-pQCT evaluation of cancellous iliac bone biopsies in patients with OI showed fewer and thinner trabeculae [13–15] The Trabecular Bone Score (TBS) as measured with HR-pQCT is related to trabecular connectivity and trabecular spacing, and low TBS in peripheral bone has a strong association with individual fracture risk [16]. In OI patients type 3 and type 4, lower TBS values were found compared to normal bone [13]. All these pathologic changes at the different architectural levels also add to the susceptibility of fractures in patients with OI.

4. Fracture Management

Fracture management in OI patients need a very tailor-made approaches, but general principles apply to all OI patients. When OI patients suffer from a fracture, emergency treatment should preferably be provided at the nearest possible institution. While some fractures do not require any treatment, some fractures need immobilization with plaster of Paris (POP), and some fractures need surgery with reinforcing intramedullary implants. Patients and family education on OI can be very beneficial in pain management, transportation, and logistics in these emergencies. Some clinics teach patients and/or parents to apply a temporary plaster or splint themselves in order to cope with the first pain before adequate professional healthcare is available. When POP is utilized, we prefer the use of flexible material over a rigid cast. Since the bone in OI is brittle, the end of a rigid cast might create a stress riser, which increases the risk of additional fractures during treatment with a cast. This risk could be minimized with more flexible cast materials.

The average time to consolidation in OI patients is lower than in controls, due to a higher bone turnover in OI bone (higher vascularity and higher cellularity). Hence, a relatively short period of immobilization is often sufficient. When surgical treatment is indicated, the authors feel that pre-existing deformity of the bone should be repaired where possible to minimize the risk of re-fracture. The simultaneous correction of deformities on the contralateral side and adjacent bone should also be considered in order to minimize frequency of surgeries and periods of immobilization for all OI patients.

5. Prevention of Fractures

5.1. Medication

As for all children, maintaining adequate vitamin D (vit D) concentrations is one of the basic pre-requisites for normal bone mineralization and bone mass [17]. Children with OI seem to be at risk for vit D deficiency, especially those with more severe OI and/or a high body mass index [18]. Therefore, children with OI should have their vit D status monitored and be supplied with a dietary vitamin D supplement to ensure optimal levels [9]. Bisphosphonate (BP) treatment is now widely employed in OI patients to improve bone mass. BP decreases bone resorption by osteoclasts, shifting the balance of bone resorption and bone formation towards more OI bone formation [19]. Based on bone mineral density (BMD) and fracture rate, BP treatment might be started early. A low BMD is not the only factor causing lower bone strength in OI. The porosity, architecture, and connectivity within bone structure, as well as the quality of collagen fibers and the collagen to mineral ratio, play important roles in decreased bone strength. BP treatment can decrease pore percentage and increase BMD, but cannot change all factors involved in the decreased bone strength in OI.

Although the impact is not completely understood yet, BPs affect osteoblast and osteocyte activity directly. The main effect of BPs in the treatment of OI lies in the modulation of osteoclast activity, altering the structure and the architecture of bone [9]. A decrease in bone turn-over is usually not a problem in children. Children with OI have a higher bone turn-over compared to children without OI. Since adults have a decrease in bone turn-over with increasing age, bisphosphonates should be used with caution in adult OI patients. Indications are stricter, and lower frequencies of BP admission is advised [20] in order to keep turnover at a minimum level, which is a prerequisite to prevent the accumulation of micro-damage and related so-called 'spontaneous' fractures [21].

Increased BMD is usually most prominent in the first year of treatment. The effect of BP is patient specific and should be monitored yearly with fracture frequency and BMD. Since BP therapy only modulates osteoclast activity, some researchers focus on new medication strategies, a phase 1 study on mesenchymal stem cell treatment [22] in which they try to create a mosaic DNA is ongoing. A phase 2a clinical trial with antisclerostin [23] together EMA and FDA approval opens the path to a phase 3 pediatric study with antisclerostin in OI. Antisclerostin increases osteoblast activity rather than decreasing osteoclast activity, as

BP do. Results from this research might change the outcomes for patients with OI in the near future.

5.2. Physical Activity

Good motor skills and physical activity are important for proper bone development and the prevention of fractures in all people. During exercise, the effect of loading has positive influences on both the quantity and quality of bone [24]. In OI, collagen type 1 affects not only the bone, but also the soft tissues in the musculoskeletal system. Increased laxity, quantified by using the Beighton score, is often found in these patients. Furthermore, muscle weakness is present more often. Muscle weakness might be directly related to the altered collagen type 1 formation [25]. Keeping the patient physically active with tailor-made activity training programs is mandatory.

5.3. Preventive Surgery

Alignment surgery with intramedullary rodding to increase bone strength should be considered to decrease the fracture risk in children with moderate to severe OI. Teamwork and clear communication with the patient and family, surgeon, and multidisciplinary team are essential for a shared decision-making process. Pre-operatively, baseline function, range of motion, muscle strength and length, pain, and quality of life should be measured, preferably using standardized and validated outcome measures [26], and re-assessed after fracture treatment. Elongating implants or constructs for stable longitudinal growth are usually preferred in growing children. The inserted intramedullary rods are left in the bones as long as possible to prevent re-fractures. However, the re-operation rate due to rod migration and telescoping failure is very high, and re-revision rates of 30% within 5 years of follow-up have been reported with the current elongating devices [27]. Fixed-length devices can be used as an alternative when bone size is small, for children with limited residual growth or when lengthening devices are not available [28]. Plates and screws as stand-alone implants should be avoided to prevent stress fractures at the edges of the plates (see Figure 4) in all OI patients.

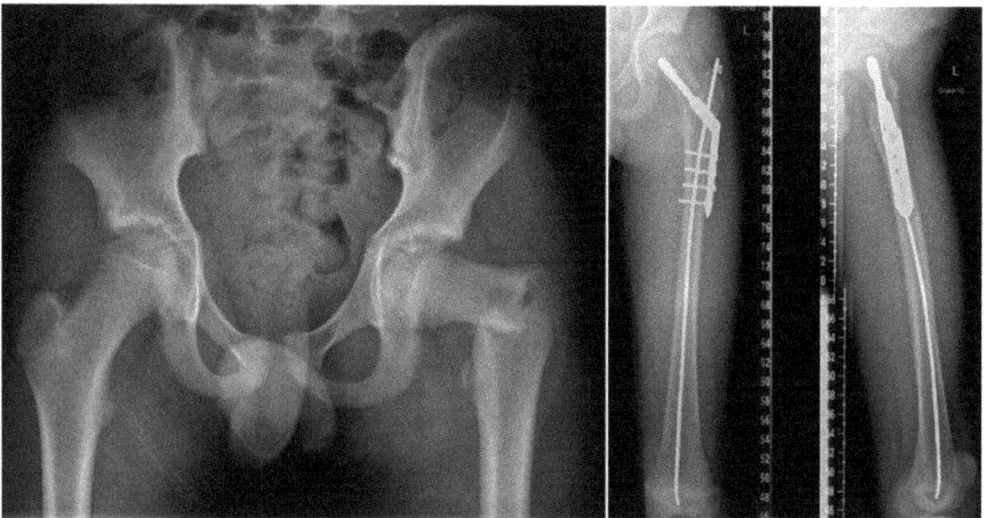

Figure 4. Adolescent patient with OI type 4 and a proximal femur fracture, treated with a dynamic hip screw and long intramedullary nail to reduce stress rising at the end of the plate. Using a monocortical distal screw would have further reduced stress rising. Note the stopper on the nail instead of a proximal bend end to prevent migration of the rod into the intramedullary canal.

Postoperative immobilization is provided with a flexible backslab or plaster cast, followed by initiation of mobilization as soon as healing permits [28].

General considerations and recommendations about surgical treatment in both fracture management and preventive surgery for both children and adults have recently been published after an international task force reached consensus in a standardized way [28].

Figures 4–6 show some illustrative cases with different surgical techniques and failures.

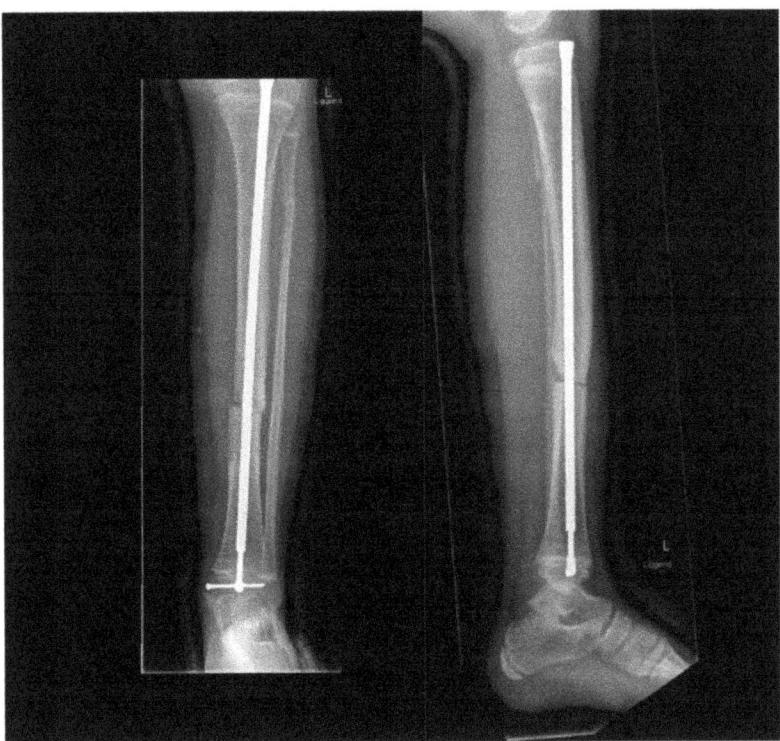

Figure 5. Eight-year-old OI type 1 patient with a delayed diagnosis presented with the fourth fracture of the tibia before OI was diagnosed. The fractures were treated conservatively and with a stand-alone plating. After removal of the last plate a third re-fracture of the tibia occurred within 1 week. To prevent any further re-fractures, a correction osteotomy at the site of the fracture was performed and stabilized with an elongating device. Note the improved distal fixation with a small screw (Peg).

5.4. Rehabilitation

After fracture management or elective surgery, patients need a personalized rehabilitation program. An early start of rehabilitation after surgery is strongly advised. The rehabilitation program should preferably be done in the patient's own environment. A multidisciplinary OI team should provide a rehabilitation program and stay connected to both patient and their local health care professionals during the rehabilitation. If the patient will wear a cast or have a partial on non-weightbearing regime, patients and their families need to learn safe methods for transfers and daily care before discharge from hospital. It is advisable to practice these transfers before surgery to become familiar with the available aids and prescribed methods. The rehabilitation program should focus on range of motion, muscle strength, and improvement of general functioning. Besides that, psychological support can be beneficial for some patients. Any rehabilitation progress should be evaluated in line with patient and family goals and surgeon's protocol.

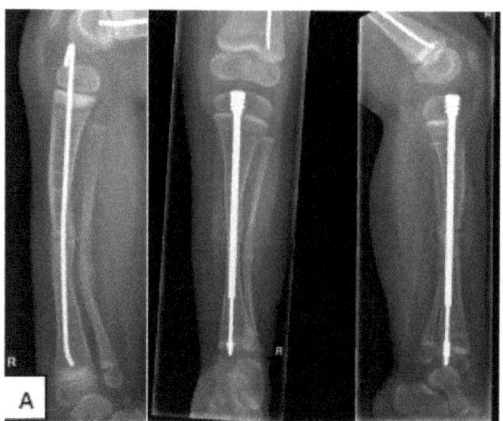 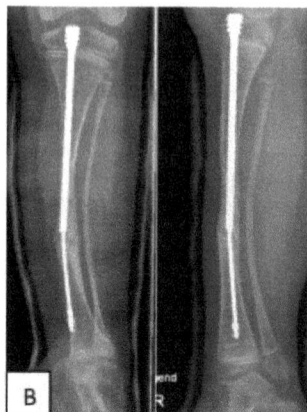

Figure 6. (A): Four-year-old OI type 3 patient after correction osteotomy of the tibia, stabilized with a flexible intramedullary nail, which was complicated with proximal nail migration causing knee pain. This complication was solved by replacing the nail with an intramedullary elongating device. **(B)**: Three years later, valgus deformation had occurred, distal fixation was lost, and the device bent, migrating out of the intramedullary canal distally.

In addition to rehabilitation care following the acute phase of fractures or surgery, continuous guidance from a rehabilitation team is important to support children with OI in optimal development and participation in society (e.g., mobility, personal care, school, and sports). The international classification of functioning, disability, and health (ICF) can be used as a framework to cover all important domains. Recently, an international interdisciplinary working group called Key4OI developed a set of global outcome measures for patients with OI using a consensus-driven modified Delphi approach. The Key4OI screening set is recommended for regular screening of daily functioning and quality of life [26].

6. Multidisciplinary Treatment Challenges

There is no cure for OI yet. Current treatment is based on increasing bone mass, prevention of fractures with alignment surgery, fracture management, and rehabilitation. The main treatment goal for children with OI is optimizing mobility, functional independency, and participation in society. The high variability in clinical severity of OI makes standard care recommendations less appropriate. Individually tailored care should therefore be the standard for OI patients. Children with OI as well as their parents often develop a fear of fractures. Health care professionals not used to treating OI patients have this fear as well. This may keep the patient from reaching their full potential in functioning. Therefore, caregivers should be educated how to handle a child with OI from birth [29]. Overprotection by both patients, their family members, and local healthcare providers may lead to a vicious cycle of fracture, immobilization, deconditioning, reduced skeletal strength and re-fracture. This needs to be addressed in a tailor-made rehabilitation program, including a psychological approach [30,31]. All treatment modalities should focus on optimal functioning of the child and family. A team with support of social workers and psychologists might be indicated.

7. Conclusions and Future Perspectives

Next to providing fracture management and prevention in patients with OI, multidisciplinary care should focus on functioning and psychosocial well-being. Despite all research and advances, the current management of fractures in OI remains a combination of surgery and medical treatment and requires a tailor-made approach from a multidisciplinary team of OI experts from different specialties.

Author Contributions: Conceptualization, W.N. and R.S.; original draft preparation, W.N.; writing—review and editing, M.V., C.v.B., H.W., R.S. All authors have read and agreed to the published version of the manuscript.

Funding: This research received no external funding.

Institutional Review Board Statement: Not applicable.

Informed Consent Statement: Not applicable.

Conflicts of Interest: The authors declare no conflict of interest.

References

1. Botor, M.; Fus-Kujawa, A.; Uroczynska, M. Osteogenesis Imperfecta: Current and Prospective Therapies. *Biomolecules* **2021**, *11*, 1493. [CrossRef] [PubMed]
2. Van Dijk, F.S.; Sillence, D.O. Osteogenesis imperfecta: Clinical diagnosis, nomenclature and severity assessment. *Am. J. Med. Genet. A* **2014**, *164A*, 1470–1481. [CrossRef]
3. Forlino, A.; Marini, J.C. Osteogenesis imperfecta. *Lancet* **2016**, *387*, 1657–1671. [CrossRef]
4. Kivirikko, K.I. Collagens and their abnormalities in a wide spectrum of diseases. *Annu. Med.* **1993**, *25*, 113–126. [CrossRef] [PubMed]
5. Byers, P.H.; Steiner, R.D. Osteogenesis imperfecta. *Annu. Rev. Med.* **1992**, *43*, 269–282. [CrossRef]
6. Prockop, D.J. Mutations that alter the primary structure of type I collagen. The perils of a system for generating large structures by the principle of nucleated growth. *J. Biol. Chem.* **1990**, *265*, 15349–15352. [CrossRef]
7. Gao, H.; Ji, B.; Jager, I.L.; Arzt, E.; Fratzl, P. Materials become insensitive to flaws at nanoscale: Lessons from nature. *Proc. Natl. Acad. Sci. USA* **2003**, *100*, 5597–5600. [CrossRef]
8. Jäger, I.; Fratzl, P. Mineralized collagen fibrils: A mechanical model with a staggered arrangement of mineral particles. *Biophys. J.* **2000**, *79*, 1737–1746. [CrossRef]
9. Nijhuis, W.H.; Eastwood, D.M.; Allgrove, J.; Hvid, I.; Weinans, H.H.; Bank, R.A.; Sakkers, R.J. Current concepts in osteogenesis imperfecta: Bone structure, biomechanics and medical management. *J. Child Orthop.* **2019**, *1*, 1–11. [CrossRef]
10. Jones, S.J.; Glorieux, F.H.; Travers, R.; Boyde, A. The microscopic structure of bone in normal children and patients with osteogenesis imperfecta: A survey using backscattered electron imaging. *Calcif. Tissue Int.* **1999**, *64*, 8–17. [CrossRef]
11. Yeni, Y.N.; Brown, C.U.; Wang, Z.; Norman, T.L. The influence of bone morphology on fracture toughness of the human femur and tibia. *Bone* **1997**, *21*, 453–459. [CrossRef]
12. Nishiyama, K.K.; Boyd, S.K. In vivo assessment of trabecular and cortical bone microstructure. *Clin. Calcium* **2011**, *21*, 1011–1019. [PubMed]
13. Kocijan, R.; Muschitz, C.; Haschka, J. Bone structure assessed by HR-pQCT, TBS and DXL in adult patients with different types of osteogenesis imperfecta. *Osteoporos. Int.* **2015**, *26*, 2431–2440. [CrossRef] [PubMed]
14. Shapiro, J.R.; McCarthy, E.F.; Rossiter, K. The effect of intravenous pamidronate on bone mineral density, bone histomorphometry, and parameters of bone turnover in adults with type IA osteogenesis imperfecta. *Calcif. Tissue Int.* **2003**, *72*, 103–112. [CrossRef] [PubMed]
15. Rauch, F.; Travers, R.; Plotkin, H.; Glorieux, F.H. The effects of intravenous pamidronate on the bone tissue of children and adolescents with osteogenesis imperfecta. *J. Clin. Investig.* **2002**, *110*, 1293–1299. [CrossRef] [PubMed]
16. Boutroy, S.; Hans, D.; Sornay-Rendu, E. Trabecular bone score improves fracture risk prediction in non-osteoporotic women: The OFELY study. *Osteoporos. Int.* **2013**, *24*, 77–85. [CrossRef] [PubMed]
17. Winzenberg, T.M.; Powell, S.; Shaw, K.; Jones, G. Vitamin D supplementation for improving bone mineral density in children. *Cochrane Database Syst. Rev.* **2010**, *10*, e23475. [CrossRef]
18. Wilsford, L.D.; Sullivan, E.; Mazur, L.J. Risk factors for vitamin D deficiency in children with osteogenesis imperfecta. *J. Pediatr. Orthop.* **2013**, *33*, 575–579. [CrossRef] [PubMed]
19. Sakkers, R.; Kok, D.; Engelbert, R.; van Dongen, A.; Jansen, M.; Pruijs, H.; Verbout, A.; Schweitzer, D.; Uiterwaal, C. Skeletal effects and functional outcome with olpadronate in children with osteogenesis imperfecta: A 2-year randomised placebo-controlled study. *Lancet* **2004**, *363*, 1427–1431. [CrossRef]
20. Scheres, L.J.J.; van Dijk, F.S.; Harsevoort, A.J.; van Dijk, A.T.H.; Dommisse, A.M.; Janus, G.J.M.; Franken, A.A.M. Adults with osteogenesis imperfecta: Clinical characteristics of 151 patients with a focus on bisphosphonate use and bone density measurements. *Bone Rep.* **2018**, *8*, 168–172. [CrossRef]
21. Chiang, C.Y.; Zebaze, R.M.; Ghasem-Zadeh, A.; Iuliano-Burns, S.; Hardidge, A.; Seeman, E. Teriparatide improves bone quality and healing of atypical femoral fractures associated with bisphosphonate therapy. *Bone* **2013**, *52*, 360–365. [CrossRef] [PubMed]
22. Götherström, C.; David, A.L.; Walther-Jallow, L.; Åström, E.; Westgren, M. Mesenchymal Stem Cell Therapy for Osteogenesis Imperfecta. *Clin. Obstet. Gynecol.* **2021**, *64*, 898–903. [CrossRef]
23. Glorieux, F.H.; Devogelaer, J.P.; Durigova, M. BPS804 anti-sclerostin antibody in adults with moderate osteogenesis imperfecta: Results of a randomized phase 2a trial. *J. Bone Miner. Res.* **2017**, *32*, 1496–1504. [CrossRef] [PubMed]
24. Brotto, M.; Bonewald, L. Bone and muscle: Interactions beyond mechanical. *Bone* **2015**, *80*, 109–114. [CrossRef] [PubMed]

25. Veilleux, L.N.; Rauch, F. Muscle-bone interactions in pediatric bone diseases. *Curr. Osteoporos. Rep.* **2017**, *15*, .425–432. [CrossRef]
26. Nijhuis, W.; Franken, A.; Ayers, K.; Damas, C.; Folkestad, L.; Forlino, A.; Fraschini, P.; Hill, C.; Janus, G.; Kruse, R.; et al. A standard set of outcome measures for the comprehensive assessment of osteogenesis imperfecta. *Orphanet. J. Rare Dis.* **2021**, *2021*, 16140. [CrossRef]
27. Azzam, K.A.; Rush, E.T.; Burke, B.R.; Nabower, A.M.; Esposito, P.W. Mid-term Results of Femoral and Tibial Osteotomies and Fassier-Duval Nailing in Children With Osteogenesis Imperfecta. *J. Pediatr. Orthop.* **2018**, *38*, 331–336. [CrossRef]
28. Sakkers, R.J.; Montpetit, K.; Tsimicalis, A.; Wirth, T.; Verhoef, M.; Hamdy, R.; Ouellet, J.A.; Castelein, R.M.; Damas, C.; Janus, G.J.; et al. A roadmap to surgery in osteogenesis imperfecta: Results of an international collaboration of patient organizations and interdisciplinary care teams. *Acta Orthop.* **2021**, *92*, 608–614. [CrossRef]
29. Mueller, B.; Engelbert, R.; Baratta-Ziska, F.; Bartels, B.; Blanc, N.; Brizola, E.; Fraschini, P.; Hill, C.; Marr, C.; Mills, L.; et al. Consensus statement on physical rehabilitation in children and adolescents with osteogenesis imperfecta. *Orphanet. J. Rare Dis.* **2018**, *13*, 158. [CrossRef]
30. Veilleux, L.N.; Pouliot-Laforte, A.; Lemay, M.; Cheung, M.S.; Glorieux, F.H.; Rauch, F. The functional muscle-bone unit in patients with osteogenesis imperfecta type I. *Bone* **2015**, *79*, 52–57. [CrossRef]
31. Tsimicalis, A.; Denis-Larocque, G.; Michalovic, A.; Lepage, C.; Williams, K.; Yao, T.R.; Palomo, T.; Dahan-Oliel, N.; Le May, S.; Rauch, F. The psychosocial experience of individuals living with osteogenesis imperfecta: A mixed-methods systematic review. *Qual. Life Res.* **2016**, *25*, 1877–1896. [CrossRef] [PubMed]

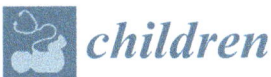

Article

Bone Fractures Numerical Analysis in a Femur Affected by Osteogenesis Imperfecta

Viridiana Ramírez-Vela [1], Luis Antonio Aguilar-Pérez [1], Juan Carlos Paredes-Rojas [2], Juan Alejandro Flores-Campos [3], Fernando ELi Ortiz-Hernández [4] and Christopher René Torres-SanMiguel [1,*]

[1] Instituto Politécnico Nacional, Escuela Superior de Ingeniería Mecánica y Eléctrica Unidad Zacatenco, Sección de Estudios de Posgrado e Investigación, Ciudad de Mexico 07738, Mexico; vramirezv0700@alumno.ipn.mx (V.R.-V.); laguilarp@ipn.mx (L.A.A.-P.)

[2] Instituto Politécnico Nacional, Centro Mexicano para la Producción más Limpia, Ciudad de Mexico 07340, Mexico; jparedes@ipn.mx

[3] Instituto Politécnico Nacional, Unidad Profesional Interdisciplinaria en Ingeniería y Tecnologías Avanzadas, Ciudad de Mexico 07340, Mexico; jaflores@ipn.mx

[4] Instituto Politécnico Nacional, Escuela Superior de Ingeniería Mecánica y Eléctrica, Unidad Culhuacán, Ciudad de Mexico 04260, Mexico; fortizh@ipn.mx

* Correspondence: ctorress@ipn.mx

Abstract: This work presents a non-invasive methodology to obtain a three-dimensional femur model of three-year-old infants affected with Osteogenesis Imperfecta (OI) type III. DICOM® Files of a femur were processed to obtain a finite element model to assess the transverse, the oblique, and the comminuted fractures. The model is evaluated under a normal walking cycle. The loads applied were considered the most critical force generated on the normal walking cycle, and the analyses considered anisotropic bone conditions. The outcome shows stress concentration areas in the central zone of the diaphysis of the femur, and the highest levels of stress occur in the case of the comminuted fracture, while the transverse fracture presents the lowest values. Thus, the method can be helpful for determining the bone fracture behavior of certain pathologies, such as osteogenesis imperfecta, osteopenia, and osteoporosis.

Keywords: biomechanics; bone fractures; osteogenesis imperfecta

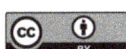

1. Introduction

The Osteogenesis Imperfecta (OI) covers a set of diseases mainly characterized by a heterogeneous connective tissue disorder correlated to collagen production. Its prevalence is estimated at 1 in 10,000–15,000 children [1]. People related to these disorders commonly present abnormal bone structures due to the increased rate of collagen production. Besides this effect, they exhibit folding and intracellular transport modifications and difficulties of incorporation in different degrees [2]. Therefore, children with OI have low bone density associated with incremental bone fragility [3].

The management of patients with OI is multidisciplinary. It requires different specialists, such as geneticists, pediatric endocrinologists, traumatologists, rehabilitators, physiotherapists, otorhinolaryngologists, neurosurgeons, psychologists, and even engineers. All the treatments currently used to counteract the effects of OI can be classified into three groups: non-surgical, surgical, and medical [4]. Within the surgical group, procedures are carried out to correct bone deformities, where the planned fracture of the bone is carried out to align it. According to medical management, a telescopic nail counteracts the incidence of fractures and supports the bone [5–8].

OI children's life is full of events that cause a fracture on their bones. The fracture usually happens with minimal or null trauma, but the injury could be equivalent to a fall from a height of one foot or less [9]. The OI affected exhibit fractures in the hip, clavicle, vertebrae, ribs, upper limbs, and lower limbs, the last of which being the area with the highest incidence of fracture, especially in long bones [10]. The femur fractures represent the third location of fractures in children [11]. The femur diaphysis fractures are frequent in males according to age, 11% affects children under two years of age, 21% between 3 and 5 years, 33% between 6 and 12 years, and 35% between 13 and 18 years [12,13]. The fracture may be incomplete, manifested by a transverse radiolucent line in the lateral cortex [14]. Some cases related to atypical femur fractures reported that the subtrochanteric area corresponds mainly to the spirals or longitudinal and transverse fractures [15].

The 3D modeling of bone tissue, in conjunction with the finite element method, has become a valuable tool in the orthopedic area since it helps to: determine the structural composition of the bone, predict the behavior of the bone subjected to various external agents, and design and optimize surgical implants [16–18]. Bone fractures can be simulated using tomography studies imported to software that computes the finite element method FEA, and they can differ from each other depending on the methodology used to carry out bone characterization and analysis [19]. The mineral density (BMD), in conjunction with finite element models, shows the possible fracture indifferent bone structures [20–22]. From another perspective, flexion and torsion tests were performed on critical areas subject to bone fracture OI [23–25]. Moreover, a numerical fracture report has been documented in 3D bone models, and various stress analyses on these models have been performed [26,27]. Additionally, other authors have performed numerical simulations to determine the behavior of the femur affected with OI considering particular case studies [28–33].

On the other hand, the OI patients are difficult to move in their normal environment, causing their parents to use temporary systems to transport them in vehicles safely. Unfortunately, these systems do not have a good design to protect children's integrity with OI efficiently. In order to evaluate prototypes of vehicle transporting devices, some researchers have tried to reproduce the biomechanical conditions of children with OI into dummies [34–36]. Implementing this kind of device necessarily needs the biomechanical properties of bones of patients with OI to increase the bio-fidelity of the dummies [37]. This eventually will be useful in the design and development of future endoprosthesis that allows for the rehabilitation of bone damage, improving the quality of children's lives with OI [38].

This work presents a 3D model of cortical and trabecular femur tissue affected by osteogenesis imperfecta disease type III. The femur was reproduced in a virtual environment using tomography images obtained from an OI patient of a three-year-old infant under the consented and informed agreement of their parents. Besides this, the biomechanical properties of the bone were determined by using Hounsfield units (HU) obtained directly from the tomographic images. Once the femur was modeled, the femur was evaluated in three ways corresponding to the most common types of fractures reported in the medical and scientific literature: transverse, oblique, and comminute. The payload and boundary conditions reproduced are computed by considering the weight of the patient. Finally, the incidences of fracture were compared through numerical analysis of the femur.

2. Materials and Methods

2.1. Methodology of 3D Modelling of an Infant's Femur with OI Type III

From a tomographic study (CT) of a three-year-old patient affected with type III OI, Digital Imaging and Communication On Medicine (DICOM®, National Electrical Manufacturers Association, Arlington, VA 22209, USA) files were obtained that provided 1569 axial slices, which were manipulated in a 3D Image Segmentation and Processing Software (Scan IP® program) to generate a virtual model femur. Initially, the area of the tomography was delimited to a section corresponding to the femur. Next, two layers were created to build the virtual model of the cortical and trabecular tissue that compose the femur. Subsequently, files with the *.stl extension were imported at the PowerShape®-e Student Edition program, which was used to create a mesh of surfaces that was part of a 3D solid model of the femur. Finally, files with the *.parasolid extension were generated, which can be identified by programs, such as Computer-aided design (CAD), that use the finite element method. Figure 1 shows the three-dimensional solid models corresponding to the cortical and trabecular tissue affected with OI.

Figure 1. Models of cortical and trabecular tissue of the femur of an infant with type III OI: (**a**) cortical tissue; (**b**) trabecular tissue.

2.2. Selection of the Minimum Unit of a 3D Image (Voxel)

In the ScanIP® program, several voxels were delimited in the tomography for both cortical and trabecular tissue that compose the bone structure of the femur. Figure 2 shows the delimitation of the minimum unit of a tomography (voxel), based on the bone model of an infant with OI.

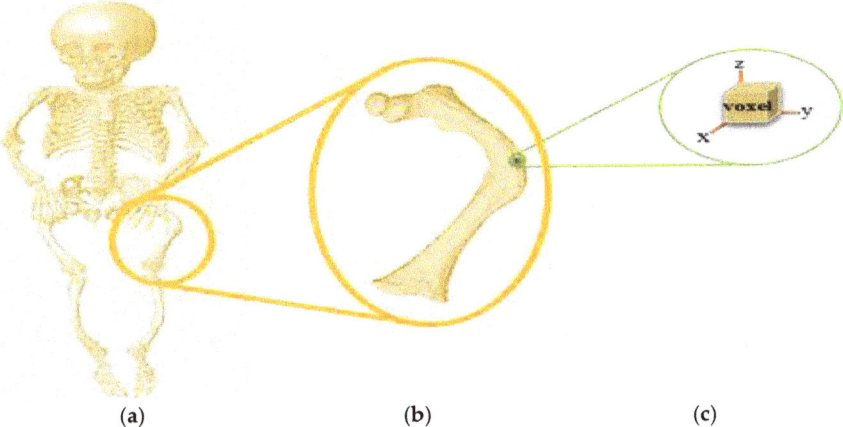

Figure 2. Determination of a voxel: (**a**) processing of all DICOM® files; (**b**) selection of the tomographic slices corresponding to the femur; (**c**) delimitation of the minimum unit of a tomography.

2.3. Hounsfield Unit (HU) Assessment and Apparent Density (ρ) Evaluations for OI Bone Type III

The Hounsfield scale has been universally adopted, assigning zero (0) to water and −1000 to air [39]. Hounsfield units and density have a linear correspondence, known as a function or calibration curve. The bone properties are modeled as a function of the apparent density, defined by mineralized mass divided by the total volume, including pores [40]. For this work, the calibration curve correction was performed using the methodology proposed by Taylor [41]. In this way, it is considered that the minimum apparent density of 0 g/cm^3 corresponds to the minimum density of the trabecular tissue, and the maximum apparent density of 2 g/cm^3 is associated with the maximum density of the cortical tissue. Fifty tomographic sections have been used to find the Hounsfield units along the femur bone, as shown in Figure 3, concentrating the highest values of HU in the central zone of the periphery of the femur diaphysis.

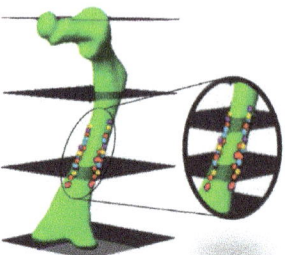

Figure 3. Obtaining HU values in different slices and areas.

Figure 4 shows the graph of HU values obtained randomly for the cortical and trabecular tissue in each of the analyzed sections. Thus, the minimum value of −96 HU was determined in the trabecular tissue, and the maximum value was 962 HU for the cortical tissue. Thus, the relationship between apparent density and HU was finally established by Equation (1).

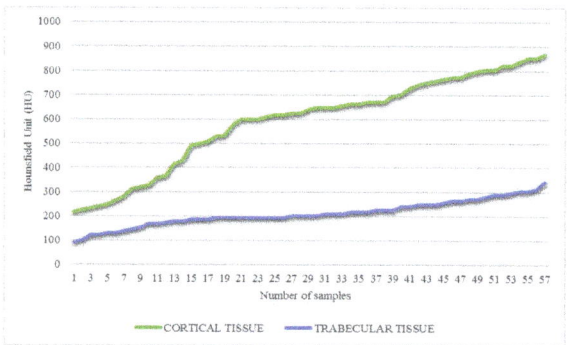

Figure 4. Values (HU) along the tomography of an affected femur with OI.

$$\rho_{ap} = \frac{2}{1058}\text{HU} + \frac{192}{1058}, \tag{1}$$

2.4. Apparent Density (ρ) Evaluations for OI Bone Type III

The bone elastic modulus is defined transversely or longitudinally, according to the direction in which a force is applied. According to Wirtz [42], the necessary equations are reported to obtain the bone elastic modulus (E) in transversal and longitudinal form by using the bone density for the cortical and trabecular tissue. Moreover, the equations that define the Poisson's coefficient (ρ) and the bone's shear modulus (G) are reported. The OI bone's biomechanical properties were computed using the apparent density values shown in Figure 3 and the Wirtz equations. Figure 5 shows the corresponding values to the relationship between the apparent density of the cortical tissue and Young's Modulus in the longitudinal and transverse direction of the femur. The relationship shown in Figure 6 concerns trabecular tissue.

The Poisson's ratio related to the bone tissue's apparent density affected by OI was also determined. Since this constant considers the relationship between linear and transverse deformation, the same coefficient is considered longitudinal and transverse. In the graphs of Figure 7, the values obtained for the cortical and trabecular tissue can be observed.

The shear modulus of the cortical and cancellous tissues in the longitudinal and transverse direction was determined by the apparent density, Young's modulus, and Poisson's ratio. Figures 8 and 9 show the values of the shear modulus for the apparent density.

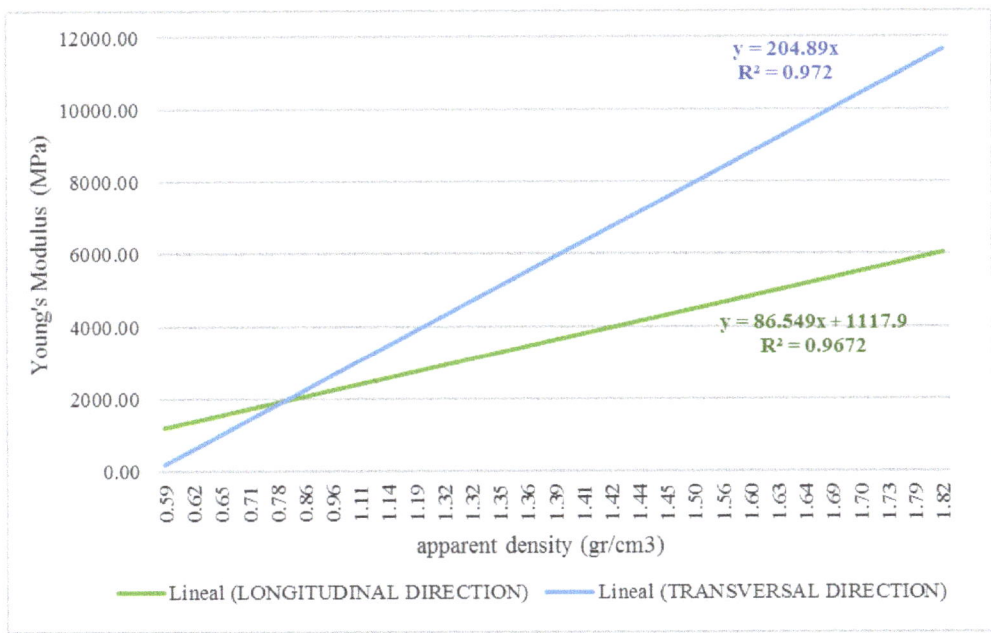

Figure 5. Relationship between apparent density and Young's modulus for cortical tissue affected with OI in the longitudinal and transversal direction.

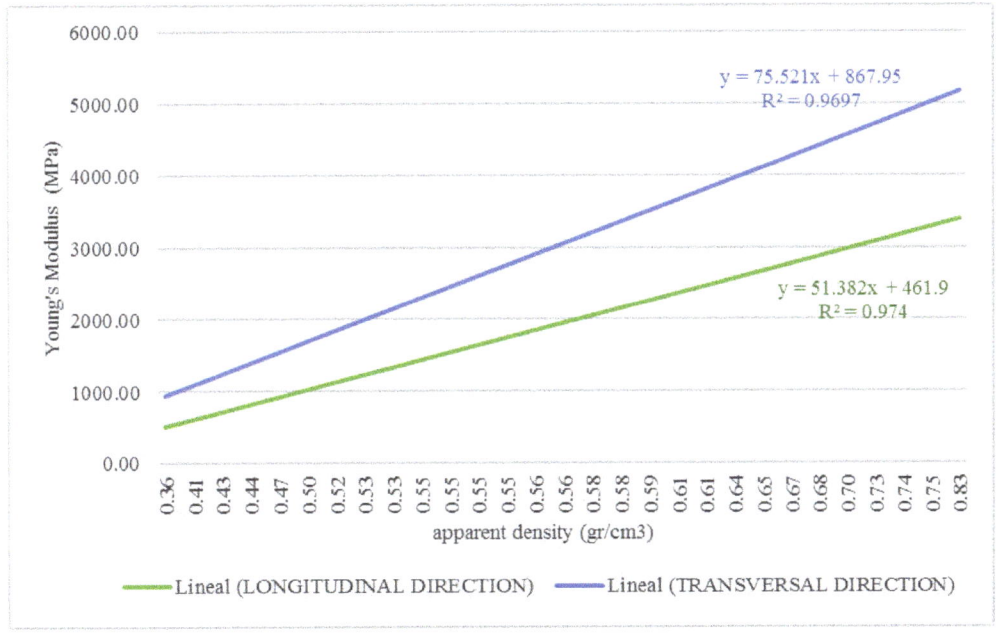

Figure 6. Relationship between apparent density and Young's modulus for trabecular tissue affected with OI in the longitudinal and transversal direction.

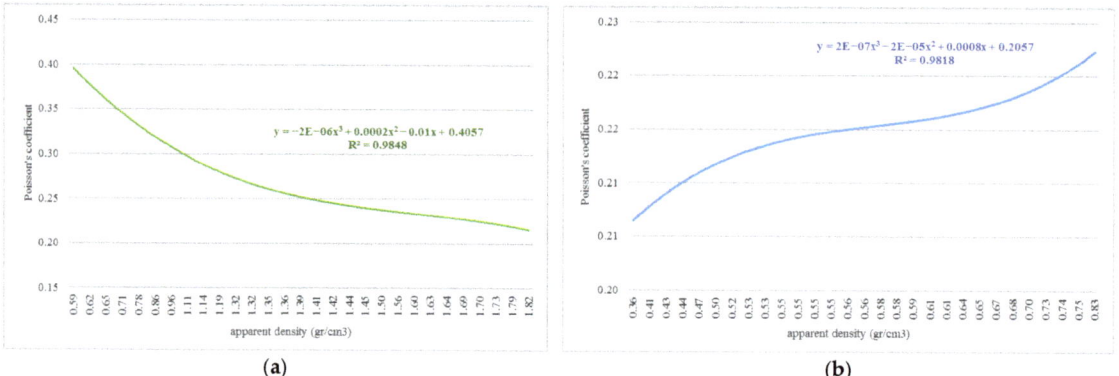

Figure 7. Relationship between apparent density and Poisson's coefficient for bone tissue affected with OI: (**a**) cortical tissue; (**b**) trabecular tissue.

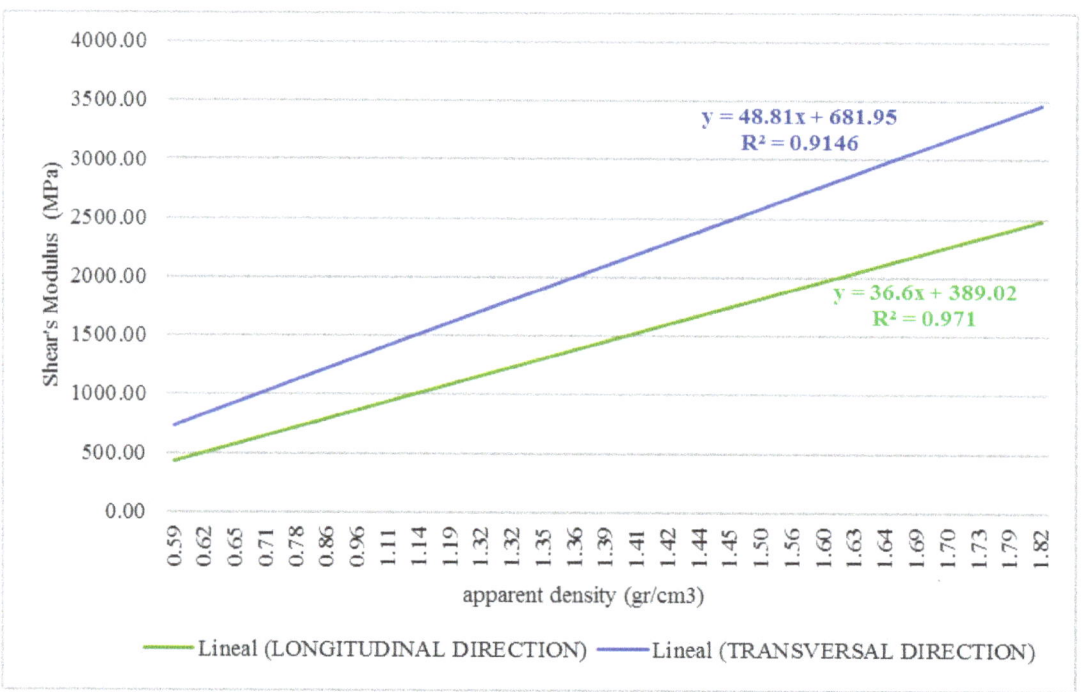

Figure 8. Relationship between apparent density and Shear's modulus for cortical tissue affected with OI in the longitudinal and transversal direction.

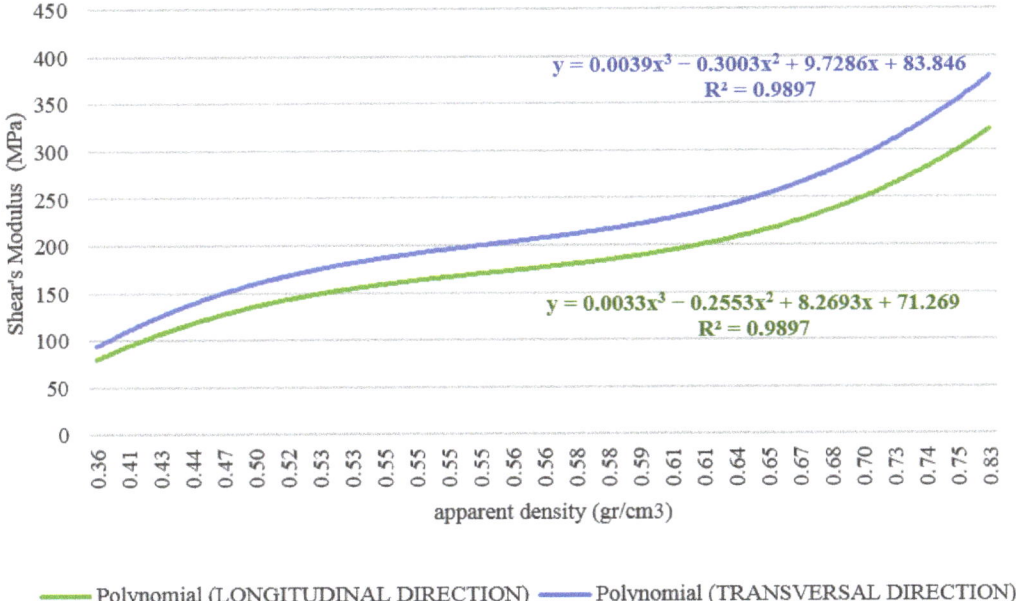

Figure 9. Relationship between apparent density and Shear's modulus for trabecular tissue affected with OI in the longitudinal and transversal direction.

2.5. Numerical 3D Model Analysis of OI Femur

The *.parasolid files were imported into ANSYS® software (Canonsburg, PA, USA) to perform an orthotropic numerical evaluation of a femur with OI. The values determined are used to set up the numerical analysis of the femur shown in Table 1.

Table 1. Bone tissue with OI properties for the cortical and trabecular.

Mechanical Property	Tissue	
	Cortical	Cortical
Modulus of elasticity transversal (E_t)	5764.54 MPa	793.88 MPa
Modulus of elasticity longitudinal (E_p)	3627.78 MPa	449.41 MPa
Shear modulus (G_t)	2097.44 MPa	217.40 MPa
Shear modulus (G_p)	1450.43 MPa	184.79 MPa
Poisson's ratio (v_{pt})	0.27	0.21

A 3D solid element of 20 nodes (SOLID186) was used to perform the mesh discretization since this element is compatible with contact elements such as TARGE170 and CONTA174. In the numerical evaluation, both elements were used to reproduce the interaction between the tissues. In general, the discretized mesh was carried out freely. According to this configuration, in total, 212,921 nodes and 142,018 elements were generated. The boundary conditions consider movement restriction and all the X, Y and Z axes' rotation on the femur distal metaphysis, as shown in Figure 10 (magenta zone).

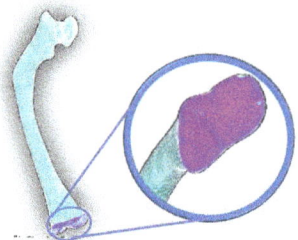

Figure 10. Border condition on the femur distal epiphysis, restricting all degrees of freedom.

The Pauwels distributed load model was used to perform a femur analysis in the frontal plane, as a hip stabilization system in the monopodial support, a more critical condition in the gait cycle. The force exerted by the abductor's muscles in this phase will be four times the infant's weight. Considering a child with an OI weight of around 11 kg, a force equivalent of 431.64 N is obtained. This force was applied to the upper part of the femur head, as shown in Figure 11 (magenta zone) [43].

Finally, the birth and death function in software ANSYS© (Canonsburg, PA, USA) was used to create transverse, comminuted, and oblique fracture types on the model.

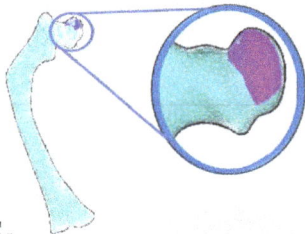

Figure 11. Force applied to the femur proximal epiphysis with a value of 431.64 N.

3. Results

Nominal stress resulting from the application of the von Mises theory is shown below. In each case, the maximum and minimum values in each analysis are indicated. In addition, the anterior and posterior of the femur model view is shown concerning the coronal anatomical axis.

3.1. Transverse Fracture Study

Figure 12a shows the transverse fracture in the medical image (radiography), and Figure 11 shows the finite element model where the fracture is generated and its appearance once the numerical analysis has been carried out.

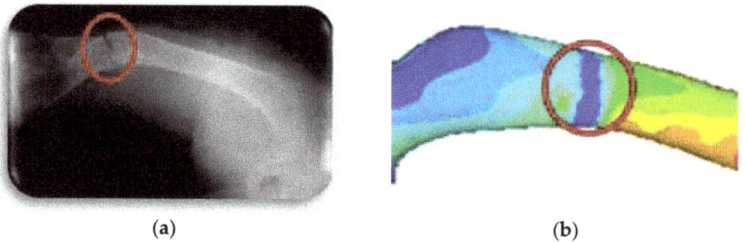

(a)   (b)

Figure 12. Transverse fracture: (**a**) medical image of bone fracture; (**b**) fracture of finite elements generated on the model.

Figure 13 shows the cuts of the model in each axis, showing the internal effect of the fracture intentionally generated in the femur bone, resulting in a high concentration of stress in the center of the femur shaft (the red areas), as this poses a significant risk when the patient's femur is subjected to critical load distribution.

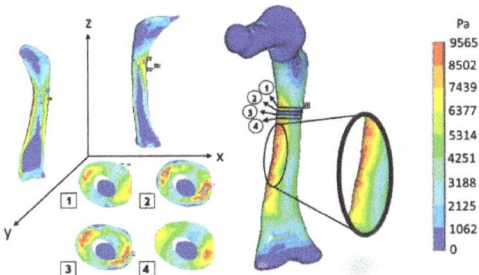

Figure 13. Orthotropic analysis. Von Mises stress showing maximum stress of 9.565 Pa.

3.2. Oblique Fracture Study

The oblique fracture in a medical image (radiography) and the finite element model fracture are generated, and their appearance after the numerical analysis is shown in Figure 14.

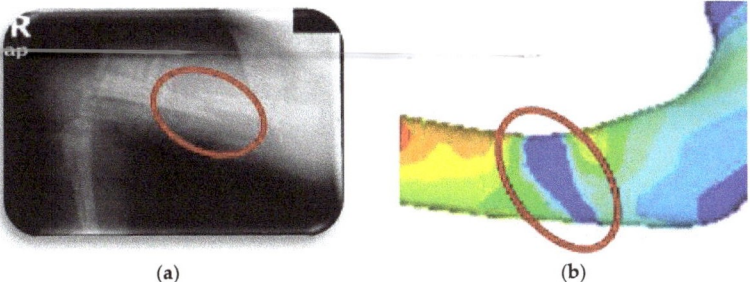

Figure 14. Oblique fracture: (**a**) medical image of bone fracture; (**b**) fracture of finite elements generated on the model.

Figure 15 shows the graphical and numerical result of the analysis carried out, where it can observe, in the first instance, the cuts of the model in each axis, showing the internal effect of the fracture intentionally generated in the femur bone, resulting in more areas with a high concentration of stress along the femoral shaft (the red areas).

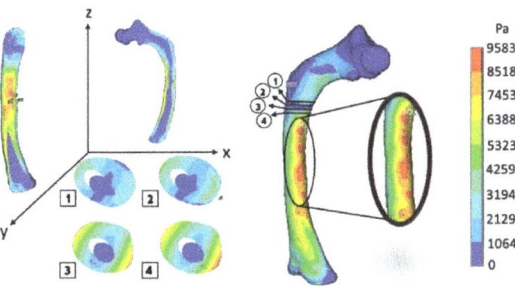

Figure 15. Orthotropic analysis. Von Mises stress showing maximum stress of 9.583 Pa.

3.3. Comminuted Fracture Study

Comminuted fracture in a medical image (radiography), the finite element model where the fracture is generated and its appearance once the numerical analysis has been carried out, is shown in Figure 16.

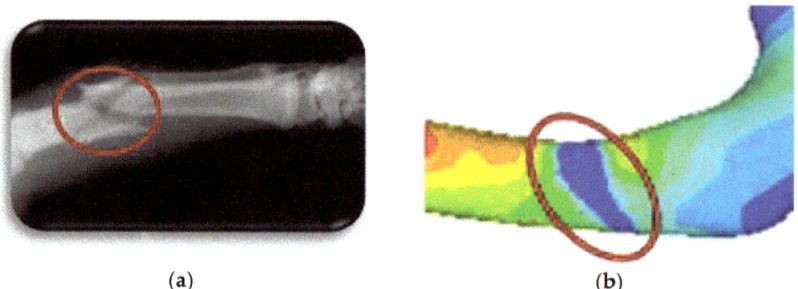

Figure 16. Comminuted fracture: (**a**) medical image of bone fracture; (**b**) fracture of finite elements generated on the model.

Figure 17 shows the graphical and numerical result of the analysis carried out, where we can observe in the first instance, the cuts of the model in each axis, showing the internal effect of the fracture intentionally generated in the femur bone, resulting in fewer areas of high-stress concentration in the upper part of the femur diaphysis (the red areas). However, the stress generated in that area is more significant than in the other analyses.

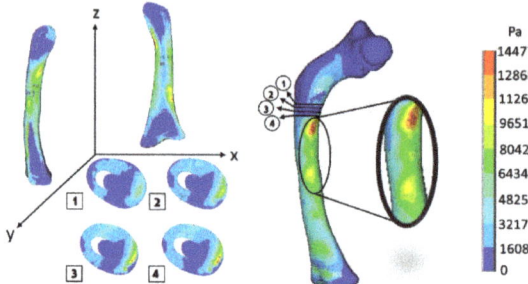

Figure 17. Orthotropic analysis. Von Mises stress showing maximum stress of 9.583 Pa.

This section may be divided into subheadings. It should provide a concise and precise description of the experimental results, their interpretation, and the experimental conclusions that can be drawn.

4. Discussion

With the development of software tools and computer hardware, the validation of bone structure models has had a great boom, allowing for a trend towards personalized finite element modeling for each patient [44]. This facilitates the study of the behavior of bones affected with OI. Although the clinical characteristics in patients affected with this disease are general, each patient's degree of bone deformation is a particular characteristic. Furthermore, the technological advancements in the area of tomography have allowed for the generation of models more attached to reality since the cortical and trabecular bone tissue can be segmented considering the grayscale, as mentioned by [33], or it can be considered by the values of the Hounsfield units, as shown in Section 2.3, and the models are shown in Figure 1. Furthermore, the finite element analysis can be performed considering both tissues, as shown by [31]. Moreover, other authors have studied femurs affected with OI from various criteria, for example, the degree of bone deformity [28], angular variation of the load application [29], increasing the load value [25,31], and influencing fracture [27]. A different method to reconstruction by tomography is shown, based on a statistical model of the shape and the appearance (SSAM) and a DXA image of the femur [26]. The use of tomography is not frequent in the diagnosis and follow-up for patients with osteoporosis. If a patient with OI has these studies, the analysis could be performed in this way. Finally, another author carries out a finite element study focused on the mechanical characterization of bone tissue affected with OI [23].

The mechanical properties of materials are an essential aspect in order to characterize them, determine their behavior, and predict under what circumstances a structural failure may present that compromises other entities within a system [24]. Derived from the above, a complete characterization of the bone tissue will define the weakest areas, where a fissure or fracture could occur under certain load conditions. Table 2 shows the values of Young's Modulus, which is a parameter that characterizes the behavior of bone with OI, obtained by different authors. Since the bone tissue affected with OI is highly heterogeneous, predominantly trabecular tissue, defining it as a fragile material with little elasticity and the ability to support expected loads, all the different authors' values are not uniform. Because performing physical tests on in vivo samples has a high cost and is difficult to reproduce, the non-invasive methodology described in this work is proposed. Indeed, the equations were described for bone tissue without any particular pathology. However, in the same way, they show that it is viable to develop this method to characterize bone tissue from a tomography performed on the limb to be analyzed, with the advantage that it can be easily reproducible and at almost zero cost compared to physical methods.

Table 2. Mechanical properties of the bone tissue with OI for the cortical and trabecular.

Author	Year	Type OI	Method of Obtaining	Cortical E (GPa)	Trabecular E (GPa)
Fan et al. [45]	2006	III	Nanoindentation	15.22 (L) 13.92 (T)	13.60
Weber et al. [46]	2006	III–IV	Nanoindentation	21.3	
Fan et al. [47]	2007	III	Nanoindentation	19.19	18.56
Fan et al. [48]	2007	III	Nanoindentation	19.67	19.23
Albert et al. [49]	2013	III	Nanoindentation	16.3	
Albert et al. [50]	2014	IV	Mechanical tests	4.4 (L) 1.6 (T)	
Imbert et al. [51]	2014	—	Nanoindentation	17.6	
Vardakastani et al. [52]	2014	—	Mechanical tests	6.8	
Imbert et al. [53]	2015	—	Mechanical tests	4.0	

T, transversal. L, longitudinal. E, Young's modulus.

The curved anatomy of the bone is a favorable condition for crack propagation. The compression and tension stress, specifically the yellow- or orange-color zones shown in Figures 13, 15 and 17, points out areas more susceptible to fracture, and the red color indicates the most critical zone. Anisotropic analysis was carried out for the same previous study cases, taking the properties of the bone tissue affected with OI obtained by Fan (2006). The analyses were configured with the same boundary conditions established previously. The results are shown in Figures 18–20 for the case of transverse, oblique, and comminuted fracture, respectively.

The isotropic analyses were compared to orthotropic analyses in the cases of transverse and oblique fracture, the stress values are remarkably similar, and the areas susceptible to fracture remain present. In contrast, in the case of comminuted fracture, the stress values and the behavior of the fabric are different.

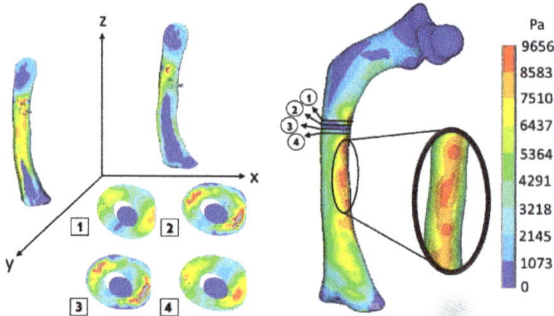

Figure 18. Isotropic analysis of the transverse fracture case. Von Mises stress showing maximum stress of 9.656 Pa.

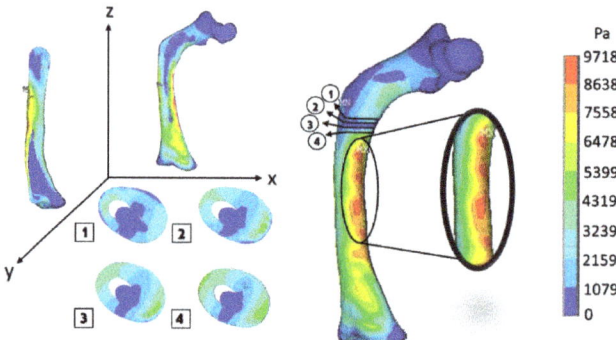

Figure 19. Isotropic analysis of the oblique fracture case. Von Mises stress showing maximum stress of 9.718 Pa.

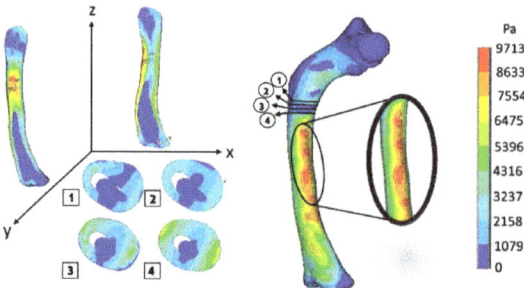

Figure 20. Isotropic analysis of the comminuted fracture case. Von Mises stress showing maximum stress of 9.713 Pa.

5. Conclusions

The importance of the method developed in this work is the facility to build biological 3D models using the DICOM® files. Likewise, this method is non-invasive because of the technology of the gadget used to obtain medical images. It can infer that the correct use of medical images due to the correct software can be helpful to determine the bone fracture behavior for certain pathologies, such as osteogenesis imperfecta, requites, osteopenia, and osteoporosis.

In most cases, the diagnostic is challenging before breaking limbs occurs. This alternative method by 3D bone models is different from the clinic method, preventing possible bone failure and fractures. For that reason, the exact image process can be helpful for OI patients. It can be perceived that the numerical analysis corresponding to the comminuted presents more significant stresses shown by the results exposed in the transverse and oblique fracture patterns; the area susceptible to failure extends in a wide radius around the crack where the fracture occurs. The transverse fracture presents minor stresses; however, it exhibits the same pattern of areas susceptible to bone failure, as in the case of the oblique fracture.

On the other hand, the results indicate that the transverse fracture presents the least stress and exposes lower critical areas. The values obtained in the different studies depend on the model achieved from the specific patient, that is, the type of OI, the patient's age, and bone quality are essential factors, and the mechanical properties, the direction of the load, and the payload are significant in the results obtained. However, the areas susceptible to fracture are similar in most studies.

This study determined how the bone type of fracture affects its integrity to a lesser or greater degree. Furthermore, several complications are reported during the healing and bone regeneration after being exposed to an osteotomy. Therefore, it is recommended that the manner in which fractures are generated is considered an essential factor in how the tissue is regenerated [5,7]. On the other hand, X-ray images of the intramedullary canal determined the adequate diameter of the intramedullary implant for patients with OI, and the implant optimization is carried out since the finite element analysis is focused on the personalized study of each patient, which is considered critical for this type of syndrome.

Lastly, FEA predicts bone remodeling, which is essential for implementing bisphosphonates in patients to consolidate fractures. Finally, determining the areas susceptible to fracture in bones affected with OI is essential to redesign implants to avoid proximal fractures and unanchored implants in the distal areas of the bone.

Author Contributions: Conceptualization, C.R.T.-S. and V.R.-V.; methodology, L.A.A.-P.; software, V.R.-V.; validation, L.A.A.-P., V.R.-V and J.C.P.-R.; formal analysis, C.R.T.-S.; investigation, V.R.-V.; resources, F.E.O.-H.; data curation, J.A.F.-C.; writing—original draft preparation, V.R.-V.; writing—review and editing, C.R.T.-S.; visualization, J.C.P.-R.; supervision, C.R.T.-S.; project administration, J.A.F.-C.; funding acquisition, F.E.O.-H. All authors have read and agreed to the published version of the manuscript.

Funding: This research received no external funding.

Institutional Review Board Statement: The Instituto Politécnico Nacional of Mexico does not have an ethics committee to evaluate this kind of research protocol that involves the use of human studies. In this case, this research does not fall within the scope of Human Rights. Therefore, we think that there is no legal obligation to be evaluated by any ethics committee. Moreover, the unique funder and publisher of this project is the Instituto Politécnico Nacional.

Informed Consent Statement: We do not carry out any clinical study in this research, and we ap-plied questionnaires to explain the final uses of tomographic studies in this scientific report. The members of the foundation Angelitos de Cristal provided the tomographic images, https://angelitosdecristal.org (accessed on 24 May 2021).

Data Availability Statement: Not applicable.

Acknowledgments: The authors acknowledge the financial support for realizing this work given to the Government of Mexico by the National Council of Science and Technology (CONACYT) and the Instituto Politécnico Nacional. In addition, the authors acknowledge partial support from project 20210282 and EDI grant, all provided by SIP/IPN.

Conflicts of Interest: The authors declare no conflict of interest.

References

1. Harrington, J.; Sochett, E.; Howard, A. Update on the Evaluation and Treatment of Osteogenesis Imperfecta. *Pediatr. Clin. N. Am.* **2014**, *61*, 1243–1257. [CrossRef]
2. Primorac, D.; Anticević, D.; Barisic, I. Osteogenesis imperfecta—Multi-systemic and life-long disease that affects whole family. *Coll. Antropol.* **2014**, *38*, 767–772.
3. Binh, H.D.; Maasalu, K.; Dung, V.C. Las características clínicas de la osteogénesis imperfecta en Vietnam. *Ortop. Int. (SICOT)* **2017**, *41*, 21–29. [CrossRef]
4. Lindahl, K.; Langdahl, B.; Ljunggren, O. Treatment of osteogenesis imperfecta in adults. *Eur. Soc. Endocrinol.* **2014**, *171*, 79–90. [CrossRef] [PubMed]
5. Munns, C.; Rauch, F.; Zeitlin, L. Delayed Osteotomy but Not Fracture Healing in Pediatric Osteogenesis Imperfecta Patients Receiving Pamidronate. *J. Bone Miner. Res.* **2004**, *19*, 1779–1986. [CrossRef]
6. Anam, E.A.; Rauch, F.; Glorieux, F.H. Osteotomy Healing in Children with Osteogenesis Imperfecta Receiving Bisphosphonate Treatment. *J. Bone Miner. Res.* **2015**, *30*, 1362–1368. [CrossRef]
7. Chotigavanichaya, C.; Jadhav, A.; Bernstein, R. Rod Diameter Prediction in Patients with Osteogenesis Imperfecta Undergoing Primary Osteotomy. *J. Pediatr. Orthop.* **2001**, *21*, 515–518. [CrossRef] [PubMed]
8. Azzam, K.; Rush, E.; Burke, B.; Nabower, A. Mid-term Results of Femoral and Tibial Osteotomies and Fassier-Duval Nailing in Children With Osteogenesis Imperfecta. *J. Pediatr. Orthop.* **2018**, *38*, 331–336. [CrossRef]
9. Gimeno, S.; Pérez, C.; Guardiola, S. Epidemiología de la osteogénesis imperfecta: Una enfermedad rara en la Comunidad Valenciana. *Rev. Esp. Salud Pública* **2017**, *91*, e201711045.
10. Alguacil, I.; Molina-Rueda, F.; Gómez, M. Tratamiento ortésico en pacientes con osteogénesis imperfecta. *An. Pediatr.* **2011**, *74*, 131.e1–131.e6. [CrossRef] [PubMed]
11. Métaizeau, J.D. Fracturas diafisarias del fémur en el niño. *EMC-Apar. Locomot.* **2015**, *48*, 1–11. [CrossRef]
12. González, P.; Rodríguez, M.; Castro, M. Fracturas diafisarias del fémur en el niño: Actualización en el tratamiento. *Rev. Esp. Cir. Ortop. Traumatol.* **2011**, *55*, 54–66. [CrossRef]
13. Bubbear, J. Atypical Femur Fractures in Patients Treated with Biphosphonates: Identification, Management, and Prevention. *Rambam Maimonides Med. J.* **2016**, *7*, e0032. [CrossRef]
14. Shane, E.; Burr, D.; Ebeling, P. Atipical subtrochanteric and diaphyseal femoral fractures: Report of a task force of the American Society for Bone and Mineral Research. *J. Bone Min. Res.* **2010**, *25*, 2267–2294. [CrossRef]
15. Guiusti, A.; Hamdy, N.; Papapoulos, S. Atypical fractures of the femur and bisphosphonate therapy. A systematic review of case/case series studies. *Bone* **2010**, *47*, 169–180. [CrossRef] [PubMed]
16. Varga, P.; Baumbach, S.; Pahr, D. Validación de un modelo anatómico de elementos finitos específico de la fractura de Colles. *J. Biomech.* **2009**, *42*, 1726–1731. [CrossRef]
17. Varga, P.; Inzana, B.; Stephan, C. Finite element analysis of bone strength in osteogenesis imperfecta. *Bone* **2020**, *133*, 115250. [CrossRef] [PubMed]
18. Aguilar, L.A.; Sánchez, J.I.; Flores, J.A.; Torres-San Miguel, C.R. Numerical and Experimental Assessment of a Novel Anchored for Intramedullary Telescopic Nails Used in Osteogenesis Imperfecta Fractures. *Appl. Sci.* **2021**, *11*, 5422. [CrossRef]
19. Li, X.; Vicenconti, M.; Cohen, M.C. Developing CT based computational models of pediatric femurs. *J. Biomech.* **2015**, *48*, 2034–2040. [CrossRef] [PubMed]
20. Helgason, B.; Perilli, E.; Schileo, E. Mathematical relationships between bone density and mechanical properties: A literature review. *Clin. Biomech.* **2008**, *23*, 135–146. [CrossRef]
21. Manhard, M.; Nyman, J.; Does, M. Advances in imaging approaches to fracture risk evaluation. *J. Lab. Clin. Med.* **2017**, *181*, 1–14. [CrossRef]
22. Caouette, C.; Ikin, N.; Villemure, I. Geometry reconstruction method for patient-specific finite element models for the assessment of tibia fracture risk in osteogenesis imperfecta. *Med. Biol. Eng. Comput.* **2017**, *55*, 549–560. [CrossRef] [PubMed]
23. Altai, Z.; Vicencoti, M.; Offiah, A. Investigating the mechanical response of paediatric bone under bending and torsion using finite element analysis. *Biomech. Model. Mechanobiol.* **2018**, *17*, 1001–1009. [CrossRef]
24. Fritz, J.; Grosland, N.; Smith, P. Finite Element Modeling and Analysis Applications in Osteogenesis Imperfecta. In *Handbook of Transitional Care in Osteogenesis Imperfecta: Advances in Biology, Technology, and Clinical Practice*, 1st ed.; Smith, P., Rauch, F., Harris, J., Eds.; Shriners Hospitals for Children Chicago: Chicago, IL, USA, 2016; pp. 149–160.
25. Fritz, J.; Guan, Y.; Wang, M. A fracture risk assessment model of the femur in children with osteogenesis imperfecta (OI) during gait. *J. Med. Eng. Phys.* **2009**, *31*, 1043–1048. [CrossRef]
26. Grassi, L.; Väänänen, S.; Ristinmaa, M. Prediction of femoral strength using 3D finite element models reconstructed from DXA images: Validation against experiments. *Biomech. Model. Mechanobiol.* **2017**, *16*, 989–1000. [CrossRef] [PubMed]
27. Cheong, V.; Masouros, S.; Bull, A. Fracture Simulation of Femoral Bone using Finite Element Method. In Proceedings of the IRCOBI Conference, Gothenburg, Sweden, 11–13 September 2013; IRC-13-96.
28. Wanna, S.B.; Basaruddin, K.; Mat Som, M.H. Prediction on fracture risk of femur with Osteogenesis Imperfecta using finite element models: Preliminary study. *J. Phys. Conf. Ser.* **2017**, *908*, 012022. [CrossRef]
29. Wanna, S.B.; Basaruddin, K.; Mat Som, M.H. Fracture risk prediction on children with Osteogenesis Imperfecta subjected to loads under activity of daily living. *IOP Conf. Ser. Mater. Sci. Eng.* **2018**, *429*, 012004. [CrossRef]

30. Wanna, S.B.; Basaruddin, K.; Mat Som, M.H. Effect of loading direction on fracture of bone with osteogénesis imperfect (OI) during standing. *AIP Conf. Proc.* **2018**, *2030*, 020094. [CrossRef]
31. Ahmad, S.F.; Mat Som, M.H.; Basaruddin, K.S. Determination of Fracture Risk on Patient-specific Model of Femur with Osteogenesis Imperfecta. *J. Phys. Conf. Ser.* **2019**, *1372*, 012042. [CrossRef]
32. Tan, L.C.; Mat Som, M.H.; Basaruddin, K.S. Biomechanical analysis of patient-specific femur model of osteogenesis imperfecta with cortical and cancellous bone. *IOP Conf. Ser. Mater. Sci. Eng.* **2019**, *670*, 012045. [CrossRef]
33. Voon, T.T.; Mat Som, M.H.; Yazid, H. Segmentation of Cortical and Cancellous Bone with Osteogenesis Imperfecta using Thresholding-based Method. *J. Phys. Conf. Ser.* **2019**, *1372*, 012006. [CrossRef]
34. Martínez, L.; García, A.; Espantaleón, M.; Monclús, J. Research to Increase Passive Safety of Affected by Osteogenesis Imperfecta. In Proceedings of the 13th International Conference, Protection of Children in Cars, Munich, Germany, 3–4 December 2015; pp. 1–22.
35. Rueda, J.L.; Torres, C.R.; Ramírez, V.; Martínez, L. Design and Comparative Numerical Analysis of Designs of Intramedular Telescopic Systems for the Rehabilitation of Patients with Osteogenesis Imperfecta (OI) Type III. In *Engineering Design Applications II Structures, Materials and Processes: Structures, Materials and Processes*; Öchsner, A., Altenbach, H., Eds.; Springer: Cham, Switzerland, 2020; Volume 113, pp. 333–341. [CrossRef]
36. Martínez, L.; Reed, M.P.; García, A. Crash Impact Dummies adapted to People Affected by Osteogenesis Imperfecta. In Proceedings of the IRCOBI Conference, Malaga, Spain, 14–16 September 2016; RC-16-97.
37. Ramírez, V.; Torres, C.R.; Rueda, J.L. Finite Element Analysis of 3D Models of Upper and Lower Limbs of Mexican Patients with Osteogenesis Imperfecta (OI) Type III. In *Engineering Design Applications II. Advanced Structured Materials*; Öchsner, A., Altenbach, H., Eds.; Springer: Cham, Switzerland, 2020; Volume 113, pp. 343–353. [CrossRef]
38. Rueda, J.L.; Torres, C.R.; Ramírez, V. Simulation by finite element method of intramedullary telescopic systems for rehabilitation of patients with osteogenesis imperfecta. *Rev. Mex. Ing. Biomed.* **2019**, *40*, e201826. [CrossRef]
39. Dellan, A.; Villarroel, M.; Hernández, A. Application of Hounsfield units in computed tomography as a diagnostic tool for intra-osseous lesions of the maxilla-mandibular complex: Diagnostic clinical study. *Rev. Odontol. Univ. Cid. Sao Paulo* **2015**, *27*, 100–111.
40. Buroni, F.C.; Commisso, P.E.; Cisilino, A.P.; Sammartino, M. Determinación De Las Constantes Elásticas Anisótropas Del Tejido Óseo Utilizando Tomografías Computadas. Aplicación a La Construcción De Modelos De Elementos Finitos. *Mec. Comput.* **2004**, *XXIII*.
41. Taylor, W.R.; Roland, E.; Ploeg, H.; Hertig, D.; Klabunde, R.; Warner, M.D.; Hobatho, M.C.; Rakotomanana, L.; Clift, S.E. Determination of orthotropic bone elastic constants using FEA and modal analysis. *J. Biomech.* **2002**, *35*, 767–773. [CrossRef]
42. Wirtz, D.C.; Schiffers, N.; Pandorf, T.; Radermacher, K.; Weichert, D.; Forst, R. Critical evaluation of known bone material properties to realize anisotropic FE-simulation of the proximal femur. *J. Biomech.* **2000**, *33*, 1325–1330. [CrossRef]
43. Houcke, J.; Khanduja, V.; Pattyn, C. The History of Biomechanics in Total Hip Arthroplasty. *Indian J. Orthop.* **2017**, *51*, 359–367. [CrossRef] [PubMed]
44. Zysset, P.K.; Dall'Ára, E.; Varga, P. Finite element analysis for prediction of bone strength. *Bonekey Rep.* **2013**, *2*, 386. [CrossRef]
45. Fan, Z.; Smith, P.A.; Eckstein, E.C.; Harris, G.F. Mechanical properties of OI type III bone tissue measured by nanoindentation. *J. Biomed. Mater. Res. A* **2006**, *79*, 71–77. [CrossRef]
46. Weber, M.; Roschger, P.; Fratzl-Zelman, N.; Schöberl, T.; Rauch, F.; Glorieux, F.H.; Fratzl, P.; Klaushofer, K. Pamidronate does not adversely affect bone intrinsic material properties in children with osteogenesis imperfecta. *Bone* **2006**, *39*, 616–622. [CrossRef] [PubMed]
47. Fan, Z.; Smith, P.A.; Harris, G.F.; Rauch, F.; Bajorunaite, R. Comparison of nanoindentation measurements between osteogenesis imperfecta Type III and Type IV and between different anatomic locations (femur/tibia versus iliac crest). *Connect Tissue Res.* **2007**, *48*, 70–75. [CrossRef] [PubMed]
48. Fan, Z.; Smith, P.; Rauch, F.; Harris, G.F. Nanoindentation as a means for distinguishing clinical type of osteogenesis imperfect. *Compos. Part B Eng.* **2007**, *38*, 411–415. [CrossRef]
49. Albert, C.; Jameson, J.; Toth, J. Bone Properties by Nanoindentation in Mild and Severe Osteogenesis Imperfecta. *Clin. Biomech.* **2013**, *28*, 110–116. [CrossRef] [PubMed]
50. Albert, C.; Jameson, J.; Smith, P.; Harris, G. Reduced diaphyseal strength associated with high intracortical vascular porosity within long bones of children with osteogenesis imperfecta. *Bone* **2014**, *66*, 121–130. [CrossRef] [PubMed]
51. Imbert, L.; Aurégan, J.C.; Pernelle, K.; Hoc, T. Mechanical and mineral properties of osteogenesis imperfecta human bones at the tissue level. *Bone* **2014**, *65*, 18–24. [CrossRef] [PubMed]
52. Vardakastani, V.; Saletti, D.; Skalli, W.; Marry, P.; Allain, J.M.; Adam, C. Increased intra-cortical porosity reduces bone stiffness and strength in pediatric patients with osteogenesis imperfecta. *Bone* **2014**, *69*, 61–67. [CrossRef]
53. Imbert, L.; Aurégan, J.; Pernelle, K. Microstructure and compressive mechanical properties of cortical bone in children with osteogenesis imperfecta treated with bisphosphonates compared with healthy children. *J. Mech. Behav. Biomed. Mater.* **2015**, *46*, 261–270. [CrossRef] [PubMed]

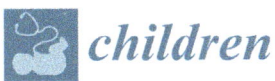

Article

Analysis of Physeal Fractures from the United States National Trauma Data Bank

Joseph R. Fuchs [1,2], Romie F. Gibly [1,3], Christopher B. Erickson [1,4], Stacey M. Thomas [1], Nancy Hadley Miller [1,5] and Karin A. Payne [1,6,*]

1. Department of Orthopedics, University of Colorado Anschutz Medical Campus, Aurora, CO 80045, USA; joseph.fuchs@cuanschutz.edu (J.R.F.); rgibly@northwestern.edu (R.F.G.); christopher.erickson@cuanschutz.edu (C.B.E.); stacey.m.thomas@cuanschutz.edu (S.M.T.); nancy.miller@childrenscolorado.org (N.H.M.)
2. McGaw Medical Center, Northwestern University, Chicago, IL 60611, USA
3. Division of Orthopaedic Surgery and Sports Medicine, Ann & Robert H. Lurie Children's Hospital of Chicago, Chicago, IL 60611, USA
4. Department of Bioengineering, University of Colorado Anschutz Medical Campus, Aurora, CO 80045, USA
5. Musculoskeletal Research Center, Children's Hospital Colorado, Aurora, CO 80045, USA
6. Gates Center for Regenerative Medicine, University of Colorado Anschutz Medical Campus, Aurora, CO 80045, USA
* Correspondence: karin.payne@cuanschutz.edu

Abstract: Background: Pediatric long-bone physeal fractures can lead to growth deformities. Previous studies have reported that physeal fractures make up 18–30% of total fractures. This study aimed to characterize physeal fractures with respect to sex, age, anatomic location, and Salter–Harris (SH) classification from a current multicenter national database. Methods: A retrospective cohort study was performed using the 2016 United States National Trauma Data Bank (NTDB). Patients ≤ 18 years of age with a fracture of the humerus, radius, ulna, femur, tibia, or fibula were included. Results: The NTDB captured 132,018 patients and 58,015 total fractures. Physeal fractures made up 5.7% (3291) of all long-bone fractures, with males accounting for 71.0% (2338). Lower extremity physeal injuries comprised 58.6% (1929) of all physeal fractures. The most common site of physeal injury was the tibia comprising 31.8% (1047), 73.9% (774) of which were distal tibia fractures. Physeal fractures were greatest at 11 years of age for females and 14 years of age for males. Most fractures were SH Type II fractures. Discussion and Conclusions: Our analysis indicates that 5.7% of pediatric long-bone fractures involved the physis, with the distal tibia being the most common. These findings suggest a lower incidence of physeal fractures than previous studies and warrant further investigation.

Keywords: physeal; physis; fracture; trauma; long-bone fractures in children

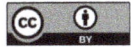

1. Introduction

It is estimated that 18% to 30% of all pediatric fractures involve the physis, a cartilaginous area at the ends of long bones [1,2]. Physeal fractures are of particular concern as they can lead to partial or complete physeal arrest, resulting in angular deformities or limb-length discrepancy. Understanding the epidemiology of physeal injuries is important for the early identification of these injuries, as late presentation can result in complex deformities that can lead to greater challenges in achieving good clinical results [3,4].

Previous epidemiology studies looking at sex differences have indicated that a predominance of physeal injuries occur in males [1–3]. The distribution of anatomic locations of physeal fractures for long bones of the appendicular skeleton has been explored as well, with most fractures occurring in the upper extremities, especially of the radius [1,3,5]. This observation has led to outcomes research analyzing the treatment of these fractures, such as outcomes based on body habitus [6]. Fractures that involve the physis are classified according to the Salter–Harris (SH) classification system, which grades fractures according to the involvement of the physis, metaphysis, and epiphysis (Figure 1). Past studies have shown that SH Type II fractures are the most common type of physeal injury [1–3].

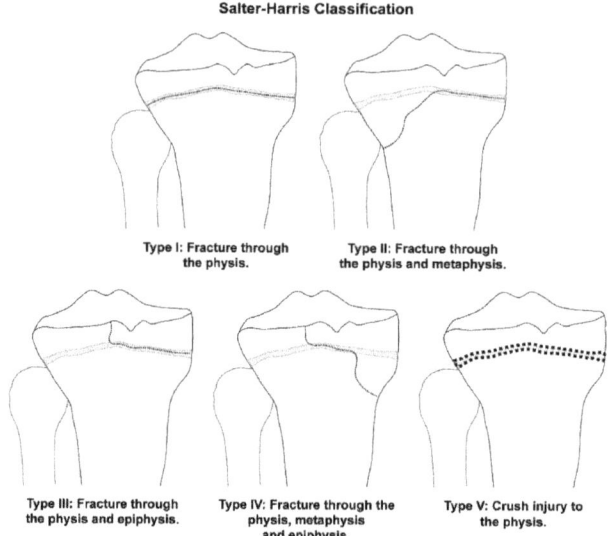

Figure 1. Salter–Harris Classification of pediatric physeal fractures. The five fracture types are shown with the fracture line represented by a dotted line.

Additional studies have analyzed trends in physeal fractures such as age and sex predominance for specific long bones and anatomic locations [7–12]. Few, however, have compared all physeal fractures and identified which anatomic locations are at a higher risk for injury [1–3]. Comparison of all long-bone fractures to physeal fractures according to age and sex has also rarely been studied [1]. While most of these studies have focused on populations from a single institution, a larger-scale study was conducted in Olmstead County, MN, between 1979–1988 [3]. This study indicated that physeal injuries peak between the ages of 12–14 years. Since that time, motor vehicle technology and sports intensity have evolved, potentially altering the prevalence and severity of physeal injuries [13]. This has been explored in previous work that has analyzed the epidemiology of pediatric fractures based on age, type, and anatomic location at a single institution over time [14]. However, analyzing a more recent and larger dataset from multiple institutions could provide a better representation of the current epidemiology of physeal fractures.

The aim of this study was to analyze trends of pediatric long-bone fractures from a current United States multicenter national database to better characterize both physeal and nonphyseal fractures with respect to sex, age, anatomic location, and SH classification.

2. Materials and Methods

Following approval from the Institutional Review Board (COMIRB 20-0020), a retrospective cohort study was performed using the American College of Surgeons (ACS) United States National Trauma Data Bank (NTDB). The NTDB consists of patient demographics, ICD-10 codes for all injuries presenting within 14 days of occurrence, trauma center designation, and population treated [15]. The NTDB is the largest aggregation of U.S. trauma registry data and was designed to establish a national standard for trauma data [16]. The NTDB has been utilized to study the epidemiology of adult patients with hip fractures and spinal injury in pediatric populations [17,18]. The ACS utilizes the National Trauma Data Standard and validates data annually to ensure incomplete and nonsensical data are not included [19].

The data, volunteered from over 740 institutions in the United States and Puerto Rico, are comprised of approximately two hundred Level I, II, III or IV trauma centers each and 36 Level I or II pediatric-only centers. Using the 2016 version of the NTDB, data given in CSV files were loaded into Microsoft Access. In the NTDB each patient is coded with a unique inclusion key and ICD-10 diagnosis code, along with demographic data. ICD-10 diagnosis codes based on the clinical presentation and incorporating clinical data are coded by the trauma registrar or data abstractor at each institution. This allowed patients ≤ 18 years to be identified. From those, records with ICD-10 diagnosis codes for long-bone fractures of the humerus, radius, ulna, femur, tibia, or fibula (S42, S49, S52, S59, S72, S79, S82, S89) were selected (Figure 2). Within the ICD-10 diagnosis codes for long-bone fractures are more specific codes for physeal injuries and SH Type classification [20]. These were utilized to categorize long-bone fractures more specifically into nonphyseal fractures or physeal fractures (excluding slipped capital femoral epiphysis). All physeal ICD-10 codes for each long bone were included. Physeal fractures were further categorized using the SH classification, when available (Figure 2). The detailed ICD-10 codes also allowed for an anatomic location such as the proximal and distal end of bones to be differentiated. For example, S49.0 codes for "physeal fracture of upper end of humerus" and S49.1 codes for "physeal fracture of lower end of humerus". The range of ICD-10 diagnosis codes analyzed ensured that all long-bone fractures were included in the study, with further granularity for anatomic location and physeal involvement based on more specific coding. Once the dataset was generated, data were analyzed based on sex, age, anatomic location, and fracture type for long-bone fractures. Age groups (0–4, 5–8, 9–12, and 13–18 years) were utilized to organize the data. These groups were determined based on groups utilized in previous studies and to highlight common ages for physeal injuries as described in the literature [2,3].

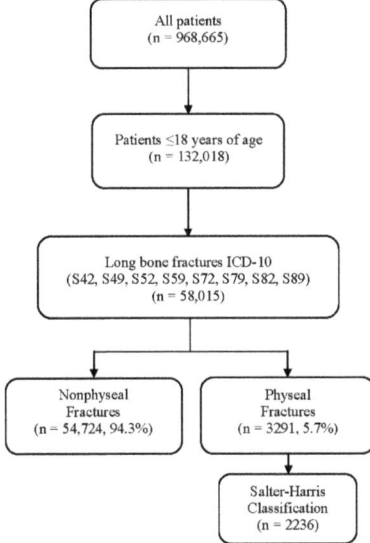

Figure 2. Flowchart of inclusion criteria using data from the NTDB.

3. Results

The 2016 version of the NTDB consisted of entries for 968,665 patients. Of those, 132,018 patients were identified to be $\leq$18 years. 42,429 of those patients had at least one long-bone fracture code associated with their entry, resulting in a total of 58,015 fractures (Figure 2).

When analyzing all long-bone fractures, regardless of physeal involvement, males accounted for 65.6% (38,053) of long bone fractures while females comprised 34.4% (19,962). The total long-bone fracture data were then categorized into nonphyseal or physeal fractures. Nonphyseal fractures comprised 94.3% (54,724) of the long-bone fractures included in this study, and males accounted for 65.3% (35,715) of all nonphyseal fractures. Fractures involving the physis made up 5.7% (3291) of the total fractures reported in this study (6.1% in males and 4.8% in females). Males accounted for 71.0% (2338) of all physeal fractures. While SH classification information was not available for all fractures, 67.9% (2236) of the overall physeal fractures were associated with an SH class by ICD-10 coding (Figure 2).

Nonphyseal fractures for each age by sex show a relative peak at the ages of 5–6 years for both males and females (Figure 3). Another peak appears for males at 13–14 years of age which is not seen for females. The distribution of nonphyseal fractures according to long bone and separated by age is represented for males in Table 1 and females in Table 2. Upper extremity nonphyseal injuries accounted for 56.6% (20,206) of all nonphyseal fractures in males and 65.6% (12,476) in females. Nonphyseal fractures occurred most frequently in the humerus, followed by the femur, radius, ulna, and tibia which all had similar occurrences. Nonphyseal fractures to the fibula occurred less frequently.

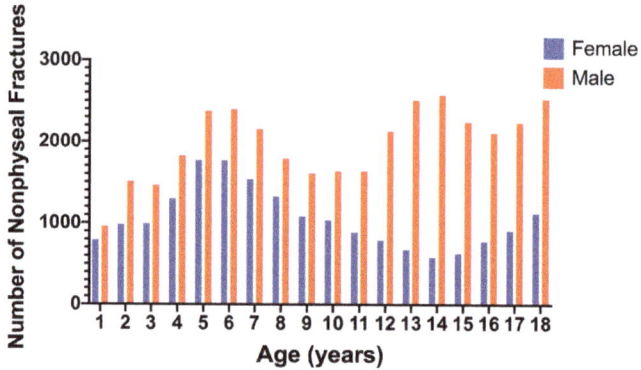

Figure 3. Number of nonphyseal fractures at each age for females (blue) and males (red).

Table 1. Nonphyseal fractures for males according to age and long bone. N = 35,715.

Age	Femur n (%)	Tibia n (%)	Fibula n (%)	Humerus n (%)	Radius n (%)	Ulna n (%)
0–4	2077 (5.8)	417 (1.2)	166 (0.5)	2190 (6.1)	461 (1.3)	450 (1.3)
5–8	987 (2.8)	485 (1.4)	296 (0.8)	3820 (10.7)	1610 (4.5)	1524 (4.3)
9–12	1012 (2.8)	873 (2.4)	616 (1.7)	1089 (3.0)	1811 (5.1)	1618 (4.5)
13–18	2657 (7.4)	3624 (10.1)	2299 (6.4)	1284 (3.6)	2290 (6.4)	2059 (5.8)
Total	6733 (18.9)	5399 (15.1)	3377 (9.5)	8383 (23.5)	6172 (17.3)	5651 (15.8)

Table 2. Nonphyseal fractures for females according to age and long bone. N = 19,009.

Age	Femur n (%)	Tibia n (%)	Fibula n (%)	Humerus n (%)	Radius n (%)	Ulna n (%)
0–4	858 (4.5)	341 (1.8)	127 (0.7)	2076 (10.9)	315 (1.7)	352 (1.9)
5–8	497 (2.6)	353 (1.9)	206 (1.1)	3308 (17.4)	1059 (5.6)	990 (5.2)
9–12	422 (2.2)	501 (2.6)	313 (1.6)	888 (4.7)	903 (4.8)	784 (4.1)
13–18	999 (5.3)	1155 (6.1)	761 (4.0)	553 (2.9)	652 (3.4)	596 (3.1)
Total	2776 (14.6)	2350 (12.4)	1407 (7.4)	6825 (35.9)	2929 (15.4)	2722 (14.3)

The number of physeal fractures at each age for males and females is shown in Figure 4. A peak occurs around the age of 11 for females and at the age of 14 for males. The number of physeal fractures is much higher for males than females after 10 years of age. The number and percentage of physeal fractures according to age, long bone, and proximal or distal location is shown for males in Table 3 and females in Table 4. In males, the largest percentage of physeal fractures were observed in the distal tibia and distal radius in the 13–18 age group (Table 3). Females also had the greatest number of physeal fractures in these locations, but they mostly occurred in the 9–12 age group (Table 4).

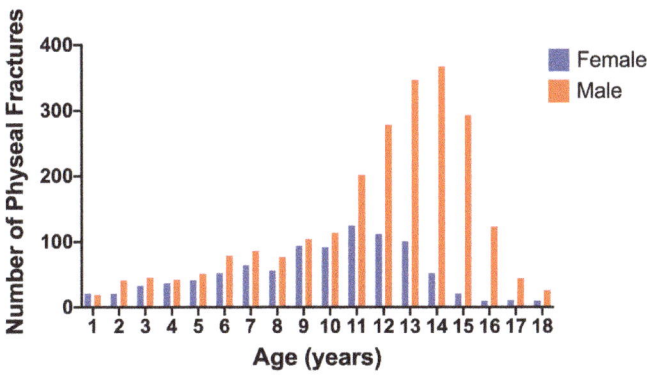

Figure 4. Number of physeal fractures at each age for females (blue) and males (red).

Table 3. Physeal fractures for males according to age, long bone, and location (proximal or distal). N = 2338.

	Bone n (%)											
	Femur		Tibia		Fibula		Humerus		Radius		Ulna	
Age	P	D	P	D	P	D	P	D	P	D	P	D
0–4	8 (0.3)	16 (0.7)	17 (0.7)	22 (0.9)	2 (0.1)	13 (0.6)	7 (0.3)	40 (1.7)	2 (0.1)	15 (0.6)	0 (0.0)	5 (0.2)
5–8	4 (0.2)	31 (1.3)	13 (0.6)	31 (1.3)	20 (0.9)	85 (3.6)	8 (0.3)	56 (2.4)	8 (0.3)	94 (4.0)	0 (0.0)	29 (1.2)
9–12	32 (1.4)	80 (3.4)	29 (1.2)	173 (7.4)	3 (0.1)	16 (0.7)	23 (1.0)	19 (0.8)	12 (0.5)	214 (9.2)	0 (0.0)	55 (2.4)
13–18	43 (1.8)	190 (8.1)	159 (6.8)	308 (13.2)	7 (0.3)	54 (2.3)	52 (2.2)	6 (0.3)	5 (0.2)	282 (12.1)	0 (0.0)	50 (2.1)

P = proximal, D = distal.

Table 4. Physeal fractures for females according to age, long bone, and location (proximal or distal). N = 953.

	Bone n (%)											
	Femur		Tibia		Fibula		Humerus		Radius		Ulna	
Age	P	D	P	D	P	D	P	D	P	D	P	D
0–4	7 (0.7)	17 (1.8)	16 (1.7)	14 (1.5)	4 (0.4)	8 (0.8)	6 (0.6)	18 (1.9)	0 (0.0)	18 (1.9)	0 (0.0)	4 (0.4)
5–8	2 (0.2)	26 (2.7)	8 (0.8)	24 (2.5)	6 (0.6)	14 (1.5)	7 (0.7)	32 (3.4)	12 (1.3)	68 (7.1)	0 (0.0)	18 (1.9)
9–12	34 (3.6)	45 (4.7)	13 (1.4)	144 (15.1)	2 (0.2)	14 (1.5)	8 (0.8)	11 (1.2)	8 (0.8)	88 (9.2)	0 (0.0)	24 (2.5)
13–18	12 (1.3)	39 (4.1)	18 (1.9)	58 (6.1)	2 (0.2)	46 (4.8)	8 (0.8)	4 (0.4)	3 (0.3)	40 (4.2)	0 (0.0)	3 (0.3)

P = proximal, D = distal.

The breakdown of all physeal fractures by bone and further separated by proximal or distal location, sex, and age can be seen in Figure 5. Lower extremity fractures comprised 58.6% (1929/3291) of physeal injuries. The most common long bone with physeal injury was the tibia, accounting for 31.8% (1047/3291) of all physeal fractures. Of these fractures, the distal tibia was predominantly injured, accounting for 71.0% (534/752) and 81.4% (240/295) of tibial physeal fractures for males and females, respectively. In females, tibial physeal fractures occurred most often between the ages of 9–12 years, while for males,

13–18 years made up the largest share. The second most common site of physeal fracture for both males and females was the radius. Similar to the tibia, the distal end of the bone was more highly affected than the proximal end. A physeal fracture affecting the distal radius occurred in 95.7% (605/632) and 90.3% (214/237) of total physeal fractures of the radius for males and females, respectively. Physeal fractures of the radius occurred most frequently for females from the ages of 9–12 and for males from ages 13–18.

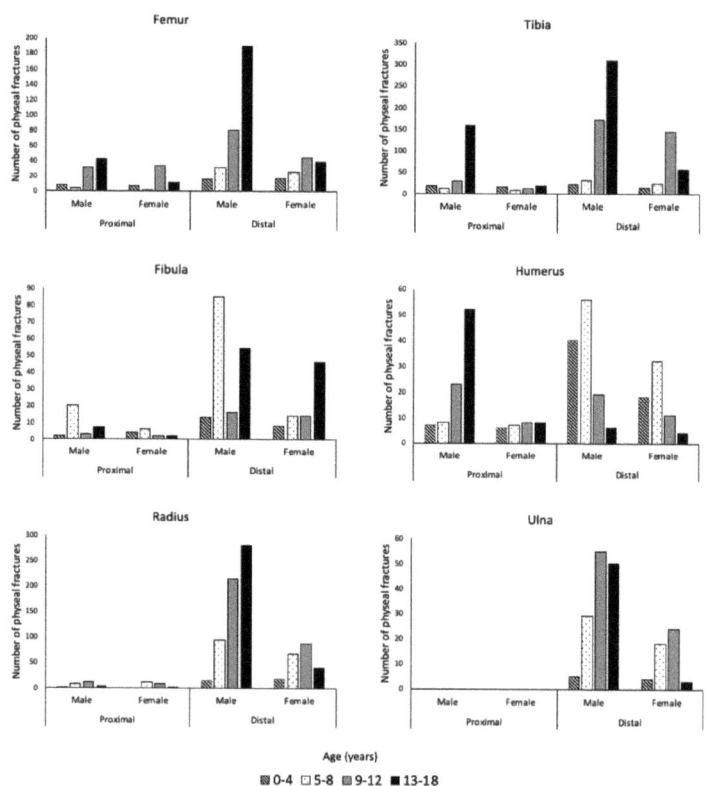

Figure 5. The number of physeal fractures for the femur, tibia, fibula, humerus, radius, and ulna, separated by sex, anatomic location (proximal and distal), and age group.

The SH classification was available for 2236 physeal fractures and analysis of these data indicated that SH class II fractures were the most common physeal fractures, comprising 69.0% (1543) of fractures (Table 5). SH class I, III, and IV each made up less than 12% of physeal fractures.

Table 5. Salter–Harris classification of physeal injuries based on long bone. N = 2236.

	SH I (%)	SH II (%)	SH III (%)	SH IV (%)
Femur	96 (4.3)	231 (10.3)	31 (1.4)	16 (0.7)
Tibia	36 (1.6)	448 (20)	119 (5.3)	204 (9.1)
Fibula	39 (1.7)	120 (5.4)	0 (0)	0 (0)
Humerus	32 (1.4)	119 (5.3)	0 (0)	20 (0.9)
Radius	50 (2.2)	546 (24.4)	13 (0.6)	16 (0.7)
Ulna	9 (0.4)	79 (3.5)	8 (0.4)	4 (0.2)
Total	262 (11.7)	1543 (69.0)	171 (7.6)	260 (11.6)

4. Discussion

Previous epidemiology studies of physeal fractures have largely been completed through an analysis of fractures at single academic institutions [1–3,21]. While this provides useful information, a more comprehensive view of physeal fractures can be obtained using data from the NTDB. The NTDB data come from 747 institutions, comprising 968,665 patient records from all regions of the United States. Therefore, this study is derived from a much larger and more varied sample of patients which allows for a better understanding of physeal fractures.

Males accounted for a majority of all fractures with peak nonphyseal fracture occurrence at 5–6 years and 13–14 years, which is similar to previous studies [21,22]. Studies have found that males generally account for 55–65% of all fractures, which is similar to our results [1,22]. In the case of nonphyseal fractures affecting females, previous studies have noted a peak at 11 years compared to the results of this study which demonstrated a peak at 5 and 6 years [2,21]. This inconsistency is possibly due to differences such as sports participation based on age and sex across times and in various countries [2,21].

In this study, the most affected long bone for nonphyseal fractures is the humerus. This deviates from studies that have found the radius to comprise 30–60% of nonphyseal fractures [1,2]. This is a unique finding that warrants further investigation to clearly establish this predominance and may relate to the subset of patients presenting to centers participating in the NTDB, with a potential for higher acuity of trauma.

Our analysis indicated that physeal fractures made up 5.7% of the total fractures, which is less than the rate of 18–30% found in previous studies [1–3,23]. One reason for this discrepancy could be that the sample was derived from long-bone fractures, while many previous studies included fractures of the phalanges. However, in Mann et al. the rate was 30% based solely on long-bone data [1]. Another factor that should be considered is the ages included in each study. For example, Peterson et al. utilized a sample of patients 0–21 years while Worlock et al. included patients 0–12 years [3,24]. However, when altering the age range analyzed using the NTDB data to include age ranges from 0–14 years, 0–15 years, 0–16 years, or 0–17 years, the maximum percentage of physeal fractures found is less than 7%. The NTDB is comprised of hundreds of institutions and thousands of patients which can be contrasted with most studies that were conducted at single institutions that are largely academic centers. It is possible that previous studies with smaller sample sizes may have seen higher rates of complicated injuries. It is also possible that not all physeal fractures would present at a trauma center. Therefore, the rate of physeal fractures compared to overall fractures may be lower than previously thought but further investigation is needed.

The most common age for physeal fractures was 14 years for males and 11 years for females. This has been noted in previous studies and has been attributed to the weakness of the growth plate during puberty [2]. Of physeal fractures, males accounted for 71.0%. This is consistent with studies that demonstrate a male predominance of 66–75% [1,3,23]. Lower extremity physeal injuries comprised a majority of injuries for both males and females. This is consistent with a previous study of long-bone physeal fractures which demonstrated that 54.78% of fractures were in the lower extremity [1]. In this study, the tibia was the long bone with the greatest percentage of physeal fractures, accounting for greater than 30% of injuries. The second most common long bone with physeal fractures was the radius with 26.4%. This deviates from previous studies, which found a predominance of physeal fractures of the radius, comprising 28–30% of long-bone physeal fractures [1,3]. This difference may be due to the NTBD being comprised of data from trauma centers that see higher acuity injuries compared to primary care settings, as tibial fractures result in difficulty with ambulation.

Tibial physeal fractures were more commonly fractured at the distal end than the proximal end. This is consistent with previous studies with distal injuries accounting for a majority (96%) of tibial physeal fractures [1]. This was also seen for the radius, with distal physeal fractures comprising greater than 90% of physeal injuries, consistent with previous estimates of 86.36% [1]. Therefore, distal tibial and radial injuries should be closely followed to ensure the physis is not impacted. A recent study of SH Type II fractures of the distal tibia suggested that fracture displacement greater than 3 mm should be treated with closed reduction and casted [25]. If displacement remains greater than 3 mm, open reduction should be performed. The study found a small risk of growth arrest after closed reduction for displaced fractures. Thus, initial recognition, treatment, and follow-up of distal tibial and radial physeal fractures by a pediatric orthopedist can help avoid long-term complications such as angular deformity and limb-length discrepancy in pediatric populations.

SH Type II fractures were the dominant type of physeal injuries observed in this study, which has been a consistent pattern throughout the decades [1–3,23]. SH Types I, III, and IV each accounted for 12% or less of physeal fractures, which has been noted previously [1].

Previous studies have looked at the incidence of physeal fractures through direct retrospective analysis of radiographs [1–3,23]. The NTDB for 2016 is the first year that contains ICD-10 codes, which have many subclassifications for physeal injuries. Previously utilized ICD-9 codes did not include specifications for proximal or distal physis, an essential piece of knowledge when addressing physeal fractures of long bones. Through proper ICD-10 coding based on radiographic reads, it is possible to have a better understanding of physeal injuries that is standardized across institutions. This is beneficial for future studies as researchers can more quickly sort through data without having to analyze numerous radiographs that will not meet study inclusion criteria. A limitation of this information, however, is that the ICD-10 diagnosis codes utilized in this analysis are reliant on radiologic reads and radiographic imaging could not be independently verified. Therefore, errors in the assignment of ICD-10 codes during data entry may have impacted our results. However, the ACS validates the NTDB by not including missing or nonsensical data. Future studies should compare ICD-10 diagnosis codes to independently verified radiographic reads to determine if differences exist.

Despite the ability of the NTDB to provide an estimate for physeal injuries across hundreds of institutions within the country, there are some limitations to the data. The most important limitation is that the data are voluntarily provided by trauma centers. Therefore, there are differences in the number of patients seen at each institution, as well as the number of institutions for each region. Thus, this study does not provide a national representation of injuries. These differences do not allow for a denominator to be determined which would provide estimates of the incidence of pediatric physeal injuries nationally. However, this is a similar limitation to previous studies that describe the occurrence of physeal injuries at singular institutions.

5. Conclusions

In conclusion, we found that 5.7% of all pediatric long-bone fractures involved the physis, with the distal tibia the most common site of injury. Utilizing this knowledge physicians should be vigilant about these injuries to prevent future complications commonly seen in physeal fractures such as bony bar formation and limb-length discrepancy.

Author Contributions: Conceptualization, J.R.F., R.F.G., K.A.P. and N.H.M.; methodology, J.R.F., R.F.G., K.A.P. and N.H.M.; validation, J.R.F. and R.F.G.; formal analysis, J.R.F., R.F.G., C.B.E. and S.M.T.; investigation, all authors; data curation, J.R.F., R.F.G., C.B.E. and S.M.T.; writing—original draft preparation, J.R.F. and R.F.G.; writing—review, and editing, all authors; visualization, J.R.F., R.F.G., C.B.E. and S.M.T.; supervision, N.H.M. and K.A.P.; project administration, N.H.M. and K.A.P.; funding acquisition, N.H.M. and K.A.P. All authors have read and agreed to the published version of the manuscript.

Funding: This research was funded by the Gates Grubstake Fund—2018 Research Award.

Institutional Review Board Statement: The study was approved by the Institutional Review Board of The University of Colorado (COMIRB 20-0020), approval date is June 2017.

Informed Consent Statement: Not applicable.

Data Availability Statement: Data available upon reasonable request.

Acknowledgments: This study was supported by the Gates Grubstake Fund.

Conflicts of Interest: The authors declare no conflict of interest. The funders had no role in the design of the study; in the collection, analyses, or interpretation of data; in the writing of the manuscript, or in the decision to publish the results.

References

1. Mann, D.C.; Rajmaira, S. Distribution of physeal and nonphyseal fractures in 2650 long-bone fractures in children aged 0–16 years. *J. Pediatr. Orthop.* **1990**, *10*, 713–716. [CrossRef] [PubMed]
2. Mizuta, T.; Benson, W.; Foster, B.K.; Pateron, D.C.; Morris, L.L. Statistical analysis of the incidence of physeal injuries. *J. Pediatr. Orthop.* **1987**, *7*, 518–523. [CrossRef] [PubMed]
3. Peterson, H.A.; Madhok, R.; Benson, J.T.; Ilstrup, D.M.; Melton, L.J. Physeal fractures: Part 1. Epidemiology in Olmsted County, Minnesota, 1979–1988. *J. Pediatr. Orthop.* **1994**, *14*, 423–430. [CrossRef] [PubMed]
4. Shaw, N.; Erickson, C.; Bryant, S.J.; Ferguson, V.L.; Krebs, M.D.; Hadley-Miller, N.; Payne, K. Regenerative Medicine Approaches for the Treatment of Pediatric Physeal Injuries. *Tissue Eng. Part B.* **2018**, *24*, 85–97. [CrossRef]
5. Naranje, S.M.; Erali, R.A.; Warner, W.C.; Sawyer, J.R.; Kelly, D.M. Epidemiology of Pediatric Fractures Presenting to Emergency Departments in the United States. *J. Pediatr. Orthop.* **2016**, *36*, e45–e48. [CrossRef]
6. Vescio, A.; Testa, G.; Sapienza, M.; Caldaci, A.; Montemagno, M.; Andreacchio, A.; Canavese, F.; Pavone, V. Is Obesity a Risk Factor for Loss of Reduction in Children with Distal Radius Fractures Treated Conservatively? *Children* **2022**, *9*, 425. [CrossRef]
7. Arkader, A.; Warner, W.C.; Horn, B.D.; Shaw, R.N.; Wells, L. Predicting the outcome of physeal fractures of the distal femur. *J. Pediatr. Orthop.* **2007**, *27*, 703–708. [CrossRef]
8. Barmada, A.; Gaynor, T.; Mubarak, S.J. Premature physeal closure following distal tibia physeal fractures: A new radiographic predictor. *J. Pediatr. Orthop.* **2003**, *23*, 733–739. [CrossRef]
9. Barr, L. Paediatric supracondylar humeral fractures: Epidemiology, mechanisms and incidence during school holidays. *J. Child. Orthop.* **2014**, *8*, 167–170. [CrossRef]
10. Larsen, M.C.; Bohm, K.C.; Rizkala, A.R.; Ward, C.M. Outcomes of nonoperative treatment of Salter-Harris II distal radius fractures: A systematic review. *Hand* **2016**, *11*, 29–35. [CrossRef]
11. Leary, J.T.; Handling, M.; Talerico, M.; Yong, L.; Bowe, A. Physeal fractures of the distal tibia: Predictive factors of premature physeal closure and growth arrest. *J. Pediatr. Orthop.* **2009**, *29*, 356–361. [CrossRef] [PubMed]
12. Rohmiller, M.T.; Gaynor, T.P.; Pawelek, J. Salter-Harris I and II fractures of the distal tibia: Does mechanism of injury relate to premature physeal closure? *J. Pediatr. Orthop.* **2006**, *26*, 322–328. [CrossRef] [PubMed]
13. 2015 Sports, Fitness and Leisure Activity Topline Participation Report. Available online: https://sfia.org/research/ (accessed on 29 May 2022).
14. Monget, F.; Sapienza, M.; McCracken, K.L.; Nectoux, E.; Fron, D.; Andreacchio, A.; Pavone, V.; Canavese, F. Clinical Characteristics and Distribution of Pediatric Fractures at a Tertiary Hospital in Northern France: A 20-Year-Distance Comparative Analysis (1999–2019). *Medicina* **2022**, *58*, 610. [CrossRef] [PubMed]
15. National Trauma Data Bank [Database]; American College of Surgeons: Chicago, IL, USA, 2016; Updated 2016.
16. Hebal, F.; Hu, Y.Y.; Raval, M.V. Resrach in using clinical registries in children's surgical care. *Semin. Pediat. Surg.* **2018**, *26*, 345–352. [CrossRef] [PubMed]
17. Belmont, P.J.; E'Stephan, J.G.; Romano, D.; Bader, J.O.; Nelson, K.J.; Schoenfeld, A.J. Risk factors for complications and in-hospital mortality following hip fractures: A study using the National Trauma Data Bank. *Arch. Orthop. Trauma Surg.* **2014**, *134*, 597–604. [CrossRef]
18. Piatt, J.H. Pediatric spinal injury in the US: Epidemiology and disparities. *J. Neurosurg. Pediatrics* **2015**, *16*, 463–471. [CrossRef]
19. Merkow, R.P.; Rademaker, A.W.; Bilimoria, K.Y. Practical guide to surgical data sets: National Cancer Database (NCDB). *JAMA Surg.* **2018**, *153*, 850–851. [CrossRef]
20. Laor, T.; Cornwall, R. Describing pediatric fractures in the era of ICD-10. *Pediatr. Radiol.* **2020**, *50*, 761–775. [CrossRef]
21. Hedström, E.M.; Svensson, O.; Bergström, U.; Michno, P. Epidemiology of fractures in children and adolescents: Increased incidence over the past decade: A population-based study from northern Sweden. *Acta Orthop.* **2010**, *81*, 148–153. [CrossRef]
22. Rennie, L.; Court-Brown, C.M.; Mok, J.Y.; Beattie, T.F. The epidemiology of fractures in children. *Injury* **2007**, *38*, 913–922. [CrossRef]
23. Kawamoto, K.; Kim, W.C.; Tsuchida, Y.; Tsuji, Y.; Fujioka, M.; Horii, M.; Mikami, Y.; Tokunaga, D.; Kubo, T. Incidence of physeal injuries in Japanese children. *J. Pediatr. Orthop. B* **2006**, *15*, 126–130. [CrossRef] [PubMed]
24. Worlock, P.; Stower, M. Fracture patterns in Nottingham children. *J. Pediatr. Orthop.* **1986**, *6*, 656–660. [CrossRef] [PubMed]
25. Thomas, R.A.; Hennrikus, W.L. Treatment and outcomes of distal tibia salter harris II fractures. *Injury* **2020**, *51*, 636–641. [CrossRef] [PubMed]

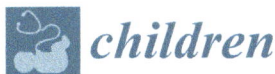

Article

Levels of Physical Activity in Children with Extremity Fractures a Dutch Observational Cross-Sectional Study

Amber Carlijn Traa [1,*], Ozcan Sir [1], Sanne W. T. Frazer [2], Brigitte van de Kerkhof-van Bon [3], Birgitte Blatter [2] and Edward C. T. H. Tan [1,4]

1. Department of Emergency Medicine, Radboud University Medical Center, Geert Grooteplein Zuid 10, 6525 GA Nijmegen, The Netherlands; ozcan.sir@radboudumc.nl (O.S.); edward.tan@radboudumc.nl (E.C.T.H.T.)
2. Consumer Safety Institute (VeiligheidNL), Overschiestraat 65, 1062 XD Amsterdam, The Netherlands; s.frazer@veiligheid.nl (S.W.T.F.); b.blatter@veiligheid.nl (B.B.)
3. Department of Emergency Medicine, Canisius Wilhelmina Hospital, Weg door Jonkerbos 100, 6532 SZ Nijmegen, The Netherlands; b.vandekerkhofvanbon@cwz.nl
4. Department of Traumasurgery, Radboud University Medical Center, Geert Grooteplein Zuid 10, 6525 GA Nijmegen, The Netherlands
* Correspondence: ambertraa@gmail.com; Tel.: +31-6361-83626

Abstract: Background: Fractures are common in children and a frequent cause of emergency department (ED) visits. Fractures can cause long-term complications, such as growth problems. Research on fractures can reveal useful areas of focus for injury prevention. Objective: To assess the role of physical activity in the occurrence of fractures, this study investigates physical activity among children with extremity fractures based on the Global Recommendations on Physical Activity for Health. Methods: A multi-center, cross-sectional study was performed at two EDs in Nijmegen, the Netherlands. Patients between 4 and 18 years of age visiting these EDs with a fracture were asked to complete a validated questionnaire. Results: Of the 188 respondents, 51% were found to adhere to the recommendations. Among participants between 13 and 18 years of age, 43% were adequately physically active, compared to participants between 4 and 12 years of age among whom 56% were adequately physically active ($p = 0.080$). Additionally, more males were found to meet the recommendations (60% versus 40%). The most common traumas were sports-related (57%). Sports-related traumas were cited more often among youth between 13 and 18 years of age, compared to those between 4 and 12 ($p < 0.001$). Conclusions: A relatively high prevalence of adherence to the Global Recommendations on Physical Activity for Health was observed among children with fractures. Most respondents obtained their fractures during participation in sports. This study emphasizes the need for more injury prevention, especially among youth between 13 and 18 years of age and children participating in sports.

Keywords: injury prevention; fracture risk; global recommendations on physical activity for health; SQUASH questionnaire; multi-center

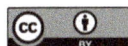

1. Introduction

The annual rate of fractures among children has been reported as ranging between 12 to 36 for every thousand children [1–3]. Fractures can result in a decrease in physical activity (PA) and long-term complications, such as growth problems. Studying fractures in children could support in developing preventive measures reducing fracture rates and avoid the possible negative consequences for children's health [4–6].

Previous studies have concluded that PA during childhood is associated with higher bone mineral density and long-term muscular benefits [7,8]. Additionally, there have been suggestions that increased PA decreases the incidence of fractures in children [9,10].

However, children's PA can also lead to injuries. Since children often take risks while playing and are thus at risk of being injured, PA could also lead to fractures [11,12].

In an effort to enhance global health systems and prevent curable diseases, the World Health Organization (WHO) developed the Global Recommendations on Physical Activity for Health in 2010. Revised in 2020, these universal recommendations for physical activity specifically target children between 5 and 17 years of age. The WHO recommends that every child exercise for at least one hour a day at a moderate-to-intensive level of intensity and also perform muscle- and bone-strengthening exercises at least three times a week. Since their publication, these recommendations have been widely adopted. For example, the United States (US) and the European Union (EU) have adopted these recommendations created by the WHO [13,14].

The WHO found that, globally, adolescents between 11 and 17 years of age attending school are insufficiently physically active in 81% of documented cases, meaning that 19% of adolescents were adhering to the WHO's recommendations [15]. In the EU, sufficient levels of PA according to the WHO's recommendations varied from 17% to 43% of cases [14]. In the Netherlands, the National Institute for Public Health and the Environment found that 42% of Dutch children between 5 and 17 years of age were sufficiently physically activity [16]. In general, the percentage of sufficient PA in children according to the WHO's recommendations is less than 50%.

Multiple studies have found fracture rates to be significantly higher among males compared to females [17,18]. Moreover, different trauma mechanisms during childhood have been observed in different age groups (1). A deeper investigation into fracture rates in children in relation to trauma mechanisms and PA could generate insights into the factors contributing to fractures. These findings would support the development of preventive measures by revealing the risk factors related to fractures during childhood.

This study explores the Global Recommendations on Physical Activity for Health created by the WHO by focusing on a population of children with extremity fractures from the Netherlands. This study aims to develop insights into levels of PA among children with extremity fractures based on the WHO's recommendations. This study also investigates the trauma mechanisms causing fractures in children.

2. Methods and Materials

2.1. Study Design and Setting

This study was designed with a multi-center, cross-sectional approach. The study was conducted at the emergency departments (EDs) of the Radboud University Medical Center (Radboudumc) and Canisius Wilhelmina Hospital (CWZ). Both centers are located in Nijmegen, the Netherlands. Radboudumc is a level 1 trauma center, and CWZ is a level 2 trauma center. Combined, the hospitals receive approximately 59,000 patient visits yearly. Both participating hospitals are located in Nijmegen, the Netherlands. Nijmegen is a mid-urbanized city in a rural environment and as such, is considered representative of the Netherlands. The Netherlands is a developed country and member of the EU. Prior to the data collection, the study was assessed and accepted by the Institutional Review Board of both Radboudumc and CWZ. Informed consent was obtained from all parents or the patient when older than 16.

2.2. Study Population

The sample for this study included all patients between 4 and 18 years of age at the time of their visit to the EDs of the Radboudumc or CWZ with a fracture acquired between November 2017 and November 2018. Patients were only included if their fracture was radiologically proven. All participating children and their parents or guardians received paper questionnaires in December 2018. In January 2019, in cases of four to six weeks non-response, the researcher called patients with a request to participate in the study in order to enlarge the response rate. Patients were excluded if they had specific diseases, were taking medications that affect bone metabolism, were involved in a high-impact trauma, or were diagnosed with more than two fractures or a fracture of the skull, face, thorax or pelvis. All exclusion criteria are specifically outlined in the questionnaire (Supplementary File S1). An a priori power size calculation indicated that, in total, 175 patients had to be included for there to be a sufficient sample size with a power of 0.8 at an alpha level of 0.05. This calculation involved the prevalence of Dutch children meeting sufficient PA levels presented in previous studies, namely 42% [16].

2.3. Data Collection

Patients received study information, an informed consent letter, and a coded questionnaire by mail. The questionnaire and informed consent letter were to be sent back to the Radboudumc for analysis. The questionnaire was developed based on previous validated questionnaires. For an evaluation of patients' level of PA, the Short Questionnaire to Assess Health Enhancing Activity (SQUASH) was used [19]. This validated questionnaire was also used for national research on the WHO's recommendations among adults and children [20]. The SQUASH questionnaire has been validated in adults and adolescents [21]. Along with the SQUASH questionnaire, patients were asked to report on the event that caused their injury and the amount of time spent behind a screen. The intensity level of the activity performed was calculated based on Metabolic Equivalents of Task (METs) (Supplementary File S1). Calculating METs is an objective way to measure the intensity of PA performed by the respondents.

2.4. Data Analysis

All data processing and analyses were performed with Microsoft Office Excel 2016 (Microsoft Corp., Redmond, WA, USA), Castor EDC (Ciwit B.V., Amsterdam, the Netherlands) and SPSS Statistics for Windows, version 25 (IBM Corp., Armonk, NY, USA). The data were described in means and percentages with standard deviations (SDs). The main variable was adherence to the recommendations created by the WHO (yes/no). This study used the same method of data analysis for the WHO's recommendations as was used for the national study on this topic performed by the National Institute for Public Health and the Environment [16]. The two sub-measurements of the norm were separately analyzed and then combined for the researcher to determine whether the recommendations were being adhered to. The sub-measurements calculated whether respondents: (1) exercise for at least one hour a day at a moderate-to-intensive level of intensity (2) perform muscle- and bone-strengthening exercises at least three times a week. Pearson χ^2 tests, ANOVAs (F), one-sample, and independent t-tests were conducted for a comparison between age groups and gender. p-values lower than 0.050 were considered statistically significant. Missing data are either mentioned separately in the results section or represented in the number of individuals (n) for each result. Analyzation of age groups 4 to 12 years and 13 to 18 years of age was performed since it was expected to find differences in PA. Therefore, calculations on solely the total study population could be misleading. Secondly, in the Netherlands, the National Institute for Public Health and the Environment also performed statistics on age subgroups making interpretations of the study results in relation to these data more insightful.

3. Results

3.1. Study Population and Baseline Characteristics

In total, 1107 potential respondents received questionnaires. Of these potential respondents, 216 had visited the ED of the Radboudumc and 891 had visited the ED of the CWZ. The total response rate was 20% (n = 216) (Radboudumc 24%, CWZ 18%). Of the respondents, 13% (n = 28) were excluded according to the exclusion criteria. In total, 188 patients were included in this study's analysis, as outlined in Figure 1.

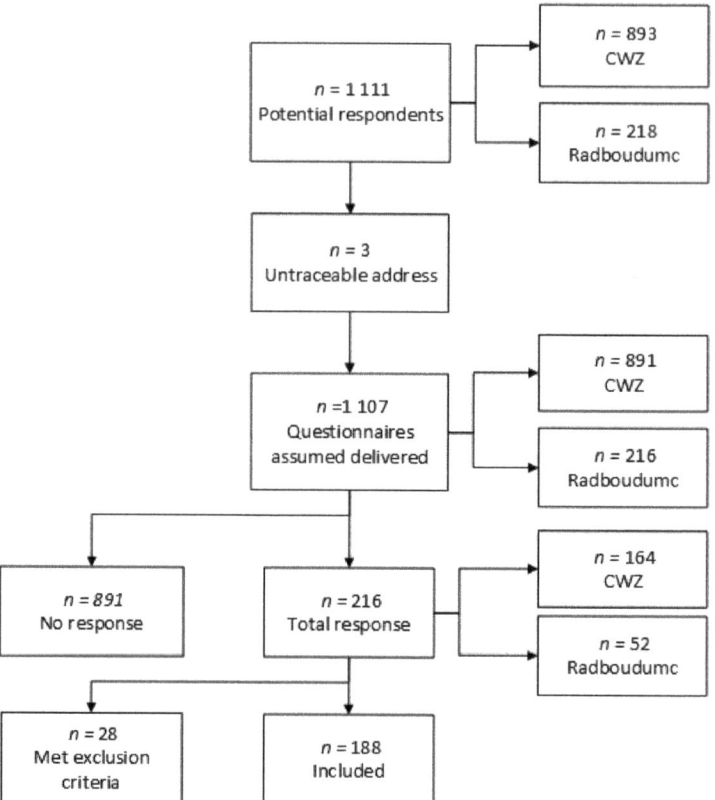

Figure 1. Flowchart of the patient inclusion process.

The mean age was 11.2 (SD = 3.7, Range 4–18), and 57.4% (n = 108) of the respondents are male. The baseline characteristics of patients included in this study are similar compared to non-respondents ($p > 0.600$). More details are included in Table 1.

Table 1. Baseline characteristics for included respondents vs. non-respondents.

Characteristics	Study Population (n = 188)	Non-Respondents (n = 891)	p-Value
	Gender–n (%) ‡		
Boys	108 (57.4%)	528 (59.3%)	0.646
Girls	80 (42.6%)	363 (40.7%)	
	Mean age–years †		
Total	11.2 (SD = 3.7, Range 4–18)	11.2 (SD = 3.9, Range 4–18)	
Boys	11.7 (SD = 3.9, Range 4–18)	11.8 (SD = 3.8, Range 4–18)	0.816
Girls	10.6 (SD = 3.37, Range 4–18)	10.2 (SD = 3.7, Range 4–18)	
	Age group–n (%) †		
4–12 years	109 (58.0%)	520 (58.4%)	0.923
13–18 years	79 (42.0%)	371 (41.6%)	

Used Statistical Test to Calculate Differences between Groups: † t-test; ‡ Chi-Square Test.

3.2. PA and the WHO's Global Recommendations on Physical Activity for Health

The mean time spent on moderate-to-intensive activities was 2.5 h daily (Table 2). With the exclusion of physical education, 84% of the children ($n = 157$) were actively participating in at least one sport at the time of the study. Moreover, children not meeting the physical activity recommendations for health spent significantly less time on sports compared to children meeting these recommendations (Table 3). Youth between 13 and 18 years of age were found to spend more time playing sports ($p < 0.001$). In contrast, young children were found to play outside more frequently than respondents between 13 and 18 years of age ($p < 0.005$).

Table 2. Comparing sufficiently physically active children vs. not-sufficiently active children.

$n = 188$ Children with Fractures	Children Meeting the Recommendations for Health ($n = 95, 50.5\%$)	Children not Meeting the Recommendations for Health ($n = 93, 49.5\%$)	p-Value
Age [†] (mean in years)	10.97 (SD = 3.6)	11.49 (SD = 3.8)	0.080
Gender [‡] (boy vs. girl n, %)	57 vs. 38 60% vs. 40%	51 vs. 42 55% vs. 45%	0.477
BMI [*,†] (mean)	18 (SD = 3.4)	17.8 (SD = 2.8)	0.332
Screentime [†] (mean min/day)	191 (SD = 131.8)	220 (SD = 171.3)	0.384
Type of fracture [‡] (Upper vs. lower extremity n, %)	79 vs. 16 83% vs. 17%	75 vs. 18 81% vs. 19%	0.654
Trauma occurred during sports [**,‡] (n, %)	56 (53%)	49 (47%)	0.337
Time spent on sports [†] (mean in hours/week)	7 (SD = 6.7)	4.5 (SD = 3.2)	**0.004**
Time playing outside [†] (Mean min/day)	26.1 (SD = 55.5)	17.8 (SD = 35.2)	0.226

[*] $n = 167$, missing data $n = 21$ not presented [**] $n = 183$, missing data $n = 5$ not presented; $p < 0.050$ are considered significant and presented in bold font. Used statistical test to calculate differences between groups: [†] t-test; [‡] chi-square test.

Of all the children included in this study, 50.5% ($n = 95$) were found to exercise for at least 1 h at a moderate-to-intensive level of intensity daily. This study also found that 99.4% ($n = 187$) of all children perform muscle- and bone-strengthening exercises at least three times a week. In total, 50.5% ($n = 95$) of the respondents were meeting the criteria outlined in the WHO's Recommendations on Physical Activity for Health. Children between 4 and 12 years of age were more likely to be adhering to the WHO's recommendations compared to those between 13 and 18 years of age; however, this was not statistically significant. More details are included in Tables 2 and 3. Table 3 presents a comparison of children meeting the recommendations for health versus children not meeting these recommendations. There are no significant differences between both groups, with only children meeting the recommendations on physical health spending more time on sports and having a decreased screen time compared to children not adhering to the recommendations. Physically active children spent 191 min per day (SD = 131) on screentime whereas physically inactive children spent 220 (SD = 171) minutes per day behind a screen.

3.3. Trauma Mechanism and Type of Fracture

Most children had acquired one fracture, namely 83% ($n = 156$). The rest of the study population acquired two fractures. Additionally, an upper extremity fracture was most often diagnosed, found in 82% ($n = 154$). Of the fractures, 56% ($n = 105$) occurred during sports. Sports-related traumas occurred significantly more often in youth between 13 and

18 years of age than children between 4 and 12 ($p < 0.001$). In contrast, a fall between 0.5 and 3 m occurred more frequently in children between 4 and 12 years of age compared to youth between 13 and 18 ($p < 0.001$) (Table 3).

Twenty-three percent ($n = 43$) of the children reported that the trauma happened while playing soccer, and 17% ($n = 32$) of the fractures were caused by a trauma involving climbing a frame, play set, or rack. Figure 2 provides more details on the trauma mechanisms found among children.

Table 3. An overview of the study population's physical activity and trauma mechanism causing fractures.

	Total Population	Boys	Girls	p-Value *	4–12 Years	13–18 Years	p-Value *
	($n = 188$)						
Trauma mechanism **							
Sports-related	105 (57.4%)	59 (55.1%)	46 (60.5%)	0.468	47 (44.8%)	58 (74.4%)	**0.001**
Fall from 0.5–3 m	52 (28.4%)	37 (34.6%)	15 (19.7%)	**0.028**	40 (38.1%)	12 (15.3%)	**0.001**
Fall from 0.5 m or less	26 (14.2%)	11 (10.3%)	15 (19.7%)	0.071	18 (17.1%)	8 (10.3%)	0.187
Physical activity							
Achieved physical activity norm	95 (50.5%)	57 (52.8%)	38 (47.5%)	0.474	61 (56%)	34 (43%)	0.080
Mean hours/day performing intensive activity	2.4 (SD = 1.5)	2.5 (SD = 1.5)	2.4 (SD = 1.5)	0.978	2.6 (SD = 1.4)	2.2 (SD = 1.6)	0.076
Mean hours/week spent on sports	5.8 (SD = 2.5)	6.3 (SD = 6.0)	5.2 (SD = 4.5)	0.165	4.5 (SD = 2.8)	7.8 (SD = 7.2)	**0.001**
Mean minutes/day playing outside	37.6 (SD = 56.2)	21.9 (SD = 51.5)	22.1 (SD = 39.6)	0.978	29.7 (SD = 56.3)	11.4 (SD = 2.9)	**0.003**

* p-values < 0.050 are considered significant and presented in bold font; ** $n = 183$, missing data $n = 5$ not presented.

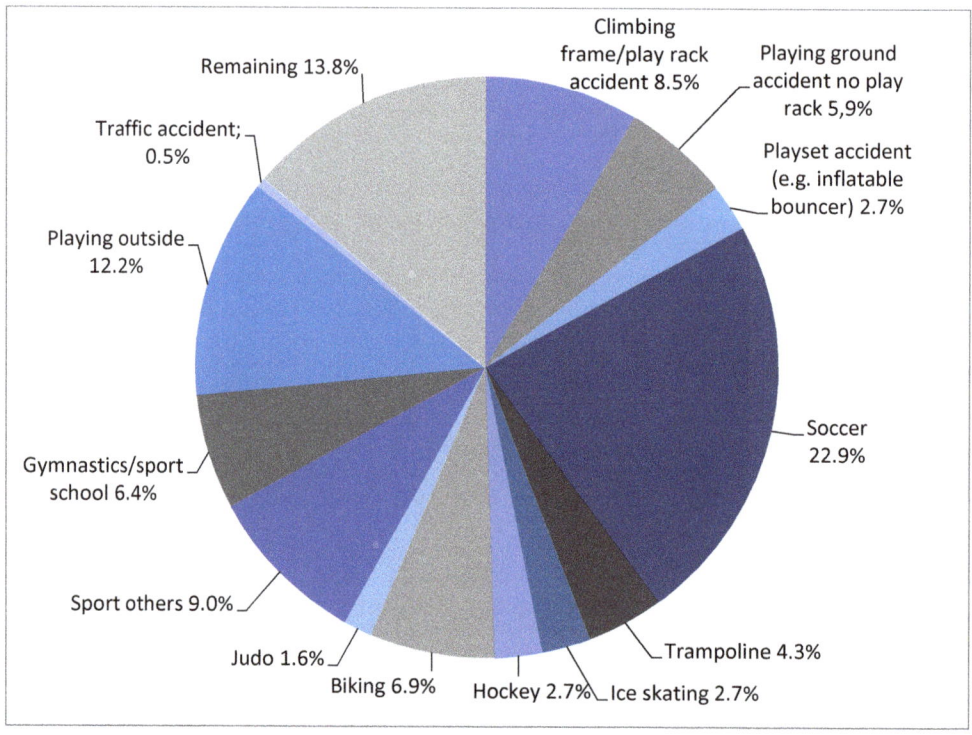

Figure 2. Most frequently occurring mechanisms of trauma ($n = 188$).

4. Discussion

This study found a relatively high prevalence of adherence to the WHO's Global Recommendations on Physical Activity for Health among children with fractures. The results demonstrate that 51% of the children with fractures involved in low to medium impact trauma adhere to the WHO's recommendations. Older children adhered to the recommendations less than younger children. The most common traumas in children with fractures were sports-related.

A comparison of this study's results and the general national study conducted on the WHO's recommendations reveals that there is an approximate 7% difference in adherence to the recommendations between Dutch children with fractures and Dutch children in general (50% versus 42%) [16]. The difference in adherence to the WHO's recommendations is even larger when this study is compared to the European and global literature which reports adherence to the WHO's recommendations in 19–43% of children [13–15,22]. However, it must be noted that differences in study methodologies between this study and the international literature with regard to response bias could have influenced the results. Overall, comparing and generalizing the study results to global literature gives insight but should be interpreted with substantial caution.

Although a relatively high prevalence of children adhering the WHO's recommendations in this study was found, this study did not find sufficient evidence to suggests that physically active children are more likely to obtain a fracture. In existing literature, contradicting results have been described regarding fracture risk and PA [9,10,12,17,23]. The differences in results could be explained by the fact that there is a contradiction in the influence of PA on fracture risk. PA both benefits bone mineral density, thus reducing fracture risk, and involves situations that potentially increase injury rates [18]. This study's results support the rationale that PA increases the exposure to risky situations, such as sports or playing [11,12]. Also, this study found boys to adhere more frequently to the WHO's recommendations compared to girls. This is in accordance with the national literature [24]. This is potentially explained by children's, especially boys', tendency to participate in risky situations as a part of their upbringing and development [11]. This is underlined in this study through a high participation in sports at an older age. Overall, this study has found a relatively high prevalence of children adhering to the WHO's recommendations, which supports the idea that PA increases exposure to the risk of injuries. However, differences in study results compared to national literature were too small to state that PA increases fracture risk.

Although PA might lead to more exposure to risky situations, it is important to acknowledge the positive effects of PA on social, psychological, and physical health [25,26]. The necessity of preventive actions is underlined by this study's finding that especially younger children with fractures are very physically active. As stated in the World report on child injury prevention, preventive measures including the redesign of playing equipment, legislative enforcements, and multifaceted community programs have been found effective in reducing injury risk [27–29]; combining these measures is even more effective. Examples of preventive measures are regulating playground equipment standards, supportive home visitation to identify fall hazards, and investment in safer routes to school [27]. Behavioral changes, such as safer playing behavior, can also prevent injuries. Evidence suggests that one of the methods for achieving behavioral changes is educating parents about their children's risky playing behavior [30]. Preventive measures and behavioral changes should be taken into account in efforts to decrease fracture rates in children. These preventive measures should, as suggested by the study results, be targeted at adolescents and children participating actively in sports.

In line with national and international literature, this study observed age differences in the percentages of adherence to the WHO's recommendations [16]. Children between 4 and 12 years of age were adequately physically active in 57% of the cases, compared to 43% among children between 13 and 18. The trend of younger children more frequently adhering to the WHO's recommendations on PA compared to older children is supported by previous studies on PA among children [14,16]. This trend can be explained by the sedentary behavior and long periods of time spent behind screens among adolescents, also found in this study [31].

Additionally, this study has found the most common traumas in low to medium impact trauma to be sports-related. This is confirmed by international literature [32,33]. Moreover, 84% of the children with fractures, in this study, were found to be active in sports. This is more than the 70.3% found in the general pediatric Dutch population [34]. Statistics also suggest that 80% of Dutch children are actively involved in sports clubs of schools [35]. The finding that children with fractures are more active in organized PA such as sports supports the idea that PA exposes children to the risk of injury and possibly increases fracture risk [11,12].

This study has also found that among younger children, a fall of 0.5 to 3 m occurred significantly more frequently, in contrast to older children, who were more frequently involved in sports traumas. This is supported by European and American literature on different fracture etiologies in different age groups [36]. Finally, 23% of the fractures described in the questionnaires were soccer related, which is, according to European literature, representative of national sport preferences [36]. In the Netherlands, soccer is a popular sport; reports have found that 22.6% of Dutch children are reported to play soccer [34]. However, it is possible that by solely including extremity fractures instead of all fractures of the body, this study has overestimated the impact of PA on fracture rates. The results on trauma mechanisms present patterns based on age and national sports preferences. As addressed before, preventive measures could help to decrease fracture incidence among children since the occurrence of trauma during sports has been found to be high [37,38].

A major limitation of this study is the low response rate of 20%. However, a sufficient sample size was achieved, and the respondent versus non-respondent analysis found similar baseline characteristics. In other survey studies, response rates vary widely, ranging from 20% to 43% [39,40]. Bias could have also influenced the results. Participation and response bias could have been present since physically active children and children in higher socio-economic classes are more likely to respond [18]. Additionally, the study's design is prone to recall bias, as it is a retrospective study which requires the respondent to fill in a questionnaire on an event that might have occurred up to one year in the past. In addition, the SQUASH questionnaire was validated for adults and adolescents yet has not been validated for younger children. It was expected that for younger children the parents or guardian filled out the questionnaire. This was also addressed in information letters provided for participants. However, response bias could have occurred. The inclusion of potential participants over one year in the past diminished the risk of seasonality impacting the results. Sequentially, bias could have been present in this study, but efforts have been made to minimize bias through a respondent versus non-respondent analysis and the use of a validated questionnaire. Based on these limitations, the study results should be interpreted with caution.

Lastly, the study design did not include a matched control group of children without fractures. By using matched controls, differences in children with and without fractures could have been measured. In this study, descriptive statistical analysis was performed. Therefore, assumptions on the differences between children with fractures compared to the pediatric population referenced in national and international literature can be described and interpreted but not measured. It is strongly advised that future researchers perform a prospective study in a case-controlled setting in order to obtain more reliable results and minimize bias.

A strength of this study was its multi-center setup. Since both a level 1 and level 2 hospital were involved, different patient populations participated in this study. The multi-center setup ensured that this study achieved a sufficient sample size. Additionally, the use of validated questionnaires as a foundation for this study's questionnaire made the results more reliable. Finally, the questionnaire was kept as simple and short as possible in order to be suitable for participants of varying ages and socio-economic statuses.

5. Conclusions

This study found a relatively high prevalence of adherence to the WHO's Global Recommendations on Physical Activity for Health among children with fractures. Most fractures were obtained during the children's participation in sports. This study suggests the need for injury prevention among youth between 13 and 18 years of age and children participating in sports. Future research in a matched case-controlled setting is essential to adequately target injury prevention programs.

Supplementary Materials: The following supporting information can be downloaded at: https://www.mdpi.com/article/10.3390/children9030325/s1, File S1: Questionnaire on physical activity in children with fractures.

Author Contributions: Conceptualization: A.C.T., S.W.T.F., B.B., and E.C.T.H.T.; Data curation: A.C.T.; Formal analysis: A.C.T. and S.W.T.F.; Project administration: A.C.T. and S.W.T.F.; Resources: O.S. and B.v.d.K.-v.B.; Writing original draft: A.C.T.; Writing–review & editing: E.C.T.H.T., S.W.T.F., B.B., O.S. and B.v.d.K.-v.B. All authors have read and agreed to the published version of the manuscript.

Funding: The authors declare that they have no funding source.

Institutional Review Board Statement: The study was conducted in accordance with the Declaration of Helsinki, and approved by the Institutional Ethics Committee of Radboud University Nijmegen Medical Centre (protocol code 2018-4766, date of approval 6 November 2018).

Informed Consent Statement: Informed consent was obtained from all subjects involved in the study. When older than sixteen informed consent was obtained from parents or the patient when older than 16.

Data Availability Statement: The data presented in this study are available on request from the corresponding author. The data are not publicly available due to privacy considerations.

Conflicts of Interest: The authors declare that the research was conducted in the absence of any commercial or financial relationships that could be construed as a potential conflict of interest.

Human Rights Statement: There were no human rights conflicts to declare.

References

1. Landin, L.A. Fracture patterns in children. Analysis of 8682 fractures with special reference to incidence, etiology and secular changes in a Swedish urban population 1950–1979. *Acta Orthop. Scand. Suppl.* **1983**, *202*, 1–109.
2. Lyons, R.A.; Delahunty, A.M.; Kraus, D.; Heaven, M.; McCabe, M.; Allen, H.; Nash, P. Children's fractures: A population based study. *Inj. Prev.* **1999**, *5*, 129–132. [CrossRef]
3. Naranje, S.M.; Erali, R.A.; Warner, W.C., Jr.; Sawyer, J.R.; Kelly, D.M. Epidemiology of Pediatric Fractures Presenting to Emergency Departments in the United States. *J. Pediatr. Orthop.* **2016**, *36*, e45–e48. [CrossRef]
4. Howe, A.S.; Asplund, C.A. General Principles of Fracture Management. Early and Late Complications. **2022**, *17*. Available online: https://www.uptodate.com/contents/general-principles-of-fracture-management-early-and-late-complications (accessed on 25 February 2022).
5. Kopjar, B.; Wickizer, T.M. Fractures among children: Incidence and impact on daily activities. *Inj. Prev.* **1998**, *4*, 194–197. [CrossRef]
6. Peterson, H.A. *Epiphyseal Growth Plate Fractures*; Springer Science & Business Media: Berlin/Heidelberg, Germany, 2007.
7. Weaver, C.; Gordon, C.; Janz, K.; Kalkwarf, H.; Lappe, J.M.; Lewis, R.; O'Karma, M.; Wallace, T.; Zemel, B. The National Osteoporosis Foundation's position statement on peak bone mass development and lifestyle factors: A systematic review and implementation recommendations. *Osteoporos. Int.* **2016**, *27*, 1281–1386. [CrossRef]
8. Löfgren, B.; Daly, R.; Nilsson, J.-Å.; Dencker, M.; Karlsson, M. An increase in school-based physical education increases muscle strength in children. *Med. Sci. Sports Exerc.* **2013**, *45*, 997–1003. [CrossRef]
9. Tveit, M.; Rosengren, B.; Nilsson, J.-Å.; Karlsson, M. Exercise in youth: High bone mass, large bone size, and low fracture risk in old age. *Scand. J. Med. Sci. Sports* **2015**, *25*, 453–461. [CrossRef]
10. Cöster, M.E.; Fritz, J.; Nilsson, J.-Å.; Karlsson, C.; Rosengren, B.E.; Dencker, M.; Karlsson, M.K. How does a physical activity programme in elementary school affect fracture risk? A prospective controlled intervention study in Malmo, Sweden. *BMJ Open* **2017**, *7*, e012513. [CrossRef]

11. Sandseter, E.B.H. Scaryfunny: A Qualitative Study of Risky Play Among Preschool Children. Ph.D. Thesis, Norwegian University of Science and Technology, Trondheim, Norway, 2010.
12. Clark, E.M.; Ness, A.R.; Tobias, J.H. Vigorous physical activity increases fracture risk in children irrespective of bone mass: A prospective study of the independent risk factors for fractures in healthy children. *J. Bone Miner. Res.* **2008**, *23*, 1012–1022. [CrossRef]
13. Piercy, K.L.; Troiano, R.P.; Ballard, R.M.; Carlson, S.A.; Fulton, J.E.; Galuska, D.A.; George, S.M.; Olson, R.D. The physical activity guidelines for Americans. *JAMA* **2018**, *320*, 2020–2028. [CrossRef]
14. World Health Organization. *Physical Activity Factsheets for the 28 European Union Member States of the WHO European Region*; World Health Organization: Geneva, Switzerland, 2018.
15. World Health Organization. *Prevalence of Insufficient Physical Activity: School Going Adolescents Aged 11–17 Years*; World Health Organization: Geneva, Switzerland, 2010.
16. Sport, Ministerie van Volksgezondheid Welzijn en Sports. *Hoeveel Mensen Voldoen aan de Door de Gezondheidsraad Geadviseerde Beweegrichtlijnen?* Rijksinstituut voor Volksgezondheid en Gezondheid (RIVM): Bilthoven, The Netherlands, 2017.
17. Randsborg, P.H.; Røtterud, J.J. No difference in the level of physical activity between children who have or have never sustained a fracture. *Scand. J. Med. Sci. Sports* **2017**, *27*, 1801–1805. [CrossRef]
18. Clark, E.M. The epidemiology of fractures in otherwise healthy children. *Curr. Osteoporos. Rep.* **2014**, *12*, 272–278. [CrossRef]
19. Wendel-Vos, W.; Schuit, J. Short Questionnaire to Assess Health Enhancing Physical Activity. *SQUASH Bilthoven Neth. Inst. Public Health Environ.* **2002**. Available online: https://meetinstrumentenzorg.nl/wp-content/uploads/instrumenten/503_2_N.pdf (accessed on 25 February 2022).
20. Wagenmakers, R.; van den Akker-Scheek, I.; Groothoff, J.W.; Zijlstra, W.; Bulstra, S.K.; Kootstra, J.W.; Wendel-Vos, G.W.; van Raaij, J.J.; Stevens, M. Reliability and validity of the short questionnaire to assess health-enhancing physical activity (SQUASH) in patients after total hip arthroplasty. *BMC Musculoskelet. Disord.* **2008**, *9*, 141. [CrossRef] [PubMed]
21. Campbell, N.; Gaston, A.; Gray, C.; Rush, E.; Maddison, R.; Prapavessis, H. The Short QUestionnaire to ASsess Health-enhancing (SQUASH) physical activity in adolescents: A validation using doubly labeled water. *J. Phys. Act. Health* **2016**, *13*, 154–158. [CrossRef]
22. Mota, J.; Coelho e Silva, M.; Raimundo, A.; Sardinha, L. Report Card on Physical Activity for Children and Youth. *J. Physical Act. Health.* **2016**, *13* (Suppl. S2), 242–245. [CrossRef] [PubMed]
23. Wren, T.A.; Shepherd, J.A.; Kalkwarf, H.J.; Zemel, B.S.; Lappe, J.M.; Oberfield, S.; Dorey, F.J.; Winer, K.K.; Gilsanz, V. Racial disparity in fracture risk between white and nonwhite children in the United States. *J. Pediatr.* **2012**, *161*, 1035–1040.e2. [CrossRef]
24. Netherlands, S. StatLine: Leefstijl en (Preventief) Gezondheidsonderzoek: Persoonskenmerken 2021. Available online: https://opendata.cbs.nl/statline/#/CBS/nl/dataset/83021NED/table?ts=1645949292480 (accessed on 25 February 2022).
25. Shanmugam, C.; Maffulli, N. Sports injuries in children. *Br. Med. Bull.* **2008**, *86*, 33–57. [CrossRef]
26. Janssen, I.; LeBlanc, A.G. Systematic review of the health benefits of physical activity and fitness in school-aged children and youth. *Int. J. Behav. Nutr. Phys. Act.* **2010**, *7*, 40. [CrossRef]
27. Branche, C.; Ozanne-Smith, J.; Oyebite, K.; Hyder, A.A. *World Report on Child Injury Prevention*; World Health Organization: Geneva, Switzerland, 2008.
28. Britton, J.W. Kids can't fly: Preventing fall injuries in children. *Off. Publ. State Med. Soc. Wis.* **2005**, *104*, 33–36.
29. Harvey, A.; Towner, E.; Peden, M.; Soori, H.; Bartolomeos, K. Injury prevention and the attainment of child and adolescent health. *Bull. World Health Organ.* **2009**, *87*, 390–394. [CrossRef]
30. Kuiper, J.; Veiligheid, N.L.; van Rooijen, M. *Position Paper Risicovol Spelen*; Universiteit voor Humanistiek: Utrecht, The Netherlands, 2017.
31. Guthold, R.; Stevens, G.A.; Riley, L.M.; Bull, F.C. Global trends in insufficient physical activity among adolescents: A pooled analysis of 298 population-based surveys with 1·6 million participants. *Lancet Child Adolesc. Health* **2020**, *4*, 23–35. [CrossRef]
32. Randsborg, P.-H.; Gulbrandsen, P.; Benth, J.Š.; Sivertsen, E.A.; Hammer, O.-L.; Fuglesang, H.F.; Årøen, A.J. Fractures in children: Epidemiology and activity-specific fracture rates. *JBJS* **2013**, *95*, e42. [CrossRef] [PubMed]
33. Wood, A.M.; Robertson, G.A.; Rennie, L.; Caesar, B.C.; Court-Brown, C.M. The epidemiology of sports-related fractures in adolescents. *Injury* **2010**, *41*, 834–838. [CrossRef] [PubMed]
34. GGD. *Gezondheidsmonitor Jeugd 2019*; GGD'en en RIVM; GGD: Amsterdam, The Netherlands, 2019.
35. GGD Gelderland Zuid. *E-MOVO in Cijfers: Tabellenboek voor de Regio Nijmegen, Behorend tot E-MOVO Onderzoek 2015/2016*; GGD: Amsterdam, The Netherlands, 2015.
36. Mäyränpää, M. *Fractures in Children: Epidemiology and Associated Bone Health Characteristics*; Helsingin Yliopisto: Helsinki, Finland, 2012.
37. Caine, D.; Maffulli, N.; Caine, C. Epidemiology of injury in child and adolescent sports: Injury rates, risk factors, and prevention. *Clin. Sports Med.* **2008**, *27*, 19–50. [CrossRef]
38. Flynn, J.M.; Lou, J.E.; Ganley, T.J. Prevention of sports injuries in children. *Clin. Sports Med.* **2002**, *14*, 719–722. [CrossRef]
39. Barry, A.R.; Egan, G.; Turgeon, R.D.; Leung, M. Evaluation of Physical Assessment Education for Practising Pharmacists: A Cross-Sectional Survey. *Can. J. Hosp. Pharm.* **2019**, *72*, 27. [CrossRef]
40. Clemen, N.M.; Blacker, B.C.; Floen, M.J.; Schweinle, W.E.; Huber, J.N. Work-life balance in women physicians in South Dakota: Results of a state-wide assessment survey. *S. D. Med.* **2018**, *71*, 550–558.

MDPI
St. Alban-Anlage 66
4052 Basel
Switzerland
Tel. +41 61 683 77 34
Fax +41 61 302 89 18
www.mdpi.com

Children Editorial Office
E-mail: children@mdpi.com
www.mdpi.com/journal/children

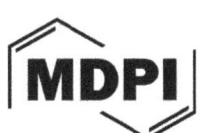

www.ingramcontent.com/pod-product-compliance
Lightning Source LLC
LaVergne TN
LVHW070434100526
838202LV00014B/1593